Undiagnosed and Rare Diseases in Critical Care

Editors

BRETT J. BORDINI
ROBERT M. KLIEGMAN

CRITICAL CARE CLINICS

www.criticalcare.theclinics.com

Consulting Editor
GREGORY S. MARTIN

April 2022 • Volume 38 • Number 2

ELSEVIER

1600 John F. Kennedy Boulevard • Suite 1800 • Philadelphia, Pennsylvania, 19103-2899

http://www.theclinics.com

CRITICAL CARE CLINICS Volume 38, Number 2
April 2022 ISSN 0749-0704, ISBN-13: 978-0-323-83604-3

Editor: Joanna Collett
Developmental Editor: Hannah Almira Lopez

Critical Care Clinics (ISSN: 0749-0704) is published quarterly by Elsevier Inc., 360 Park Avenue South, New York, NY 10010-1710. Months of issue are January, April, July, and October. Business and Editorial Offices: 1600 John F. Kennedy Blvd., Suite 1800, Philadelphia, PA 19103-2899. Customer Service Office: 6277 Sea Harbor Drive, Orlando, FL 32887-4800. Periodicals postage paid at New York, NY and additional mailing offices. Subscription prices are $266.00 per year for US individuals, $921.00 per year for US institutions, $100.00 per year for US students and residents, $296.00 per year for Canadian individuals, $953.00 per year for Canadian institutions, $338.00 per year for international individuals, $953.00 per year for international institutions, $100.00 per year for Canadian students/residents, and $150.00 per year for foreign students/residents. To receive student/resident rate, orders must be accompanied by name of affiliated institution, date of term, and the signature of program/residency coordinator on institution letterhead. Orders will be billed at individual rate until proof of status is received. Foreign air speed delivery is included in all *Clinics* subscription prices. All prices are subject to change without notice. POSTMASTER: Send address changes to *Critical Care Clinics*, Elsevier Periodicals Customer Service, 11830 Westline Industrial Drive, St. Louis, MO 63146. **Customer Service: 1-800-654-2452 (US). From outside of the US, call 1-314-447-8871. Fax: 1-314-447-8029. E-mail: journalscustomerservice-usa@elsevier.com (for print support) or journalsonlinesupport-usa@elsevier.com (for online support).**

Reprints. For copies of 100 or more of articles in this publication, please contact the Commercial Reprints Department, Elsevier Inc., 360 Park Avenue South, New York, NY 10010-1710. Tel.: 212-633-3874; Fax: 212-633-3820; E-mail: reprints@elsevier.com.

Critical Care Clinics is also published in Spanish by Editorial Inter-Medica, Junin 917, 1er A, 1113, Buenos Aires, Argentina.

Critical Care Clinics is covered in *MEDLINE/PubMed (Index Medicus), EMBASE/Excerpta Medica, Current Concepts/ Clinical Medicine, ISI/BIOMED, and Chemical Abstracts.*

Contributors

CONSULTING EDITOR

GREGORY S. MARTIN, MD, MSC
Professor, Division of Pulmonary, Allergy, Critical Care and Sleep Medicine, Research
Director, Emory Critical Care Center, Director, Emory/Georgia Tech Predictive Health
Institute, Co-Director, Atlanta Center for Microsystems Engineered Point-of-Care
Technologies (ACME POCT), President, Society of Critical Care Medicine, Atlanta,
Georgia, USA

EDITORS

BRETT J. BORDINI, MD
Associate Professor of Pediatrics, Division of Hospital Medicine, Medical College of
Wisconsin, Children's Wisconsin, Children's Corporate Center, Milwaukee, Wisconsin,
USA

ROBERT M. KLIEGMAN, MD
Professor of Pediatrics, Department of Pediatrics, Medical College of Wisconsin,
Children's Wisconsin, Children's Corporate Center, Milwaukee, Wisconsin, USA

AUTHORS

SAMUEL ADAMS, MD
Assistant Professor of Neurology, Department of Neurology, Division of Child Neurology,
Children's Wisconsin, Medical College of Wisconsin, Milwaukee, Wisconsin, USA

DONALD BASEL, MBBCh
Professor, Genetics, Department of Pediatrics, Medical College of Wisconsin, Milwaukee,
Wisconsin, USA

BRETT J. BORDINI, MD
Associate Professor of Pediatrics, Division of Hospital Medicine, Medical College of
Wisconsin, Children's Wisconsin, Children's Corporate Center, Milwaukee, Wisconsin,
USA

JOSEPH A. CARCILLO, MD
Center for Critical Care Nephrology, University of Pittsburgh, Department of Critical Care
Medicine, University of Pittsburgh School of Medicine, UPMC Children's Hospital of
Pittsburgh, Pittsburgh, Pennsylvania, USA

ASRIANI M. CHIU, MD
Department of Pediatrics (Allergy and Immunology) and Medicine, Medical College of
Wisconsin, Milwaukee, Wisconsin, USA

YVONNE E. CHIU, MD
Professor, Departments of Dermatology and Pediatrics, Medical College of Wisconsin, Milwaukee, Wisconsin, USA

ERICA Y. CHOU, MD
Department of Pediatrics, Medical College of Wisconsin, Milwaukee, Wisconsin, USA

DOMINIC O. CO, MD, PhD
Assistant Professor, Division of Allergy, Immunology and Rheumatology, Department of Pediatrics, University of Wisconsin–Madison, Clinical Science Center, Madison, Wisconsin, USA

SUSAN COHEN, MD
Associate Professor of Pediatrics, Division of Neonatology, Medical College of Wisconsin, Children's Corporate Center, Milwaukee, Wisconsin, USA

RAQUEL FARIAS-MOELLER, MD
Assistant Professor of Neurology and Pediatrics, Department of Neurology and Pediatrics, Division of Child Neurology, Children's Wisconsin, Medical College of Wisconsin, Milwaukee, Wisconsin, USA

CASSANDRA L. FORMECK, MD, MS
Assistant Professor of Pediatrics, Division of Nephrology, Department of Pediatrics, University of Pittsburgh School of Medicine, UPMC Children's Hospital of Pittsburgh, Center for Critical Care Nephrology, University of Pittsburgh, Pittsburgh, Pennsylvania, USA

HERNANDO GÓMEZ, MD
Assistant Professor of Critical Care Medicine, Center for Critical Care Nephrology, University of Pittsburgh, Department of Critical Care Medicine, University of Pittsburgh School of Medicine, Pittsburgh, Pennsylvania, USA

MATTHEW HARMELINK, MD
Assistant Professor, Department of Neurology, Medical College of Wisconsin, Milwaukee, Wisconsin, USA

DANA HARRAR, MD, PhD
Assistant Professor of Neurology and Pediatrics, Division of Neurology, Department of Neurology and Pediatrics, Children's National Hospital, George Washington University, Washington, DC, USA

JOHN A. KELLUM, MD, MCCM
Center for Critical Care Nephrology, University of Pittsburgh, Department of Critical Care Medicine, University of Pittsburgh School of Medicine, Professor of Critical Care Medicine, Medicine, Bioengineering, and Translational and Clinical Science, Director, Center for Critical Care Nephrology, Pittsburgh, Pennsylvania, USA

KATE F. KERNAN, MD
Center for Critical Care Nephrology, University of Pittsburgh, Department of Critical Care Medicine, University of Pittsburgh School of Medicine, UPMC Children's Hospital of Pittsburgh, Pittsburgh, Pennsylvania, USA

JENNIFER M. KWON, MD
Professor, Department of Neurology, University of Wisconsin–Madison, Madison, Wisconsin, USA

CATHERINE LARSON-NATH, MD
Assistant Professor, Department of Pediatrics, Division of Pediatric Gastroenterology, Hepatology, and Nutrition, University of Minnesota, Minneapolis, Minnesota, USA

CARLOS L. MANRIQUE-CABALLERO, MD
Center for Critical Care Nephrology, University of Pittsburgh, Post-Doc Associate, Renal-Electrolyte Division, Department of Medicine, University of Pittsburgh, Pittsburgh, Pennsylvania, USA

LILETH MONDOK, MD
Assistant Professor of Neurology, Department of Neurology, Division of Child Neurology, Children's Wisconsin, Medical College of Wisconsin, Milwaukee, Wisconsin, USA

MICHAEL MURIELLO, MD
Assistant Professor, Genetics, Department of Pediatrics, Medical College of Wisconsin, Milwaukee, Wisconsin, USA

SHILPA NARAYAN, MD
Assistant Professor of Pediatrics (Critical Care), Medical College of Wisconsin, Milwaukee, Wisconsin, USA

CYNTHIA G. PAN, MD
Professor, Department of Pediatrics, Medical College of Wisconsin, Milwaukee, Wisconsin, USA

BARRY J. PELZ, MD
Department of Pediatrics (Allergy and Immunology) and Medicine, Medical College of Wisconsin, Milwaukee, Wisconsin, USA

TARA L. PETERSEN, MD, MSEd
Associate Professor of Pediatrics (Critical Care), The Medical College of Wisconsin, Milwaukee, Wisconsin, USA

JOHN P. SCOTT, MD
Associate Professor, Departments of Anesthesiology and Pediatrics, Sections of Pediatric Anesthesiology and Pediatric Critical Care, Medical College of Wisconsin, Milwaukee, Wisconsin, USA

BRIDGET E. SHIELDS, MD
Assistant Professor, Department of Dermatology, University of Wisconsin–Madison, Madison, Wisconsin, USA

ANOOP KUMAR SINGH, MB BCh
Associate Professor of Pediatrics, Medical College of Wisconsin, Director of Cardiac Electrophysiology, Children's Wisconsin, Milwaukee, Wisconsin, USA

PAULA J. SOUNG, MD
Department of Pediatrics, Medical College of Wisconsin, Milwaukee, Wisconsin, USA

JUSTINN M. TANEM, MD
Assistant Professor, Departments of Anesthesiology and Pediatrics, Sections of Pediatric Anesthesiology and Pediatric Critical Care, Medical College of Wisconsin, Milwaukee, Wisconsin, USA

ROBERT CHARLES TASKER, MBBS, MD, FRCP
Professor, Department of Anesthesiology, Critical Care and Pain Medicine, Boston Children's Hospital, Boston, Massachusetts, USA; Fellow, College Lecturer in Medicine and Postgraduates' Tutor, Selwyn College, Cambridge University, United Kingdom

SCOTT K. VAN WHY, MD
Professor, Department of Pediatrics, Medical College of Wisconsin, Milwaukee, Wisconsin, USA

JAMES VERBSKY, MD, PhD
Professor of Pediatrics and Microbiology/Immunology, Medical College of Wisconsin, Milwaukee, Wisconsin, USA

BERNADETTE VITOLA, MD, MPH
Associate Professor, Transplant Institute, MedStar Georgetown University Hospital, Washington, DC, USA

KAROLYN A. WANAT, MD
Assistant Professor, Departments of Dermatology and Pathology, Medical College of Wisconsin, Milwaukee, Wisconsin, USA

SARAH YALE, MD
Assistant Professor of Pediatrics, Division of Hospital Medicine, Medical College of Wisconsin, Children's Corporate Center, Milwaukee, Wisconsin, USA

Contents

> Critically ill patients with undiagnosed and rare diseases are at high risk for cognitive diagnostic errors as well as delays in diagnosis that are the result of impaired diagnostic access. Local evaluation teams dedicated to undiagnosed and rare diseases can address both the risk and actuality of diagnostic error, as well as shortfalls in diagnostic access, particularly for patients whose diminished access is a result of critical illness. Features of successful teams are discussed.

> Rapid genomic sequencing has become a powerful diagnostic tool for critically ill children. Accumulated data support clinical utility. Advances in sequencing technology have improved reliability of rapid results and reduced turnaround times. Cost savings to health care institutions are not only the result of reduced sequencing charges (which have paralleled advances in sequencing technology), but also and more specifically the impact on diagnosis-specific medical management and reduced length of hospitalization. The use of genomic sequencing in critical care is still primarily limited to academic centers but will ultimately become the widespread standard of care for select patients.

> Diagnostic errors harm patients. While the underlying causes of diagnostic error and the settings in which they occur are diverse, the use of a cognitive forcing function in the form of a diagnostic time-out can mitigate the risk of diagnostic error. Barriers to the implementation of diagnostic time-outs remain. In our survey of neonatal intensive care unit (NICU) providers, perceived time constraints were universally cited as a barrier. Attending neonatologists and neonatology nurse practitioners reported decreased perception of the risk of diagnostic error impacting patient outcomes, relative to the perception among neonatology fellowship trainees. Future directions include addressing concerns over the perceived time investment required for a diagnostic time-out and increasing provider appreciation of the nature and impact of diagnostic error on patient outcomes.

that may have gone unnoticed until fulminant deterioration with respiratory failure.

Shock is a state in which the cardiovascular system fails to adequately deliver required substrates to maintain end-organ perfusion, tissue homeostasis, and cellular metabolism. Rapid recognition of shock and intervention is of utmost importance to reverse the shock state. This article reviews uncommon etiologies of shock classified in the following categories: distributive, hypovolemic, cardiogenic, and dissociative shock.

Viral immunity is a complex, multistep process involving both the innate and adaptive immune systems. Genetic defects in the immune system known as primary immune deficiency disorders (PIDDs) can result in viral infections that are severe, recurrent, or recalcitrant to therapy. These infections can lead to respiratory tract disease and pneumonitis, skin disease, and disseminated viral syndromes that affect multiple organs and even the brain. This review will provide a brief overview of immunity to viruses, an overview of PIDDs that result in significant viral susceptibility, as well as a diagnostic approach to these infections with a focus on defects that are severe and may require intensivist care.

CRITICAL CARE CLINICS

FORTHCOMING ISSUES

July 2022
Covid-19
Michelle N. Gong and Gregory S. Martin,
Editors

October 2022
Global Health and Critical Care Medicine
Kristina Elizabeth Rudd and Wangari
Waweru-Siika, *Editors*

January 2023
Neurocritical Care
Lori Shutter and Deepa Malaiyandi,
Editors

RECENT ISSUES

January 2022
**Diagnostic Excellence in the ICU: Thinking
Critically and Masterfully**
Paul A. Bergl and Rahul S. Nanchal, *Editors*

October 2021
Acute Respiratory Distress Syndrome
Michael A. Matthay and Kathleen D. Liu,
Editors

July 2021
Toxicology
Janice L. Zimmerman, *Editor*

SERIES OF RELATED INTEREST

Emergency Medicine Clinics
https://www.emed.theclinics.com/

THE CLINICS ARE AVAILABLE ONLINE!
Access your subscription at:
www.theclinics.com

Preface

Undiagnosed and Rare Diseases in Critical Care

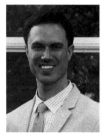 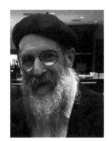

Brett J. Bordini, MD   Robert M. Kliegman, MD
Editors

Over the last several decades, advances in patient safety as well as diagnostics and therapeutics have led to dramatic improvements in outcomes for patients admitted to the intensive care unit. Nonetheless, many critically ill patients continue to experience adverse outcomes, oftentimes as a result of diagnostic error.[1] While some patients may present with atypical manifestations of a common disorder and elude diagnosis, others may have a rare disease whose signs and symptoms mimic a more common disorder or whose features are sufficiently nonspecific so as to preclude accurate and timely diagnosis. With more than 8000 rare diseases now known to the scientific community and an additional 250 or more described annually,[2] there are now more individual rare diseases than there are common diseases, collectively impacting more than 25 million people.[3] In addition to being at high risk for diagnostic error, patients with undiagnosed and rare diseases face additional barriers to diagnosis, key among them the access to diagnostic information and resources.

In this issue of *Critical Care Clinics*, we present a variety of rare disorders that may manifest with critical illness and that may confound diagnosis by virtue of mimicking more common diseases, as well as an overview of atypical presentations of common disorders that result in critical illness. In doing so, we leverage the experience of a predominantly single center's undiagnosed and rare disease program in creating an environment and a process that mitigates the risk of diagnostic error and improves diagnostic access for critically ill patients. The principles discussed herein provide a framework for evaluating and managing undiagnosed and rare diseases in critically

Crit Care Clin 38 (2022) xiii–xiv
https://doi.org/10.1016/j.ccc.2021.12.001
0749-0704/22/© 2021 Published by Elsevier Inc.

ill patients, as well as highlight general concepts in the approach to diagnostic error, undiagnosed disease, and rare disorders.

Brett J. Bordini, MD
Medical College of Wisconsin
Children's Wisconsin
Children's Corporate Center
999 North 92nd Street–Suite C560
Milwaukee, WI 53226, USA

Robert M. Kliegman, MD
Medical College of Wisconsin
Children's Wisconsin
Children's Corporate Center
999 North 92nd Street–Suite C450
Milwaukee, WI 53226, USA

E-mail addresses:
bbordini@mcw.edu (B.J. Bordini)
rkliegma@mcw.edu (R.M. Kliegman)

REFERENCES

1. Bergl PA, Nanchal RS, Singh H. Diagnostic error in the critically ill: defining the problem and exploring next steps to advance intensive care unit safety. Ann Am Thorac Soc 2018;15(8):903–7.
2. Gainotti S, Mascalzoni D, Bros-Facer V, et al. Meeting patients' right to the correct diagnosis: ongoing international initiatives on undiagnosed rare diseases and ethical and social issues. Int J Environ Res Public Health 2018;15(10). https://doi.org/10.3390/ijerph15102072.
3. Tifft CJ, Adams DR. The National Institutes of Health undiagnosed diseases program. Curr Opin Pediatr 2014;26(6):626–33.

Undiagnosed and Rare Diseases in Critical Care

The Role of Diagnostic Access

Brett J. Bordini, MD

KEYWORDS

- Bias • Critically ill • Diagnostic error • URD

KEY POINTS

- Diagnostic errors are common, harm patients, and are most frequently related to cognitive biases that impact medical reasoning and decision making.
- Patients with undiagnosed or rare diseases (URD) are at high risk for diagnostic error; critically ill patients with URD face additional shortfalls in diagnostic access that compound the risk of error.
- Diagnostic access is the ability to be evaluated in a health care environment with the requisite knowledge, experience, and resources capable of producing a timely, accurate, and satisfactory explanation for patient signs and symptoms.
- Local teams dedicated to patients with URD can address shortfalls in diagnostic access while mitigating the risk of diagnostic error.
- URD teams should be compromised of generalists and specialists from a wide array of disciplines, should engage in a structured evaluation, and should employ cognitive forcing functions to produce high-quality phenotypic data, guide diagnostic testing, and ensure rigor.

In the years following the 2015 publication of *Improving Diagnosis in Health Care* by the National Academies of Science-Engineering-Medicine, diagnostic error has become a central focus in improving patient outcomes. Although a lack of precise metrics leaves the exact scope unknown, diagnostic error is estimated to occur in approximately 15% of all medical encounters[1] and in up to 20% to 30% of intensive care unit deaths.[2–4] Cognitive psychology has provided a strong conceptual framework for understanding the causes of diagnostic error; evidence-based solutions remain nascent. Both the understanding and mitigation of diagnostic error rely on appreciating how the context of a diagnostic evaluation can influence its outcome.[5,6] In the intensive care unit, critically ill patients require simultaneous efforts to stabilize

Division of Hospital Medicine, Medical College of Wisconsin, Children's Corporate Center Suite 560, 999 N 92nd Street, Milwaukee, WI 53226, USA
E-mail address: bbordini@mcw.edu

Crit Care Clin 38 (2022) 159–171
https://doi.org/10.1016/j.ccc.2021.12.002   **criticalcare.theclinics.com**

tenuous physiology and to establish a working diagnosis sufficient for goal-directed therapy. These challenges, and the very context of the intensive care unit itself, increase cognitive burden and compound the risk of diagnostic error.[3,5,7] Patients with undiagnosed and rare diseases (URDs) face additional barriers to timely and accurate diagnosis when presenting with critical illness: in addition to the risk of diagnostic error, critically ill patients with URD, by virtue of their physiologic instability, often confront challenges in *diagnostic access*, the ability to be evaluated in a health care environment with the requisite resources capable of producing a timely, accurate, and satisfactory explanation for a patient's signs and symptoms.[8] Improving outcomes for critically ill patients with URD requires recognizing the possibility of an undiagnosed or rare condition leading to critical illness, mitigating the risk of diagnostic error, and reducing inequities in diagnostic access.

A FRAMEWORK FOR DIAGNOSTIC ERROR

Errors consist of missed, wrong, or delayed diagnoses. The causes are diverse, although they are broadly categorized as systems related, in which technical or organizational factors impede diagnosis, such as the unavailability of a particular testing modality or subspecialty service; no fault, in which diseases present with masked or unusual manifestations or in which diagnosis is obscured secondary to the patient being unable or unwilling to participate in the evaluation; or cognitive, in which shortfalls in clinician knowledge, data gathering, or medical reasoning and decision making produce errors.[9] Cognitive errors, either alone or in combination with systems-related errors, comprise approximately 75% of all diagnostic errors; most are related not to deficits in knowledge or data gathering, but rather to the ways in which various cognitive biases can confound medical reasoning and decision making.[9–11]

According to dual process theory, clinicians engaging in medical reasoning use either a predominantly intuitive approach, termed a *system 1 process*, or a more analytical approach, termed a *system 2 process*.[11,12] System 1 processes are based in heuristics, in which pattern recognition and rules of thumb are used to rapidly sort large amounts of clinical information into an illness script, a preformed cognitive representation of a specific disease, that allows for the quick formulation of a specific diagnosis or a limited differential diagnosis. On the other hand, system 2 processes rely on deliberate counterfactual reasoning and hypothesis generation based on individual patient data to arrive at a more robust differential diagnosis that attempts to unify patient problems via shared pathophysiologic mechanisms. Clinicians primarily use system 1 processes and achieve relatively accurate diagnoses for most patients under most circumstances,[11] although system 1 processes can fail when patient presentations are multisystem, complex, or evolving, instead becoming a form of cognitive bias that can result in diagnostic error.[13,14]

Cognitive biases affecting medical reasoning and decision making can be classified as heuristic failure, errors of attribution, and context-related. In heuristic failure, the very rules of thumb and quick pattern recognition that physicians use to arrive at a diagnosis fail to account for the entire scope of patient information or fail to adapt to new information as it becomes available.[14] While there are many examples of how heuristics can fail (**Table 1**), several are of particular importance for critically ill patients with undiagnosed or rare diseases. Diagnostic error can be a result of anchoring, wherein a clinician locks into a diagnosis based on the initial presenting features, failing to adjust diagnostic impressions as new information becomes available. With a wealth of diagnostic technology available, the proper probabilistic application and interpretation of testing can be challenging and can make clinicians susceptible to

Table 1	
Cognitive biases related to heuristic failure	
Bias	**Definition**
Anchoring	Locking into a diagnosis based on initial presenting features, failing to adjust diagnostic impressions when new information becomes available
Confirmation bias	Looking for and accepting only evidence that confirms a diagnostic impression, rejecting or not seeking contradictory evidence
Diagnostic momentum	Perpetuating a diagnostic label over time, usually by multiple providers both within and across health care systems, despite the label being incomplete or inaccurate
Expertise bias/yin-yang out	Believing that a patient who has already undergone an extensive evaluation will have nothing more to gain from further investigations, despite the possibility that the disease process or diagnostic techniques may have evolved so as to allow for appropriate diagnosis
Overconfidence bias	Believing one knows more than one does, acting on incomplete information or hunches, and prioritizing opinion or authority, as opposed to evidence
Premature closure	Accepting the first plausible diagnosis before obtaining confirmatory evidence or considering all available evidence. *"When the diagnosis is made, thinking stops"*
Unpacking principle	Failing to explore primary evidence or data in its entirety and subsequently failing to uncover important facts or findings, such as accepting a biopsy report or imaging study report without reviewing the actual specimen or image

From Bordini BJ, Stephany A, Kliegman R. Overcoming Diagnostic Errors in Medical Practice. J Pediatr. 2017;185:19-25.e1. https://doi:10.1016/j.jpeds.2017.02.065; with permission.

confirmation bias, wherein one looks only for evidence that confirms diagnostic impressions, to the neglect of contradictory evidence. Finally, diagnostic momentum is a significant source of cognitive bias, especially in the era of electronic medical records, wherein diagnostic labels are copied forward and perpetuated over time without being questioned, despite those labels oftentimes being outdated, incomplete, or even inaccurate.

Cognitive bias related to errors of attribution occurs when perceived characteristics of patients, family members, or members of the medical evaluation team are given undue weight in the diagnostic formulation (**Table 2**). These factors can influence the affective state of the clinician and the integrity of cognition, increasing the likelihood of error.[15] Important examples in the evaluation of URD include the appeal to authority, wherein senior, supervising, or otherwise expert recommendations are treated as authoritative, independent of whether evidence supports those recommendations. Statements such as "I've never seen that disease present in this way," when coming from a senior, experienced clinician, can be given undue emphasis and remove certain diagnoses from consideration. Outcome biases may occur when clinicians deemphasize the importance of certain results by labeling them as "slightly" or "mildly" abnormal, rather than treating them as objective data points to be interpreted within the context of the patient's physiology and pathophysiology. Finally, patients with a history of mental illness, or with symptoms that do not immediately suggest organic pathology, can be labeled as having symptoms secondary to a psychiatric diagnosis when organic pathology may be the sole cause of their symptoms.

Table 2 Cognitive biases related to errors of attribution	
Bias	**Definition**
Affective bias	Allowing emotions to interfere with a diagnosis, either positively or negatively; dislikes of patient types (e.g., "frequent flyers")
Appeal to authority	Deferring to authoritative recommendations from senior, supervising, or "expert" clinicians, independent of the evidentiary support for such recommendations
Ascertainment bias	Maintaining preconceived expectations based on patient or disease stereotypes
Countertransference	Being influenced by positive or negative subjective feelings toward a specific patient
Outcome bias	Minimizing or overemphasizing the significance of a finding or result, often based on subjective feelings about a patient, a desired outcome, or personal confidence in one's own clinical skills; the use of "slightly" to describe abnormal results
Psych-out bias	Maintaining biases about people with presumed mental illness

From Bordini BJ, Stephany A, Kliegman R. Overcoming diagnostic errors in medical practice. J Pediatr 2017;185:19–25.e1. doi:10.1016/j.jpeds.2017.02.065; with permission.

With context-related biases, the setting of the diagnostic evaluation influences how clinicians perceive and process the information used in medical decision making (**Table 3**). External factors, such as increased patient volumes, higher patient acuity, or staffing shortages, as well as internal factors, such as sleep deprivation, stress, and physician burnout, can amplify individual cognitive burden and increase the likelihood of diagnostic error.[7,16,17] Independent of and in addition to cognitive burden, context can introduce bias by causing clinicians to consciously or subconsciously deemphasize relevant information and amplify impertinent information while formulating a diagnosis. Important examples of context-related biases include the availability bias, in which recent previous cases that are more easily recalled influence the differential diagnosis of the present case. Not every infant with respiratory distress in the middle of viral season has bronchiolitis; some may indeed have heart failure, for example. The *framing effect* produces bias when the manner or setting in which a patient is presented influences the perception of information. For example, a patient presenting with abdominal pain may have drastically different differential diagnoses generated for their pain depending on whether they are evaluated in an emergency department, a primary care office, or a gastroenterology clinic. Finally, patients with URDs who are evaluated in fragmented specialty settings are often susceptible to thinking in silo, in which the patient's complaints are only considered within the spectrum of pathophysiology relevant to that specialty.

For critically ill patients with unstable physiology, efforts to re-establish homeostasis may succeed despite the lack of an established, accurate diagnosis, leading to a hindsight bias in which clinicians overestimate the efficacy of their diagnostic reasoning and therapeutic interventions. Examples include patients with self-limited viral or noninfectious inflammatory disorders whose symptoms resolve despite and not due to interventions like parenteral antibacterials. Such illnesses are often inaccurately labeled "culture-negative" bacterial sepsis, which may preclude consideration of treatable viral, autoimmune, or autoinflammatory disorders. For other patients, interventions may merely stabilize patient signs or symptoms while failing to recognize or correct critical pathophysiology. In these circumstances, the underlying illness fails

Table 3
Cognitive biases related to errors of context

Bias	Definition
Availability bias	Basing decisions on the most recent patient with similar symptoms, preferentially recalling recent and more common diseases
Base-rate neglect	Overestimating or underestimating the prevalence of a disease, typically overestimating the prevalence of common diseases and underestimating the prevalence of rare diseases
Framing effect	Being influenced by how or by whom a problem is described, or by the setting in which the evaluation takes place
Frequency bias	Believing that common things happen commonly and are usually benign in general practice
Hindsight bias	Reinforcing diagnostic errors once a diagnosis is discovered in spite of these errors. May lead to a clinician overestimating the efficacy of his or her clinical reasoning and may reinforce ineffective techniques
Posterior probability error	Considering the likelihood of a particular diagnosis in light of a patient's prior or chronic illnesses. New headaches in a patient with a history of migraines may in fact be a tumor
Representative bias	Basing decisions on an expected typical presentation. Not effective for atypical presentations. Overemphasis on disease diagnostic criteria or "classic" presentations. "Looks like a duck, quacks like a duck"
Sutton's slip	Ignoring alternate explanations for "obvious" diagnoses (Sutton law is that one should first consider the obvious)
Thinking in silo	Restricting diagnostic considerations to a particular specialty or organ system. Each discipline has a set of diseases within its comfort zone, which reduces diagnostic flexibility or team-based communication
Zebra retreat	Lacking conviction to pursue rare disorders even when suggested by evidence

From Bordini BJ, Stephany A, Kliegman R. Overcoming Diagnostic Errors in Medical Practice. J Pediatr. 2017;185:19-25.e1. https://doi.org/10.1016/j.jpeds.2017.02.065; with permission.

to resolve, although its presenting features are now being normalized such that ongoing disease is no longer appreciated; common examples include the failure to consider or comprehensively evaluate for secondary causes of hypertension or chronic headache, leading to disorders such as pheochromocytoma or a brain mass not being diagnosed in a timely fashion.

THE ROLE OF DIAGNOSTIC ACCESS

Patients with URDs frequently experience delays in diagnosis. Rare Diseases Europe (EURORDIS) conducted a survey among 6000 patients with a selection of rare diseases that included, among others, Duchenne muscular dystrophy, Prader-Willi syndrome, tuberous sclerosis, and fragile X syndrome, finding that 25% of respondents experienced waits varying between 5 and 30 years from the time of symptom onset to diagnosis and that 40% of respondents were given at least one erroneous diagnosis.[18] Furthermore, 25% of respondents had to travel to a different region to obtain diagnosis, with 2% having to travel to a different country.[18] For rarer disorders, wait times and limitations in local diagnostic resources can be even more pronounced, resulting in limited access to diagnosis that compounds diagnostic errors.

Diagnostic access is the ability to be evaluated in a health care environment with the requisite knowledge, experience, and resources capable of producing a timely, accurate, and satisfactory explanation for patient signs and symptoms. Diagnostic access may consist of the relative availability of disease-specific knowledge to patients[19] or clinicians,[20] as well as the affordability or availability of advanced diagnostic modalities such as genomic sequencing, metabolomics, or proteomics. However, access to information and advanced diagnostic technologies alone is not enough. With increasing parity in terms of access to diagnostic technology, many primary care or specialty clinicians can order advanced diagnostic assays for their patients when facing a diagnostic dilemma. Patients often present for evaluation to a rare disease program already having obtained at least one or more gene panels, if not having exome sequencing already completed, and yet persisting without a diagnosis. Next-generation molecular genetic technologies, if not paired with high-quality next-generation phenotypic data, may not only fail to attain diagnosis but also can confound the diagnostic formulation.[21] As such, the final critical component of diagnostic access is the availability of a coordinated and collaborative team of clinicians that can provide high-quality and refined phenotyping to inform the ordering and interpretation of advanced diagnostic modalities such as genomic sequencing.

Understanding diagnostic access first requires an understanding of how patients with rare or undiagnosed disorders can present for medical evaluation and hopefully attain diagnosis. *First, not all rare disorders pose a diagnostic dilemma.* Some present with pathognomonic historical, physical, laboratory, or imaging findings that facilitate diagnosis shortly after presentation. Disorders in children like cystic fibrosis are now routinely detected on newborn screening, or in fortunately increasingly rarer instances, upon symptom presentation. In adults, the characteristic findings of Huntington disease allow for expedited diagnosis. Not all rare disorders remain undiagnosed for long.

Second, not all patients with an undiagnosed disease have a rare disease. Some may have atypical manifestations of a common disorder, others may have more than one underlying common disease process, while others may have iatrogenic symptoms that confound the presentation of a common disease. An example from our own program was a patient who was hospitalized with typhoid fever who subsequently developed neurologic symptoms that were initially labeled as acute disseminated encephalomyelitis secondary to the infection, who was instead ultimately diagnosed with an invasive T-cell lymphoma.

Finally, some rare diseases can closely mimic more common disorders, whereas others may have multisystem, complex, and slowly evolving symptoms that make the appreciation of a single, unifying diagnosis elusive. Within our own program, we evaluated a patient who was hospitalized initially with a presumptive diagnosis of acute cerebellar ataxia, who would improve after being administered steroids, only to have symptoms recur once the steroids were tapered. Over time, the patient manifested additional concerning physical and laboratory findings, although did so slowly and incompletely, and it was not until exome sequencing revealed a diagnosis of familial hemophagocytic lymphohistiocytosis that we were able to retroactively appreciate the patient gradually satisfying clinical criteria for diagnosis over time before our involvement.

Patients with URDs are not homogeneous. Regardless of how symptoms manifest, though, one theme is common: patients with rare or undiagnosed disorders frequently find themselves on a diagnostic odyssey (**Fig. 1**),[21,22] the journey of developing

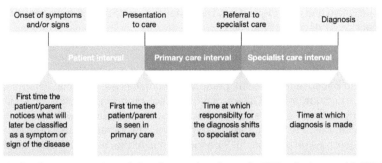

Fig. 1. A visual representation of the diagnostic odyssey in URDs. Patients with URDs may develop critical illness and present to an intensive care unit at any of the 3 intervals, which may limit or interrupt access to URD-focused evaluation. (*From* Black, N; Martineau, F; Manacorda, Tommaso; (2015) Diagnostic odyssey for rare diseases: exploration of potential indicators. Policy Innovation Research Unit (PIRU). %%%https://piru.ac.uk/assets/files/Rare% 20diseases%20Final%20report.pdf; with permission.)

symptoms, seeking evaluation, experiencing symptom evolution, and seeking further evaluation, all in the attempt to finally obtain an accurate diagnosis.

The diagnostic odyssey can last months, years, or even decades, and can be thought of as occurring in several distinct phases. First, as symptoms develop, patients or their families start to notice the findings that will ultimately be recognized as a manifestation of the underlying disease. As those symptoms fail to resolve, most patients first seek evaluation within the context of their primary care relationship. Often, this phase can last for quite some time, as round after round of "routine" tests are obtained and fail to yield conclusive evidence of an underlying disorder. However, over time, if symptoms persist and evaluation with the primary care physician fails to reveal a diagnosis, patients are typically referred to a specialist based on the involved organ system suggested by the patient's symptoms. Under ideal circumstances, diagnosis occurs within either the primary care or specialist care intervals, and the odyssey ends. For patients who remain undiagnosed, if a referral is made, these phases of primary and specialty care evaluation can be the entry points from which someone will access the rare and undiagnosed disease space, but there can be many delays, detours, and disruptions along the path to diagnosis, and despite best intentions, sometimes patients remain undiagnosed after months or even years of evaluation.

Patients on diagnostic odysseys may remain undiagnosed for a variety of reasons related to access that can broadly be divided into 3 categories. First, some patients may remain in diagnostic stasis, engaging in a plan of symptom management that may result in the ability to function day-to-day, but without a specific diagnosis and properly tailored management plan. These patients may persist without a satisfactory diagnosis because their symptomatic management plan is sufficient to allow them to continue living their daily lives, despite ultimately being suboptimal or improperly matched to their true disease process. These patients remain within the primary and specialty care intervals of the diagnostic odyssey and fail to access the URD diagnostic space altogether. Examples include patients with iron-resistant iron deficiency anemia who end up on staggeringly high doses of enteral iron supplementation or chronic transfusion with the attendant side effects and risks involved, or one patient with a presumptive diagnosis of static encephalopathy being managed symptomatically for seizures and spasticity who was referred to our program for rapidly progressive and profound neurodegeneration. By the time the diagnosis of cerebral folate deficiency was established, the disease was so advanced that the family opted to pursue palliative and end-of-life care. These patients have an undiagnosed or rare disease, but do not necessarily know it.

In contrast, there are patients who know they are on a diagnostic odyssey, are referred for evaluation to a rare and undiagnosed disease evaluation program, but are not accepted for or are unable to participate in the evaluation. Some may be unable to do so because their health, personal circumstances, or social determinants of health may preclude travel. Others may not meet program selection criteria. Fortunately, many national evaluation programs provide assistance with travel, lodging, and evaluation costs to ameliorate these barriers. The increased use of telemedicine during the coronavirus disease 2019 pandemic has further allowed many rare disease programs to engage in distance-based evaluations for patients who are unable to travel for evaluation, instead providing recommendations to local clinicians who have the resources to perform the prescribed evaluation locally. Nonetheless, many patients on a diagnostic odyssey are unable to satisfactorily obtain timely or comprehensive evaluation.

Finally, there are patients with rare or undiagnosed diseases who present acutely or critically ill and require urgent evaluation. Owing to physiologic instability and the need for rapid evaluation and diagnosis, these patients require a team of expert diagnosticians who can mobilize rapidly around them, where they are, and evaluate them directly at the bedside.

All these patients benefit from an evaluation team that can meet them at these challenged points of access, particularly when it comes to pediatric patients, considering that approximately half of rare diseases present in children.[21,23] These hospital-based programs, often affiliated with academic institutions, can address the diagnostic needs of acutely and critically ill patients, serve as a complimentary referral pipeline for patients unable to participate in national referral network evaluations, and meet the diagnostic needs of patients emerging from stasis in the primary and specialty care evaluation phases of their diagnostic odyssey. The goal of local institution-based URD evaluation teams is to rapidly and collaboratively provide high-quality phenotype clarification to inform the diagnostic process and the interpretation of advanced diagnostic modalities.

UNDIAGNOSED AND RARE DISEASES IN CRITICAL CARE

Patients with undiagnosed or rare diseases may experience episodic critical illness or may even have their first symptom presentation consist of a critical illness. Despite wider appreciation of its role in adverse patient outcomes, the risk of diagnostic error for critically ill patients remains high.[3] At least one misdiagnosis is identified in approximately 30% of adult intensive care unit autopsies, and estimates suggest that up to 7% of intensive care unit deaths are due to lethal misdiagnoses[24]; pediatric autopsy data have identified major diagnostic errors in up to 20% of patients.[2] Patients experiencing diagnostic error in the intensive care unit may have a rare disease presenting in extremis, such as febrile infection-related epilepsy syndrome or new-onset refractory status epilepticus, or may have an atypical manifestation of a common disease that leaves them undiagnosed.

Critically ill patients with undiagnosed or rare diseases are no different with respect to being on a diagnostic odyssey; however, by virtue of the severity of their presentation, they have limitations in their access to diagnosis, whether it be limited ability for in-person evaluation with rare disease specialists or larger referral-based programs, limited time for the primary team to engage in expanded diagnostic reasoning, or limited availability of certain advanced diagnostic modalities at the institution in which they are being treated. Local, in-house URD teams can improve access to diagnosis in critically ill patients with undiagnosed or rare diseases by identifying and minimizing the risk and actuality of diagnostic error, and in doing so, can produce a high-quality next-generation phenotype that can enhance the utility of advanced diagnostic modalities such as genetic sequencing. URD teams should operate under several guiding principles: the team-based approach, the structured evaluation, and the use of cognitive forcing functions such as diagnostic time-outs to ensure rigor.

The Team-Based Approach

A *team-based approach* enhances diagnostic accuracy beyond that achieved by individual senior expert clinicians. The primary aphorism that has driven the evaluation of each patient in our program is that "none of us is as smart as all of us"; indeed, collective intelligence-based medical decision making has consistently and significantly outperformed even the most accurate diagnosticians in certain clinical contexts.[25] Each patient evaluation team should be composed not only of generalists and those specialists whose area of expertise is directly related to the patient's primary concerns but also of additional specialists from a wide breadth of disciplines. Doing so fosters a collective knowledge base that mitigates context-related biases by soliciting perspectives on pathophysiology and differential diagnoses that may not have otherwise been considered were the patient evaluated within the silos of individual specialty settings. This collaborative and more deliberate approach to diagnosis additionally encourages the use of system 2 processes by actively promoting the generation of multiple diagnostic hypotheses and testing strategies. The end goal and product of this process is the group phenotype, in which the evaluation team has collectively—as a group—analyzed the patient's primary concerns, physical findings, and objective data into discrete phenotypic phenomena. These phenomena can then be explored further in attempts to uncover underlying and unifying pathophysiologic mechanisms—a differential pathophysiology—and can additionally serve as high-quality phenotypic data that can better inform the interpretation of molecular genetic studies.[26]

The Structured Evaluation

Following referral, URD evaluation begins by obtaining and comprehensively reviewing the entirety of the medical record, inclusive of any institutions that have evaluated the patient previously. The review should be conducted objectively and in a manner that consciously avoids potential sources of bias that may perpetuate inaccurate diagnostic labels. Such labels are removed and replaced with descriptions of the clinical phenomena in question: for example, recurrent Guillain-Barré syndrome becomes episodic extremity weakness, dysesthesia, and hyporeflexia. Doing so interrupts diagnostic momentum, avoids premature closure, and allows for consideration of alternate hypotheses, such as inherited neuropathies, channelopathies, or infectious myelitis.[27–30] Any imaging studies and pathology specimens from other institutions are obtained and directly reviewed by a team member whose area of expertise is pertinent to the study. Previous written interpretations of these studies are never accepted at face value, so as to avoid the unpacking principle, in which failure to elicit all available information leads to an incomplete understanding of the patient's concerns. Rereviewing this clinical information with "another set of eyes" will sometimes lead to the detection of previously overlooked critical findings.

The next step in the structured evaluation is to distill the patient's history, results of previous diagnostic testing, and physical examination findings into a clearly defined phenotype of the disease to generate hypotheses about underlying pathophysiology. When defining the phenotype, it is critical to consider which findings are likely to represent primary pathology, which represent morbidity secondary to that pathology, which findings may be true though unrelated to the underlying disease, and which may be consequences of therapy or otherwise iatrogenic. For example, recurrent pneumonias may be a direct manifestation of primary ciliary dyskinesia or immunodeficiency or may be secondary to restrictive lung disease from neuromuscular weakness. Defining the phenotype is further aided by emphasizing the symptoms and signs over specific diagnostic labels, so as to avoid any cognitive biases that such labels would introduce. Emphasizing symptoms is more likely to engage hypothetical and counterfactual reasoning, whereas using diagnostic labels engages heuristics. Instead of thinking "what illness script or disease process can I make this fit?" the clinician instead generates the differential pathophysiology by which the symptom could have occurred, which allows for the recognition of common processes that may be impacting numerous organ systems, thereby linking findings together in a unifying mechanism.[27–30]

After all relevant clinical data have been gathered and analyzed, and hypotheses regarding the underlying pathophysiology of the URD have been generated, a testing strategy that will maximize the yield while minimizing the burden on the patient and the family should be developed. If noninvasive diagnostic measures will yield accurate and reliable results, they should be favored, but one should never shy away from invasive measures if they are going to prove critical in establishing the diagnosis. The turn-around time of various diagnostic modalities should be considered as well. Under certain circumstances, genetic sequencing results can be obtained in as little as 1 to 2 weeks, or even as little as 26 hours,[31] although most instances still require several months. If a functional assay can provide a diagnosis with a similar degree of certainty, although in a shorter amount of time than a molecular genetic assay, then that assay should be ordered in place of or in addition to genetic testing, in which case the genetic testing results become confirmatory and assist further in prognosis and therapy planning. For example, a perforin granzyme assay may indicate a diagnosis of hemophagocytic lymphohistiocytosis more rapidly than a gene panel or exome sequencing.

Cognitive Forcing Functions and Diagnostic Time-Outs

The context of each diagnostic evaluation is unique and includes not only the cognitive and affective circumstances of the clinician in that moment but also the circumstances of the patient, the patient's family, and other members of the evaluation team, as well as those of the clinic or hospital unit in which the evaluation is being conducted. This combination of factors invariably carries the risk of producing bias, although most physicians maintain a bias blind spot, perceiving themselves as being less susceptible to bias despite bias being a universal "operating characteristic of the diagnosing brain."[11,32–35] Operationalizing an awareness of bias into improved patient outcomes remains challenging,[11,35] although primary among successful strategies are cognitive forcing functions,[36] structured opportunities to pause, re-evaluate data and diagnostic impressions, and question the appropriateness of any diagnostic labels that have accumulated in the course of a patient evaluation. Mirroring the patient safety movement and the use of interventions such as procedural time-outs, diagnostic checklists such as a diagnostic time-out can be used at regular intervals, following any diagnostic test or therapeutic intervention, with any change in patient status, and—perhaps most importantly—with any patient handoff or change in attending provider or team members. These structured opportunities allow for the interruption of diagnostic momentum and form part of a feedback system that over time improves individual and collective diagnostic performance.[25,36,37] Over the course of evaluation of each patient with URD, we regularly use the following checklist[38]:

1. Have we gathered sufficient information upon which to base our analysis?
2. Have we unpacked that information and processed it in an objective and bias-free manner?
3. What is the ultimate phenotype suggested by the patient's complaints and findings?
4. Does that phenotype suggest one underlying disease process or multiple disease processes occurring simultaneously?
5. Have we generated plausible hypotheses regarding the pathophysiology of these complaints and findings?
6. Have we implemented a directed diagnostic testing strategy using sufficiently sensitive and specific diagnostic assays that will allow us to discern among these diagnostic hypotheses in a Bayesian probabilistic fashion, as opposed to a dichotomous, "rule in, rule out" fashion?
7. Have we checked for additional sources of bias?
8. Have we considered alternate diagnoses sufficiently, and in particular, "do-not-miss" diagnoses?

SUMMARY

Critically ill patients with URDs are at high risk for cognitive diagnostic errors as well as delays in diagnosis that are the result of impaired diagnostic access. Local evaluation teams dedicated to URDs can address both the risk and actuality of diagnostic error, as well as shortfalls in diagnostic access, particularly for patients whose diminished diagnostic access is a result of critical illness. Teams that draw on a breadth of specialty representation and work in a structured fashion toward the creation of a group phenotype, a differential pathophysiology, and robust diagnostic hypotheses can produce a directed testing strategy that can expedite the evaluation of critically ill patients with URDs.

CLINICS CARE POINTS

- Critically ill patients are at high risk of diagnostic error.
- Patients with undiagnosed or rare diseases (URD) may experience episodic critical illness or may have their first symptomatic presentation consist of a critical illness.
- Critical illness can impair diagnostic access; local, in-house URD evaluation teams can improve diagnostic access and minimize the risk of diagnostic error.

REFERENCES

1. Committee on Diagnostic Error in Health Care, Board on Health Care Services, Institute of Medicine, The National Academies of Sciences, Engineering, and Medicine.. In: Balogh EP, Miller BT, Ball JR, editors. Improving diagnosis in health care. National Academies Press; 2015. Available at: http://www.nap.edu/catalog/21794. July 18, 2016.
2. Custer JW, Winters BD, Goode V, et al. Diagnostic errors in the pediatric and neonatal ICU: a systematic review. Pediatr Crit Care Med 2015;16(1):29–36.
3. Bergl PA, Nanchal RS, Singh H. Diagnostic error in the critically iii: defining the problem and exploring next steps to advance intensive care unit safety. Ann ATS 2018;15(8):903–7.
4. Cifra CL, Eyck PT, Dawson JD, et al. Factors associated with diagnostic error on admission to a pediatric intensive care unit: a Pilot Study. Pediatr Crit Care Med 2020;21(5):e311–5.

5. Shafer GJ, Suresh G. Diagnostic errors in the neonatal intensive care unit: a case series. AJP Rep 2018;08(4):e379–83.

6. Bordini BJ, Kliegman RM, Basel D, et al. Undiagnosed and rare diseases in perinatal medicine. Clin Perinatology 2020;47(1):1–14.

7. Sweller J. Cognitive load theory, learning difficulty, and instructional design. Learn Instruction 1994;4(4):295–312.

8. Bordini BJ. Addressing undiagnosed and rare disease in 2020 and beyond. In: Undiagnosed and rare diseases in children and adolescents: translation to clinic and society. Barcelona (Spain): Hospital Sant Joan de Déu; 2019. Available at: https://www.fundacionareces.es/fundacionareces/en/events/undiagnosed-and-rare-diseases-in-children-and-adolescents-translation-to-clinic-and-society.html#pestanas-programa1.

9. Graber ML, Franklin N, Gordon R. Diagnostic error in internal medicine. Arch Intern Med 2005;165(13):1493–9.

10. Zwaan L, de Bruijne M, Wagner C, et al. Patient record review of the incidence, consequences, and causes of diagnostic adverse events. Arch Intern Med 2010; 170(12):1015–21.

11. Croskerry P. Bias: a normal operating characteristic of the diagnosing brain. Diagnosis 2014;1(1):23–7.

12. Norman G. Dual processing and diagnostic errors. Adv Health Sci Educ Theory Pract 2009;14(Suppl 1):37–49.

13. Slonim AD, LaFleur BJ, Ahmed W, et al. Hospital-reported medical errors in children. Pediatrics 2003;111(3):617–21.

14. McDonald CJ. Medical heuristics: the silent adjudicators of clinical practice. Ann Intern Med 1996;124(1 Pt 1):56–62.

15. Croskerry P. Diagnostic failure: a cognitive and affective approach. In: Henriksen K, Battles JB, Marks ES, et al, editors. Advances in patient safety: from Research to implementation (volume 2: concepts and methodology). Advances in patient safety. Rockville (MD): Agency for Healthcare Research and Quality; 2005. p. 241–54. Available at: http://www.ncbi.nlm.nih.gov/books/NBK20487/. August 1, 2021.

16. Patel VL, Buchman TG. Cognitive overload in the ICU. Available at: https://psnet.ahrq.gov/web-mm/cognitive-overload-icu. August 1, 2021.

17. Patel VL, Zhang J, Yoskowitz NA, et al. Translational cognition for decision support in critical care environments: a review. J Biomed Inform 2008;41(3):413–31.

18. EURORDIS.. Survey of the delay in diagnosis for 8 rare diseases in Europe (EurordisCare2). Paris, France: EURORDIS; 2007.

19. Dong D, Chung RYN, Chan RHW, et al. Why is misdiagnosis more likely among some people with rare diseases than others? Insights from a population-based cross-sectional study in China. Orphanet J Rare Dis 2020;15(1):307.

20. Faviez C, Chen X, Garcelon N, et al. Diagnosis support systems for rare diseases: a scoping review. Orphanet J Rare Dis 2020;15(1):94.

21. Gainotti S, Mascalzoni D, Bros-Facer V, et al. Meeting patients' right to the correct diagnosis: ongoing International Initiatives on undiagnosed rare diseases and ethical and social Issues. Int J Environ Res Public Health 2018;15(10). https://doi.org/10.3390/ijerph15102072.

22. Black N, Martineau F, Manacorda T. Diagnostic odyssey for rare diseases: exploration of potential indicators. London: Policy Innovation Research Unit, LSHTM; 2015.

23. Richter T, Nestler-Parr S, Babela R, et al. Rare disease terminology and definitions—a systematic global review: report of the ISPOR rare disease special interest group. Value Health 2015;18(6):906–14.
24. Winters B, Custer J, Galvagno SM, et al. Diagnostic errors in the intensive care unit: a systematic review of autopsy studies. BMJ Qual Saf 2012;21(11):894–902.
25. Wolf M, Krause J, Carney PA, et al. Collective intelligence meets medical decision-making: the collective outperforms the best radiologist. PLoS ONE 2015;10(8):e0134269.
26. Lu JT, Campeau PM, Lee BH. Genotype-phenotype correlation–promiscuity in the era of next-generation sequencing. N Engl J Med 2014;371(7):593-596. doi:10.1056/NEJMp1400788.
27. Schiff GD, Hasan O, Kim S, et al. Diagnostic error in medicine: analysis of 583 physician-reported errors. Arch Intern Med 2009;169(20):1881–7.
28. Ely JW, Kaldjian LC, D'Alessandro DM. Diagnostic errors in primary care: lessons learned. J Am Board Fam Med 2012;25(1):87–97.
29. Kostopoulou O, Oudhoff J, Nath R, et al. Predictors of diagnostic accuracy and safe management in difficult diagnostic problems in family medicine. Med Decis Making 2008;28(5):668–80.
30. Kostopoulou O, Devereaux-Walsh C, Delaney BC. Missing celiac disease in family medicine: the importance of hypothesis generation. Med Decis Making 2009;29(3):282–90.
31. Miller NA, Farrow EG, Gibson M, et al. A 26-hour system of highly sensitive whole genome sequencing for emergency management of genetic diseases. Genome Med 2015;7(1):100.
32. National Academies of Sciences E. Improving diagnosis in health care.; 2015. doi:10.17226/21794
33. Schiff GD, Kim S, Abrams R, et al. Diagnosing diagnosis errors: lessons from a multi-institutional collaborative project. Rockville (MD): Agency for Healthcare Research and Quality; 2005. Available at: https://www.ncbi.nlm.nih.gov/books/NBK20492/. September 19, 2016.
34. Holmboe ES, Durning SJ. Assessing clinical reasoning: moving from in vitro to in vivo. Diagnosis 2014;1(1):111–7.
35. West RF, Meserve RJ, Stanovich KE. Cognitive sophistication does not attenuate the bias blind spot. J Personal Social Psychol 2012;103(3):506–19.
36. Ely JW, Graber ML, Croskerry P. Checklists to reduce diagnostic errors. Acad Med 2011;86(3):307.
37. Berner ES, Graber ML. Overconfidence as a cause of diagnostic error in medicine. Am J Med 2008;121(5 Suppl):S2–23.
38. Bordini BJ, Stephany A, Kliegman R. Overcoming diagnostic errors in medical practice. J Pediatr 2017;185:19–25.e1.

Rapid Exome and Genome Sequencing in the Intensive Care Unit

Michael Muriello, MD, Donald Basel, MBBCh*

KEYWORDS

- Rapid genome sequencing • Rapid exome sequencing • Genomics in critical care

KEY POINTS

- Congenital malformations are a leading cause of morbidity and mortality, and children with genetic disorders are at higher risk for requiring acute care than children without a known diagnosis.
- Genetic disorders can manifest at any age with various acute symptoms.
- Cost savings are not necessarily due to the acquired data but rather the expediency at which the data can be provided, supporting rapid sequencing.
- Cumulative data from several studies support clinical utility, with specific management changes recommended in 65% of diagnosed patients and 26% of patients tested overall.

Genetic sequencing plays an established and important role in the diagnosis of heritable disorders in the outpatient setting. Historically, inpatient genetic sequencing has had little to no role in acute medical decision making, as the turnaround time for results has typically exceeded the duration of the index hospitalization. The neonatal intensive care unit has been an exception, where extended hospitalizations for neonates with complex disease manifestations, many of which are heritable, are more common. The advent of rapid genomic sequencing offers the opportunity to apply this technology in the setting of an acute or critical illness hospitalization. Although most critically ill children in the intensive care unit (ICU) do not have an undiagnosed genetic condition causing their hospitalization, many genetic disorders can present with critical illness, and making a diagnosis may dictate the outcome of the acute presentation. Genetic disorders can manifest at any age with various acute symptoms including hypoglycemia, acidosis, hyperammonemia, encephalopathy, refractory seizures, liver failure, cardiomyopathy, and progressive central nervous system dysfunction, among others. A high index of suspicion for genetic etiologies is essential, as quick initiation of

Genetics, Department of Pediatrics, Medical College of Wisconsin, 9000 W. Wisconsin Avenue, MC 716, Milwaukee, WI 53226, USA
* Corresponding author.
E-mail address: dbasel@mcw.edu

Crit Care Clin 38 (2022) 173–184
https://doi.org/10.1016/j.ccc.2021.11.001
0749-0704/22/© 2021 Elsevier Inc. All rights reserved.

additional investigations, which could include rapid sequencing, may be the only way to improve outcomes. Other clues to the presence of an underlying genetic disorder may include a history of developmental delay or intellectual disability, hypotonia, exercise intolerance, failure to thrive, or a family history of symptoms suggestive of a Mendelian disorder. It is always important to review the newborn screening results (in the case of pediatric patients and younger adults born after the initiation of widespread newborn screening programs) and any other available diagnostic data to help guide the appropriate additional evaluation of a patient in critical care. Biochemical and functional results can often be obtained in a shorter period of time and should not be delayed if considering genomic sequencing. However, many disorders present nonspecifically or atypically and can only be diagnosed by genomic sequencing.

THE TECHNOLOGY

Medical genetics has made unprecedented advances in the last half-century (**Fig. 1**), from chromosome visualization and banding in 1959, Sanger sequencing in 1977, fluorescence in situ hybridization (FISH) in 1982, and massively parallel sequencing (developed in 1992), which allowed the evolution of genomic medicine. The human genome project launched in 1990, and the first publication of the core sequence was completed in 2003. Clinical exome sequencing was validated in the research setting for the diagnosis of rare or undiagnosed disease late in the first decade of the 2000s. The first clinical genetic diagnosis was made by exome sequencing in 2009,[1] and the technology began to be used widely in clinical practice after 2010.

Genomic sequencing technology has continued to evolve equally rapidly in the decades since the first sequence of the human genome was completed. This evolution, combined with increased utilization, has resulted in a precipitous drop in cost.[2] Genomic sequencing is no longer cost-prohibitive and is used in routine clinical

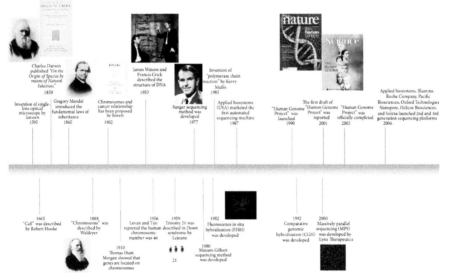

Fig. 1. Key landmarks in the history of genomic science. (*From* Durmaz AA, Karaca E, Demkow U, et al. Evolution of genetic techniques: past, present, and beyond. Biomed Res Int 2015;2015:461524. https://doi.org/10.1155/2015/461524; with permission)

care in both the inpatient and outpatient setting for the diagnosis of rare genetic disorders. The turnaround time to complete sequencing has fallen alongside overall cost (**Fig. 2**). What once took several months can now be achieved in a few days. The technology has arrived at the point at which it makes practical sense to consider its use in critical care management, and since 2012 the work of many groups has accumulated data supporting exome sequencing and genome sequencing in the ICU (**Table 1**).

EXOME SEQUENCING VERSUS GENOME SEQUENCING

Exome sequencing (ES) targets exons, which represent approximately 1% of all DNA and harbor over 99% of all known disease-causing variants. Genome sequencing (GS) is untargeted and generates sequence data for the entire genome. GS and ES generate similar quality data and have some of the same limitations. Copy number variants (CNVs), deletions, or duplications of genetic material can be more readily and directly detected by GS, owing to relatively even read depth coverage across all genomic regions. Some studies have shown that GS provides better coverage of exons, especially for the first exons of genes.[3] CNVs can be extrapolated from ES data, but there are still reservations regarding absolute accuracy when compared with true microarray/comparative genomic hybridization and GS. As there is no required target capture step for sample preparation with GS, it can be initiated and completed more rapidly than ES. Rapid GS (rGS) generally has 2- to 4-day turnaround time from receipt of sample but many laboratories still work on 10- to 14-day turnaround. The fastest published clinical GS turnaround time is 19 hours.[4] GS is more expensive than ES because of the need to generate, store, and bioinformatically process more data.

GS provides between a 5% to a 10% increase in the diagnostic yield compared with ES, primarily by detection of deep intronic and intergenic variation.[3] GS data can be used to identify some pathogenic repeat expansions.[5,6] Other studies have shown no increase in diagnostic utility of GS over ES.[7] Including both parents in sequencing (termed a trio analysis) allows for immediate segregation of variants and confirmation that putative pathogenic variants are de novo or inherited, further increasing diagnostic yield. Such segregation of variants can allow for richer analysis when the

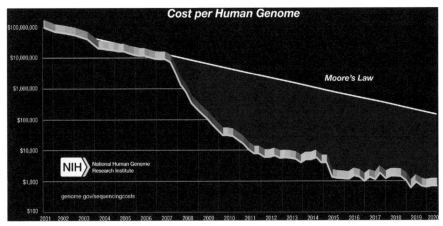

Fig. 2. Down-trending cost of genome sequencing. (*From* Wetterstrand KA. DNA sequencing costs: data from the NHGRI genome sequencing program (GSP). Available at: www.genome.gov/sequencingcostsdata. Accessed [November 30, 2020])

Table 1
Summary of key genomic studies in pediatric critical care setting and impact on decision making

Publication	year	Study Population[a]	Study Type	Test[b]	Turn-Around Time	Diagnostic Rate	Change in Management[c]
Willig et al	2015	n = 35, infants; NICU, PICU	Retrospective	GS	23 d (median)	57%	65% of diagnosed (37% of tested)
van Diemen	2017	n = 23, infants; ICU	Prospective	GS	12 d (median)	30%	71% of diagnosed (22% of tested)
Meng	2017	n = 63, infants; ICU	Retrospective	ES	13 d (median)	37%	52% of diagnosed (19% of tested)
Petrikin	2018	n = 32, infants; NICU/PICU	RCT	GS	14 d (median)	31%	48% of diagnosed (15% of tested)
Farnaes	2018	n = 42, infants; ICU/Inpatient	Retrospective	GS	23 d (median); 7d median for those with change in management	43%	72% of diagnosed (31% of tested)
Mestek-Boukhibar	2018	n = 24, infants; PICU	Prospective	GS (trio)	8.5 d (median)	42%	100% of diagnosed (24% of tested)
Clark	2019	n = 7, neonates; NICU	Prospective	GS (trio)	20 h (median)	43%	100% of diagnosed (43% of tested)
Elliot	2019	n = 25, neonates; NICU	Prospective	ES (trio)	7 d (mean)	60%	83% of diagnosed (60% of tested)
French	2019	n = 195, pediatric; pediatric ICU (PICU)/NICU	Prospective	GS (trio)	4.5 weeks (median; 21 d fastest)	21%	65% of diagnosed (13% of tested)
Sanford	2019	n = 33, pediatric; PICU	Retrospective	GS	13 d (mean)	45%	24% of diagnosed (12% of tested)
Wu	2019	n = 40, pediatric; PICU	Prospective	ES	6 d (mean)	53%	81% of diagnosed (25% of tested)
Wang, Qian	2020	n = 33, infants; ICU	prospective	ES	24 h (median)	69%	43% of diagnosed (30% of tested)

Wang, Lu	2020	n = 130, pediatric; PICU/NICU	Prospective	GS (trio)	3.75 d (median)	48%	48% of diagnosed (23% of tested)
Chung	2020	n = 102, pediatric; PICU/NICU	Prospective	ES	11 d (median)	31%	88% of diagnosed (27% of tested)
Lunke	2020	n = 108, neonates; ICU	Prospective	ES	3 d (range 2–7)	51%	76% with and 11% without diagnosis (44% of all tested)
Freed	2020	n = 46, neonates; NICU	prospective	ES (trio)	9 d (mean)	43%	95% of diagnosed (52% of tested)
Wu	2021	n = 202, pediatric; PICU	prospective	GS (trio)	7 d (median)	36%	21% of diagnosed (immediate changes only) (8% of total)
Sweeney	2021	n = 24, infants; NICU/CICU	retrospective	GS	5–10 d	43%	45% of diagnosed (20% of total)

[a] Inclusion criteria and patient populations were not uniform across studies. In general, "neonate" is <2 months of age, "infant" less than 12 months, and "pediatric" less than 10 y. Most patient populations had wide variety of organ system involvement. Amount of prior genetic workup also varied.
[b] If not noted, sequencing either proband-only or a mix of proband-only, trio, and other familial approaches.
[c] Excluding cases where the only change was genetic counseling, familial risk assessment, outpatient referrals, or long-term management change. Not including impact of negative cases or variants of uncertain significance, except where specified.

proband and a parent share the same putative pathogenic variant yet lack shared phenotypic features, suggesting against pathogenicity with respect to the proband's phenotype. However, several studies have demonstrated that proband-only (singleton) ES and GS have a diagnostic yield either equivalent to or only moderately diminished in comparison to trio, including rapid testing in the ICU.[7–10] Trio sequencing is more expensive, as it involves testing more individuals, and may slow the testing process if parents are not immediately available. It should be remembered that uninformative genomic sequencing results can also provide value to parents and families[11] through the exclusion of suspected disease processes with well-defined genetic etiologies.

GENOMIC TESTING IN CRITICAL CARE

In addition to directing appropriate long-term management, there are several ways in which establishing an underlying genetic diagnosis might influence more immediate critical care decisions: identifying specific or targeted therapies, identifying risks to other organ systems, and providing prognostic information could help direct the goals of care. As an example, a child with congenital-onset spondyloepiphyseal dysplasia is at risk for increased intracranial pressure and cervical spine instability. A patient with a known mitochondrial disorder would be at risk for cardiac decompensation if medications that are known to negatively impact mitochondrial energy metabolism are selected for the treatment of the original cause of his or her hospitalization. Children with inborn errors of metabolism are at greater risk for catabolic decompensation when under the increased physiologic stress of illness; appropriately managing their energy metabolism needs impacts outcomes. A child presenting with acute status epilepticus or rapid-onset cardiomyopathy can be managed in a more targeted manner with the knowledge of an underlying gene pathway to consider. Pharmacogenomics allows for the optimal management of an illness with medications known to be effective in the child being treated. Many of these circumstances, however, require prior knowledge of the genetic data to be impactful. The appropriate time to consider genome sequencing in critical care remains a subjective decision dependent on the experience of the care team and the access to sequencing. A general guide would be to consider rapid genome sequencing for any patient in a critical decompensated state who has no clear etiology for their circumstance. Occasionally there may be certain phenotypic clues or a family history suggestive of a Mendelian disorder. Clinical situations that should raise this concern are listed in **Box 1**. Of particular concern in an ICU setting is the severity and course of illness; time is often a limited resource for the critically ill patient, and shortening the time to diagnosis by any means may have outsized impact compared with an outpatient diagnostic odyssey.

Genetic counseling by a certified professional and, whenever possible, consultation with a medical geneticist are highly recommended when ordering genomic testing. Given the potential negative impact that certain genomic testing results can have on families, informed consent is crucial. Genetic counseling aids in setting expectations regarding potentially confusing results, as well as understanding cost, turnaround time, diagnoses unrelated to the indication for testing (i.e., incidental findings), and deciding whether secondary findings are going to be reported. Medical genetics expertise is especially useful when deciding how to interpret and follow up on variants of uncertain significance.

There are several considerations when selecting the most appropriate test:

First is the availability of genetic testing for hospitalized patients. This is not a universal option, especially outside of an academic medical center where a genetics

> **Box 1**
> **Phenotypic red flags for considering genomic sequencing in critical care**
>
> Indications for Genomic Sequencing
>   Phenotype and/or family history strongly suggest unexplained congenital or
>   neurodevelopmental disorder
>   • Multiple congenital anomalies highly suggestive of a genetic etiology
>   • Metabolic abnormalities (i.e., hyperammonemia, lactic acidosis) that suggest an inborn
>   error of metabolism
>   • Neurologic abnormalities (severe hypotonia, seizures) unexplained by hypoxic ischemic
>   encephalopathy
>   • First-degree relative with sudden unexplained death in infancy or childhood
>   • Unexplained dysfunction of multiple organ systems
>   • Intellectual disability or developmental regression
>   Clinical features not specific to single genetic disorder (e.g., trisomies, VACTERL would be
>   excluded)
>   Atypical disease course (severity, duration, failure of or abnormal response to therapy)
>   Atypical or complex combinations of signs, symptoms, laboratory findings not explained by
>   clinical presentation
>   More than 1 genetic test is justifiable based on differential diagnosis
>
> These are general guidelines, and the decision to initiate ES/GS is often subjective, taking into
> consideration other clinical factors not listed here.

consultative service is often not available. In circumstances where such a service is not available, the choice to implement genetic testing must be purposeful and through an institutional agreement with large genomic centers. Clear protocols should be established to guide decision support.

Second is the acuity of illness. In critically ill neonates and children, the choice between rapid exome or genome sequencing is the difference between a 3- to 7-day turnaround for GS and a 14- to 21-day turnaround for ES, which could potentially impact outcomes significantly. When there is little risk of decompensation, death, or progressive morbidity, or in the setting of subacute or chronic medical concerns, exome-based testing would be an appropriate choice to reduce the overall burden to health care expenditure.

Third is the specific disease process and prior genetic testing. Some differential diagnoses are better evaluated by non-genomic sequencing (e.g., spinocerebellar ataxias caused by repeat expansions, imprinting disorders). If both genome-wide CNV analysis and genomic testing are indicated, either GS, or alternately, ES with CNV analysis is advisable, although the latter is not always available through every ES laboratory. If there is negative prior testing (especially large gene panels or ES), GS should be considered. If ES or GS has been completed in the past (>1 year) and the patient remains undiagnosed, reanalysis is recommended.

EVIDENCE FOR IMPACTING DECISION MAKING

Congenital malformations are a leading cause of morbidity and mortality; children with genetic disorders are at higher risk for requiring acute care than children without a known diagnosis.[12–14] The proportion of children in an ICU with a clinically significant underlying yet undiagnosed genetic condition is less well understood, as is the quantifiable impact of establishing a diagnosis on management decisions and outcomes. There have been many studies that have tried to assess these important questions over the past decade, and as technology has evolved, so too has the ability to extract data to support the use of rapid genomic sequencing in critical care. The summative data have been compiled in **Box 1**.

These studies are not directly comparable; either ES or GS was selected, and turn-around times varied from 24 hours to 40 days, with a averaged median across all studies of approximately 10 days. In general, inclusion criteria were similar to the indications for genomic testing laid out in **Box 1**. Diagnostic yield ranged from 21% to 69% (average 43%), and the management was reported to be impacted in 21% to 100% (average of 65% in patients with a diagnosis and 26% overall) of patients tested. A meta-analysis of 18 studies (1049 patients) found a diagnostic yield of 43% (95% confidence interval [CI] 36%–50%), with no significant difference between ES and GS.[15] This reported impact depended on the study, and there was, in general, a greater impact on neonatal ICU (NICU) patients. Despite methodologic heterogeneity, the data clearly support the notion that among diagnosed patients, immediate management change (e.g., diet, procedures, surgical planning, medication, and goals of care) is common. Several studies additionally noted the immediate management impact of negative testing.[16,17]

It is important to review these reported data in the context of critically ill infants or children, especially as related to impact on medical decision making. Impact ranged widely and depended on the diagnosis; the most commonly-reported changes in management included implementing targeted medical therapy, avoiding surgery or altering the choice of surgical approach, undertaking curative bone marrow transplant, and transitioning from high-intensity intervention to palliative care. Furthermore, those with a clear diagnosis underwent fewer invasive investigations and had shorter lengths of stay. Of note, the first randomized-controlled trial of rapid GS versus standard care in the NICU[18,19] was terminated because of lack of equipoise, with all investigators considering standard care inferior. Qualitative outcomes include positive survey feedback from critical care faculty and parents, with only a minority of parents endorsing distress as a result of the testing.[20] Manickam and colleagues reported high value on negative results, emphasizing that diagnostic yield is not a predictor of perceived utility.[21] Several studies supported the finding that the clinical phenotype or differential diagnosis was frequently not aligned with the molecular diagnosis, and in a minority of cases, dual diagnoses led to a confounding phenotype.[17,20,22] In 1 study, the analysis was expanded to all genomic content (i.e., metagenomics) if sepsis was suspected; pathogenic microbial DNA was identified, confirming the diagnosis of sepsis and identifying the specific pathogen in 6 critically ill infants.[23] All studies that have performed cost analysis found a significant reduction in health care costs attributable to inpatient genomic sequencing, even when accounting for the cost of all sequenced patients.[9,10,15,19,20,24] The cost savings varied between reports but mostly related to reduced length of hospitalization stay and decreased invasive interventions. Of interest, Dimmock and colleagues reported that the cost differential was not because of the acquired data but the expediency at which the data could be provided.[20] Their control study arm that followed conventional genetic and molecular work-up did not show the same cost savings as the study group that underwent rapid genome sequencing.

FRONTIERS IN GENOMIC MEDICINE: LONG-READ TECHNOLOGIES AND RNA SEQUENCING

There are several technologies that increase the diagnostic ability of molecular sequencing. Of 54 participants diagnosed by the Undiagnosed Disease Network before May 2019, 68% were diagnosed through detection of coding variants on ES, while 28% required additional testing (e.g., GS, repeat expansion testing, or methylation profiling) to reach a final diagnosis.[25]

RNA sequencing, or RNA-seq, is especially powerful when combined with GS to allow for correlation of rare noncoding variants and their effect on transcript levels or splicing. The challenges of assessing tissue-specific expression of many genes remains a limitation (i.e., RNA-seq must be performed on affected muscle tissue to assess for myopathy or muscular dystrophy, or on brain biopsy specimens for neuronal tissue in cases with epilepsy or brain malformations); however, several studies have demonstrated that RNA-seq from nonaffected tissues (blood) can be diagnostically useful despite the tissue of interest not being amenable to collection clinically.[26,27] Other limitations of RNA-seq include the presence of multiple transcripts from a gene, which can make interpretation challenging, as well as the notion that some deleterious effects on RNA may only occur at particular stages in development or embryogenesis. These limitations indicate that normal RNA-seq cannot definitively rule out an effect on the gene expression of a rare variant. Convincing evidence from several studies has shown the diagnostic utility of RNA-seq; in undiagnosed patients suspected to have rare Mendelian disorders who had prior nondiagnostic ES or GS, the diagnostic yield of transcriptome sequencing ranged between 7% and 36%.[26–30] Increased utilization of RNA-seq for cases with negative GS can be anticipated as the next phase of genomic exploration in undiagnosed and rare disease investigation. Combining GS and RNA-seq may provide the highest yield of any approach to date.

Long-read sequencing using either fluorescence-based or nanopore-based technology generates reads of up to 20,000 base pairs from unamplified DNA. These technologies can provide accurate sequencing of previously untestable repetitive regions of the genome. In the rare disease context, they allow detection of complex structural variation (e.g., inversions, rearrangements, or repetitive element insertions), resolution of dark genomic regions that are difficult to map because of high homology with other regions of the genome, and accurate analysis of large repetitive elements, such as repeat expansions. The use of long-read sequencing for rare diseases has not been systematically studied, but holds promise.

CONCLUDING REMARKS

Rapid genomic testing in critically ill patients has high diagnostic yield and clinical utility, with frequent impacts on medication choice, surgical planning, diagnostic formulation, and prognosis determination to direct goals of care. The outcomes of past and ongoing studies regarding the role of rapid genomic sequencing serve as a foundation on which to base decisions for critically ill patients that meet the guidelines for considering genomic sequencing in the context of their disease presentation. Further improvements in sequencing technology and reductions in cost will increase the universal accessibility to this testing modality such that rapid genomic testing should be considered as a component in the arsenal of diagnostic tools to help guide management of patients admitted to critical care.

CLINICS CARE POINTS

- Rapid genomic testing in critically ill pediatric patients has high diagnostic yield and clinical utility with impact on optimal medications, surgical planning, diagnostic process, and informing prognosis to direct goals of care.

- Rapid genomic testing should be considered to help guide management of children admitted to critical care.

DISCLOSURE

The authors have nothing to disclose.

REFERENCES

1. Choi M, Scholl UI, Ji W, et al. Genetic diagnosis by whole exome capture and massively parallel DNA sequencing. Proc Natl Acad Sci U S A 2009;106(45): 19096–101.
2. van Dijk EL, Auger H, Jaszczyszyn Y, et al. Ten years of next-generation sequencing technology. Trends Genet 2014;30(9):418–26.
3. Bick D, Jones M, Taylor SL, et al. Case for genome sequencing in infants and children with rare, undiagnosed or genetic diseases. J Med Genet 2019;56:783–91.
4. Clark MM, Hildreth A, Batalov S, et al. Diagnosis of genetic diseases in seriously ill children by rapid whole-genome sequencing and automated phenotyping and interpretation. Sci Transl Med 2019;11:eaat6177.
5. Dolzhenko E, van Vugt JJFA, Shaw RJ, et al. Detection of long repeat expansions from PCR-free whole-genome sequence data. Genome Res 2017;27:1895–903.
6. Tankard RM, Bennett MF, Degorski P, et al. Detecting expansions of tandem repeats in cohorts sequenced with short-read sequencing data. Am J Hum Genet 2018;103:858–73.
7. Clark MM, Stark Z, Farnaes L, et al. Meta-analysis of the diagnostic and clinical utility of genome and exome sequencing and chromosomal microarray in children with suspected genetic diseases. NPJ Genom Med 2018;3:16.
8. Brockman DG, Austin-Tse CA, Pelletier RC, et al. Randomized prospective evaluation of genome sequencing versus standard-of-care as a first molecular diagnostic test. Genet Med 2021;23(9):1689–96.
9. Stark Z, Lunke S, Brett GR, et al. Meeting the challenges of implementing rapid genomic testing in acute pediatric care. Genet Med 2018;20:1554–63.
10. Yeung A, Tan NB, Tan TY, et al. A cost-effectiveness analysis of genomic sequencing in a prospective versus historical cohort of complex pediatric patients. Genet Med 2020;22:1986–93.
11. Mollison L, O'Daniel JM, Henderson GE, et al. Parents' perceptions of personal utility of exome sequencing results. Genet Med 2020;22(4):752–7.
12. Brooten D, Youngblut JM, Caicedo C, et al. Cause of death of infants and children in the intensive care unit: parents' recall vs chart review. Am J Crit Care 2016;25: 235–42.
13. Hagen CM, Hansen TW. Deaths in a neonatal intensive care unit: a 10-year perspective. Pediatr Crit Care Med 2004;5:463–8.
14. Weiner J, Sharma J, Lantos J, et al. How infants die in the neonatal intensive care unit: trends from 1999 through 2008. Arch Pediatr Adolesc Med 2011;165:630–4.
15. Chung CCY, Leung GKC, Mak CCY, et al. Rapid whole-exome sequencing facilitates precision medicine in paediatric rare disease patients and reduces healthcare costs. Lancet Reg Health – West Pac 2020;1:100001.
16. Wu E-T, Hwu W-L, Chien Y-H, et al. Critical trio exome benefits in-time decision-making for pediatric patients with severe illnesses. Pediatr Crit Care Med 2019; 20:1021–6.

17. Lunke S, Eggers S, Wilson M, et al. Feasibility of ultra-rapid exome sequencing in critically ill infants and children with suspected monogenic conditions in the australian public health care system. JAMA 2020;323:2503–11.
18. Petrikin JE, Cakici JA, Clark MM, et al. The NSIGHT1-randomized controlled trial: rapid whole-genome sequencing for accelerated etiologic diagnosis in critically ill infants. NPJ Genom Med 2018;3:6.
19. Farnaes L, Hildreth A, Sweeney NM, et al. Rapid whole-genome sequencing decreases infant morbidity and cost of hospitalization. NPJ Genom Med 2018;3:10.
20. Dimmock DP, Clark MM, Gaughran M, et al. An RCT of rapid genomic sequencing among seriously ill infants results in high clinical utility, changes in management, and low perceived harm. Am J Hum Genet 2020;107:942–52.
21. Manickam K, McClain MR, Demmer LA, et al. Exome and genome sequencing for pediatric patients with congenital anomalies or intellectual disability: an evidence-based clinical guideline of the American College of Medical Genetics and Genomics (ACMG). Genet Med 2021;23(11):2029–37.
22. Freed AS, Clowes Candadai SV, Sikes MC, et al. The impact of rapid exome sequencing on medical management of critically ill children. J Pediatr 2020; 226:202–12.e1.
23. Wu B, Kang W, Wang Y, et al. Application of full-spectrum rapid clinical genome sequencing improves diagnostic rate and clinical outcomes in critically ill infants in the China neonatal genomes project. Crit Care Med 2021;49(10):1674–83.
24. Sweeney NM, Nahas SA, Chowdhury S, et al. Rapid whole genome sequencing impacts care and resource utilization in infants with congenital heart disease. NPJ Genom Med 2021;6:1–10.
25. Burdick KJ, Cogan JD, Rives LC, et al. Limitations of exome sequencing in detecting rare and undiagnosed diseases. Am J Med Genet A 2020;182:1400–6.
26. Frésard L, Smail C, Ferraro NM, et al. Identification of rare-disease genes using blood transcriptome sequencing and large control cohorts. Nat Med 2019;25: 911–9.
27. Gonorazky HD, Naumenko S, Ramani AK, et al. Expanding the boundaries of RNA sequencing as a diagnostic tool for rare mendelian disease. Am J Hum Genet 2019;104:466–83.
28. Cummings BB, Marshall JL, Tukiainen T, et al. Improving genetic diagnosis in Mendelian disease with transcriptome sequencing. Sci Transl Med 2017;9: eaal5209.
29. Maddirevula S, Kuwahara H, Ewida N, et al. Analysis of transcript-deleterious variants in Mendelian disorders: implications for RNA-based diagnostics. Genome Biol 2020;21:145.
30. Lee H, Huang AY, Wang L, et al. Diagnostic utility of transcriptome sequencing for rare Mendelian diseases. Genet Med 2019;22(3):490–9.

ADDITIONAL READING

Bourchany A, Thauvin-Robinet C, Lehalle D, et al. Reducing diagnostic turnaround times of exome sequencing for families requiring timely diagnoses. Eur J Med Genet 2017;60:595–604.
van Diemen CC, Kerstjens-Frederikse WS, Bergman KA, et al. Rapid targeted genomics in critically ill newborns. Pediatrics 2017;140:e20162854.
Elliott AM, du Souich C, Lehman A, et al. RAPIDOMICS: rapid genome-wide sequencing in a neonatal intensive care unit—successes and challenges. Eur J Pediatr 2019;178:1207–18.

French CE, Delon I, Dolling H, et al. Whole genome sequencing reveals that genetic conditions are frequent in intensively ill children. Intensive Care Med 2019;45: 627–36.

Kamolvisit W, Phowthongkum P, Boonsimma P, et al. Rapid exome sequencing as the first-tier investigation for diagnosis of acutely and severely ill children and adults in Thailand. Clinical Genetics 2021;100:100–5.

Kingsmore SF, Cakici JA, Clark MM, et al. A randomized, controlled trial of the analytic and diagnostic performance of singleton and trio, rapid genome and exome sequencing in ill infants. Am J Hum Genet 2019;105:719–33.

Meng L, Pammi M, Saronwala A, et al. Use of exome sequencing for infants in intensive care units: ascertainment of severe single-gene disorders and effect on medical management. JAMA Pediatr 2017;171:e173438.

Mestek-Boukhibar L, Clement E, Jones WD, et al. Rapid Paediatric Sequencing (RaPS): comprehensive real-life workflow for rapid diagnosis of critically ill children. J Med Genet 2018;55:721–8.

Powis Z, Farwell Hagman KD, Speare V, et al. Exome sequencing in neonates: diagnostic rates, characteristics, and time to diagnosis. Genet Med 2018;20:1468–71.

Saunders CJ, Miller NA, Soden SE, et al. Rapid whole-genome sequencing for genetic disease diagnosis in neonatal intensive care units. Sci Transl Med 2012;4: 154ra135.

Sanford EF, Clark MM, Farnaes L, et al. Rapid whole genome sequencing has clinical utility in children in the PICU. Pediatr Crit Care Med 2019;20:1007–20.

Śmigiel R, Biela M, Szmyd K, et al. Rapid whole-exome sequencing as a diagnostic tool in a neonatal/pediatric intensive care unit. J Clin Med 2020;9:2220.

Wang H, Qian Y, Lu Y, et al. Clinical utility of 24-h rapid trio-exome sequencing for critically ill infants. NPJ Genom Med 2020;5:1–6.

Wang H, Lu Y, Dong X, et al. Optimized trio genome sequencing (OTGS) as a first-tier genetic test in critically ill infants: practice in China. Hum Genet 2020;139:473–82.

Willig LK, Petrikin JE, Smith LD, et al. Whole-genome sequencing for identification of Mendelian disorders in critically ill infants: a retrospective analysis of diagnostic and clinical findings. Lancet Respir Med 2015;3:377–87.

Diagnostic Time-Outs to Improve Diagnosis

Sarah Yale, MD[a,*], Susan Cohen, MD[b], Brett J. Bordini, MD[a]

KEYWORDS

- Diagnostic error • Diagnostic time-out • Cognitive bias

KEY POINTS

- Diagnostic errors are common, cause direct harm to patients, and are implicated in up to 20% of intensive care unit deaths.
- Most diagnostic errors are related to the impact of various cognitive biases on medical reasoning and decision-making.
- Diagnostic time-outs are an essential cognitive forcing function that can mitigate the role of cognitive bias in leading to diagnostic error.
- Diagnostic time-outs can be implemented in a structured fashion during transitions of care, or as needed in times of diagnostic uncertainty or therapeutic stasis.
- Common barriers to implementation among survey respondents include perceived time constraints and decreased perception of the role of diagnostic error leading to patient harm.

INTRODUCTION

Diagnostic errors harm patients. While estimated to occur in approximately 15% of medical encounters[1] and up to 20% or more of intensive care unit deaths,[2,3] a lack of precise metrics leaves the exact magnitude of this harm unknown, despite attempts to refine measurement by incorporating autopsy data and error reporting systems. The fields of quality improvement and patient safety have made significant progress in reducing systems-related medical errors over the past 20 years, yet far fewer advances have occurred with respect to diagnostic error. Diagnostic errors are often multi-factorial; although cognitive errors, in isolation or in combination with systems-based errors, comprise up to 75% of all diagnostic errors.[4] Most of these errors are attributable to the various cognitive biases inherent in medical reasoning and clinical decision making.[4,5] While awareness of cognitive biases has improved

[a] Division of Hospital Medicine, Medical College of Wisconsin, Children's Corporate Center, Suite 560, 999 North 92nd Street, Milwaukee, WI 53226, USA; [b] Division of Neonatology, Medical College of Wisconsin, Children's Corporate Center, Suite 410, 999 North 92nd Street, Milwaukee, WI 53226, USA
* Corresponding author.
E-mail address: syale@mcw.edu

Crit Care Clin 38 (2022) 185–194
https://doi.org/10.1016/j.ccc.2021.11.008
0749-0704/22/© 2021 Elsevier Inc. All rights reserved.

and has been increasingly incorporated into medical education, practical solutions to mitigate the risk of cognitive diagnostic error at the patient bedside remain nascent and faced with numerous barriers to implementation. In this article, we describe the taxonomy of diagnostic errors and present a framework for understanding cognitive bias as it relates to medical reasoning. In addition, using survey data, we report medical provider perceptions regarding the awareness of diagnostic error and its impact on patient outcomes. We further assessed provider readiness to implement a practical solution—the diagnostic time-out—at the patient bedside in a patient population at high risk for diagnostic error: neonates status-post primary gastroschisis closure in a tertiary care, level IV neonatal intensive care unit (NICU).

UNDERSTANDING DIAGNOSTIC ERROR

Diagnostic errors include wrong, missed, or delayed diagnoses. They may represent a systems-based error, a no-fault error—in which presenting features either mimic another disease process or are so subtle as to preclude accurate diagnosis, or a cognitive error related to improper data gathering, knowledge application, or the confounding effects of cognitive biases. Up to 75% of all diagnostic errors are attributable to a cognitive error or a combination of cognitive and systems-based errors.[4,6,7] While improper data gathering or knowledge application may contribute to cognitive diagnostic error, the majority is caused by the impact of cognitive bias on medical reasoning. *Dual process theory* holds that individuals engaging in medical decision-making use one of 2 distinct cognitive processes: a *system 1 process* based on *heuristics*—the use of rapid pattern recognition and rules of thumb—or a *system 2 process*, based on deliberate analytical modeling and hypothesis generation. While invoking system 1 processes, individuals can think fast and reflexively and can even operate at a subconscious level, using pattern recognition to sort vast amounts of clinical information quickly to form an *illness script* that allows for the rapid elaboration of a differential diagnosis. In contrast, system 2 processes require focused attention and are purposefully analytical, relying on deliberate counter-factual reasoning to generate hypotheses regarding the pathophysiologic mechanisms by which a patient's symptoms are produced.[8]

While clinicians predominantly engage system 1 processes and achieve relatively accurate diagnoses for most patients under most circumstances,[5] heuristics can fail when patient presentations are multisystem, complex, or evolving, instead becoming a form of *cognitive bias* that can result in diagnostic error (**Table 1** for cognitive biases related to *heuristic failure*). Cognitive biases can additionally result from *errors of attribution* (**Table 2**), in which providers attribute greater weight in the diagnostic formulation to perceived characteristics of the patient or members of the care team, potentially altering the affective state and cognition of the medical provider and increasing the likelihood of error.[9] Lastly, cognitive biases may result from *errors of context*, wherein the context or setting in which a diagnostic evaluation takes place alters how information is perceived and interpreted. Context-related errors can affect how providers triage and categorize information; for example, the differential diagnosis generated for lower abdominal pain may be vastly different depending on whether the patient is evaluated in the emergency department, primary care office, urology clinic, or gastroenterology clinic. Furthermore, context can influence the *cognitive burden* of the provider: internal factors—stress, provider burnout, poor nutrition, or sleep deficit—or external factors—higher patient volumes or acuity, changes in hospital policy or practice—can intensify a provider's cognitive load and increase diagnostic error.[10-12] The context-induced improper triaging and categorizing of

Table 1
Cognitive biases related to heuristic failure

Bias	Definition
Anchoring	Locking into a diagnosis based on initial presenting features, failing to adjust diagnostic impressions when new information becomes available.
Confirmation bias	Looking for and accepting only evidence that confirms a diagnostic impression, rejecting or not seeking contradictory evidence.
Diagnostic momentum	Perpetuating a diagnostic label over time, usually by multiple providers both within and across health care systems, despite the label being incomplete or inaccurate.
Expertise bias/yin-yang out	Believing that a patient who has already undergone an extensive evaluation will have nothing more to gain from further investigations, despite the possibility that the disease process or diagnostic techniques may have evolved so as to allow for appropriate diagnosis.
Overconfidence bias	Believing one knows more than one does, acting on incomplete information or hunches, and prioritizing opinion or authority, as opposed to evidence.
Premature closure	Accepting the first plausible diagnosis before obtaining confirmatory evidence or considering all available evidence. *"When the diagnosis is made, thinking stops."*
Unpacking principle	Failing to explore primary evidence or data in its entirety and subsequently failing to uncover important facts or findings, such as accepting a biopsy report or imaging study report without reviewing the actual specimen or image.

From Bordini BJ, Stephany A, Kliegman R. Overcoming Diagnostic Errors in Medical Practice. J Pediatr. 2017;185:19-25.e1. doi:10.1016/j.jpeds.2017.02.065; with permission

Table 2
Cognitive biases related to errors of attribution

Bias	Definition
Affective bias	Allowing emotions to interfere with a diagnosis, either positively or negatively; dislikes of patient types (e.g., "frequent flyers").
Appeal to authority	Deferring to authoritative recommendations from senior, supervising, or "expert" clinicians, independent of the evidentiary support for such recommendations.
Ascertainment bias	Maintaining preconceived expectations based on patient or disease stereotypes.
Countertransference	Being influenced by positive or negative subjective feelings toward a specific patient.
Outcome bias	Minimizing or over-emphasizing the significance of a finding or result, often based on subjective feelings about a patient, a desired outcome, or personal confidence in one's own clinical skills; the use of "slightly" to describe abnormal results.
Psych-out bias	Maintaining biases about people with presumed mental illness.

From Bordini BJ, Stephany A, Kliegman R. Overcoming Diagnostic Errors in Medical Practice. J Pediatr. 2017;185:19-25.e1. doi:10.1016/j.jpeds.2017.02.065; with permission

information, as well as increased cognitive burden, introduce bias by leading providers to increasingly focus on impertinent information or deemphasize pertinent information during the diagnostic evaluation (**Table 3** for cognitive biases related to errors of context).

MITIGATING DIAGNOSTIC ERROR

Given the degree to which system 1 processes are susceptible to cognitive biases, it would seem as though solutions to mitigate diagnostic error should focus on training clinicians to universally use system 2 processes in diagnostic reasoning; indeed, certain aspects of the patient safety movement have begun to cast system 1 processes in a negative light.[13] However, in the daily practice of medicine it is not feasible to make all decisions analytically, as it is both time and resource intensive.[14] Heuristic thinking is a necessary and integral part of clinical decision-making, particularly in circumstances of high patient acuity, such as the intensive care unit. The critical point of intervention may instead be training clinicians to recognize when system 1 processes

Table 3
Cognitive biases related to errors of context

Bias	Definition
Availability bias	Basing decisions on the most recent patient with similar symptoms, preferentially recalling recent and more common diseases.
Base-rate neglect	Over- or underestimating the prevalence of a disease, typically overestimating the prevalence of common diseases and underestimating the prevalence of rare diseases.
Framing effect	Being influenced by how or by whom a problem is described, or by the setting in which the evaluation takes place.
Frequency bias	Believing that common things happen commonly and are usually benign in general practice.
Hindsight bias	Reinforcing diagnostic errors once a diagnosis is discovered in spite of these errors. May lead to a clinician overestimating the efficacy of his or her clinical reasoning and may reinforce ineffective techniques.
Posterior probability error	Considering the likelihood of a particular diagnosis in light of a patient's prior or chronic illnesses. New headaches in a patient with a history of migraines may in fact be a tumor.
Representative bias	Basing decisions on an expected typical presentation. Not effective for atypical presentations. Overemphasis on disease diagnostic criteria or "classic" presentations. "Looks like a duck, quacks like a duck".
Sutton's slip	Ignoring alternate explanations for "obvious" diagnoses (Sutton's law is that one should first consider the obvious).
Thinking in silo	Restricting diagnostic considerations to a particular specialty or organ system. Each discipline has a set of diseases within its comfort zone, which reduces diagnostic flexibility or team-based communication.
Zebra retreat	Lacking conviction to pursue rare disorders even when suggested by evidence.

From Bordini BJ, Stephany A, Kliegman R. Overcoming Diagnostic Errors in Medical Practice. J Pediatr. 2017;185:19-25.e1. doi:10.1016/j.jpeds.2017.02.065; with permission

may be increasing the risk of diagnostic error, and when it may be appropriate to engage system 2 processes to mitigate that risk. It can be difficult to recognize when this shift in mindset is needed, as well as when biases are inhibiting accurate and timely diagnosis. *Diagnostic calibration* refers to the degree of concordance between diagnostic confidence and diagnostic accuracy.[15] The context of the intensive care unit can readily create circumstances in which diagnostic calibration can be compromised, whether through cognitive bias-induced overconfidence in a working diagnosis, or cognitive burden-related acceptance of a poorly-fitting working diagnosis wherein a provider may underestimate the risk or impact of a diagnostic error,[15] particularly if interventions to normalize tenuous physiology seem to be working.

Despite an increasingly sophisticated appreciation of the myriad forms of cognitive bias, evidence-based solutions to mitigate their role in diagnostic error are lacking. Patient safety and quality improvement initiatives have demonstrated the value of incorporating checklists and procedural time-outs into clinical care in a variety of settings,[6,12,16,17] providing a potential model for structured interventions to address diagnostic error. The challenges lie in identifying how to adapt such a model for improving diagnosis in real time, minimizing barriers to implementation, and demonstrating both enhanced diagnostic calibration and patient outcomes.

Checklists and procedural time-outs serve as *cognitive forcing functions*[6] meant to engage a specific set of mental tasks to ensure that proper and comprehensive care is being provided under the appropriate circumstances. Examples of these cognitive forcing functions include verifying that a surgical procedure is being performed on the correct site in the correct patient, or that a central line is being placed with the proper technique and with the appropriate precautions and equipment in place to minimize the risk of introducing a bloodstream infection. The same concept underlies the *diagnostic time-out*, a structured opportunity for the care team to purposefully question whether system 1 processes or other factors have introduced cognitive bias and the risk of diagnostic error into the diagnostic formulation and identify whether engaging a more analytical system 2 process can counteract those risks.[18] A secondary benefit of regularly implementing diagnostic time-outs is retrospectively identifying missed or delayed diagnoses, thereby enhancing diagnostic calibration by allowing providers to become more familiar with both specific and general circumstances that lead to diagnostic error.

THE DIAGNOSTIC TIME-OUT
Timing and Format

The diagnostic time-out is not meant to simply generate a longer differential diagnosis, but rather is intended to serve as a cognitive forcing function, allowing providers to question whether the current diagnostic formulation has become biased or otherwise at risk for error, and to redirect diagnostic and therapeutic efforts prospectively in real time, as opposed to retrospectively, after a patient may have already incurred harm.[6,19] While appropriate as an individual exercise, the diagnostic time-out is best implemented among the entire care team, as collective medical reasoning has been shown in certain settings to outperform even the most experienced individual diagnosticians.[20]

There are many circumstances under which the timing and setting of a diagnostic time-out are optimal. Oftentimes, clinicians only pause to reevaluate a diagnosis when the patient seems to be in a "diagnostic dilemma." However, additional opportunities for a diagnostic time-out include deteriorations in patient acuity, clinician intuition, failure to follow an anticipated clinical course or to respond to therapy as expected, provider handoffs, or patient transfer between hospital or clinical care settings. For example, when a patient is being transferred from the emergency department to the inpatient unit with a proposed admitting diagnostic label, a diagnostic time-out could be implemented as part of the overall admission process. Furthermore, when attending providers go "off service" and are handing off their patient census, a diagnostic time-out could be implemented with the oncoming attending provider for any patients without firmly established diagnoses.[21]

The format of the diagnostic time-out is as follows:

---

1. Name the clinical concern or diagnostic dilemma

2. Remove diagnostic labels and instead list out signs and symptoms

3. Do we currently have a leading diagnosis? If so...
   - What clinical data cannot be explained with the provisional diagnosis?
   - What are the "cannot miss" or "worst case scenario" diagnoses?

4. Broaden the differential using an anatomic (or age-based if pediatric patient) approach

5. Decide on next steps:
   - Obtain further history and repeat physical examination
   - Review laboratories and actual images (not just the reports)
   - Discuss with other team members (consultants, nurses) and family
   - Obtain further laboratories /imaging (using pre and posttest probability)

Implementation with Trainees

To prepare trainees to provide accurate yet timely care, medical education necessarily involves the development and refinement of system 1-based diagnostic reasoning. Before attaining these skills, most trainees approach diagnosis via a more analytical system 2-based approach, yet as trainees progress through their education, they become less and less reliant on analytical thinking.[22,23] To prevent the attrition of analytical reasoning, regular modeling of diagnostic time-outs by more senior clinicians can help demonstrate the worth of well-honed system 2 skills in preventing diagnostic error and increasing diagnostic calibration.

Barriers to Implementation

Both internal and external factors create barriers to implementing diagnostic time-outs. Many providers maintain a *bias blind spot*, wherein they feel they are less susceptible to bias, despite bias being a universal "operating characteristic of the diagnosing brain".[5,24,25] In busy clinical settings such as the intensive care unit, there may be perceived time constraints that create additional hesitancy. Finally, in the era of value-based care, providers may be resistant to engage in a diagnostic time-out that may potentially lead to an expanded diagnostic evaluation.[21] Simple changes have been previously proposed to help with this culture shift and remove stigmatization of uncertainty, including changing of name from "diagnostic error" to "missed opportunities in diagnosis"[5] and from "differential diagnosis" to "list of hypotheses".[26] Identification of a local leader or champion to help with implementation of the diagnostic time-out is recommended to ease feelings of discomfort and the barrier of perceived time constraints.

Application in Specific Settings: a Pilot Survey

We investigated barriers to implementation of a diagnostic time-out among providers caring for the postprimary closure gastroschisis population in our NICU. Mortality rates are as high as 10% in neonates with gastroschisis, and outcomes from surgical intervention depend on timely identification and management of postsurgical complications.[16,27] Furthermore, the need for gastroschisis-related surgeries in later childhood in up to 30% of these patients may be related to delayed identification of severe complications.[17] Data on the impact of cognitive bias on clinical decision-making among neonatologists have been less well studied relative to other provider populations.[5] We sought to evaluate how cognitive bias may play a role in the timeliness of accurately diagnosing serious postsurgical complications in neonates requiring complex gastroschisis-related surgical intervention; to explore these relationships, we first conducted a survey regarding provider knowledge of and attitudes toward diagnostic error and readiness to implement diagnostic time-outs at the patient bedside.

To measure awareness of diagnostic error and cognitive bias in the NICU, we conducted 2 surveys of neonatal providers, 1 among neonatology fellowship trainees, and another among attending neonatologists and neonatology nurse practitioners. Neonatology fellowship trainees are the primary stakeholders at our institution that respond to clinical concerns at the bedside associated with postsurgical complications in this population. Of the fellowship trainee respondents (n = 8), there was a feeling that there was a 67% likelihood that diagnostic error due to cognitive bias occurs in the NICU. None of the respondents stated they would refuse to use a tool to address diagnostic error, although half responded that they "maybe" would use it. Nearly all (7 of 8 respondents) reported feeling a tool to address diagnostic error would be most valuable in a case conference atmosphere, 25% responded they would use it on daily rounds, and 50% responded that it could be valuable once weekly separate from daily rounds. To capture enthusiasm for a tool to address diagnostic error, we allowed for a sliding response from 0 to 100. The mean enthusiasm response score was 66, with a standard deviation of 22, suggesting a lukewarm response. Representative narrative comments included, "It should not take time away from daily rounding time and should not be a very time-consuming process"; "I've been less excited about this idea because I feel we do often do something similar naturally when things aren't making sense"; and "For me, a specified format feels less helpful, but may be desired by others." The overwhelming response was that any tool implemented should not delay the daily routine of patient care in the NICU.

When we surveyed attending neonatologists and neonatology nurse practitioners (n = 27), there was overall less enthusiasm. Respondents felt that there was a 48% likelihood that diagnostic errors occur in the NICU due to cognitive bias. There was a mixed response to whether and in what setting diagnostic time-outs would be useful, suggesting no strong preference to any one scenario. On the sliding scale, the mean enthusiasm response was less than 60% for tool implementation, although no respondents said they would refuse to use one if available. The comments from this cohort highlighted time pressures and external constraints for patient care would be the barriers for a tool of this sort.

DISCUSSION

Diagnostic errors harm patients. While the underlying causes of diagnostic error and the settings in which they occur are diverse, the use of a cognitive forcing function in the form of a diagnostic time-out can mitigate the risk of diagnostic error despite this variability in cause and context. The purposeful engagement of system 2-based analytical reasoning via the use of a standardized tool during transitions of care or changes in patient status can quickly refocus diagnostic and therapeutic interventions for the benefit of the patient, and as a secondary benefit to providers, can enhance diagnostic calibration. While medical education aims to train clinicians to be highly adaptable in complex high-stakes clinical scenarios,[13] the same skills used to address acuity and complexity can lead to cognitive bias and diagnostic error.[8,28] The use of the diagnostic time-out can serve as a "second opinion" from oneself and from others directly involved in the care of the patient[7] and can help shift thinking from solely preventing errors to that of managing complexity.[13]

Despite these benefits, barriers to implementation of diagnostic time-outs remain. In our survey populations, perceived time constraints were universally cited as a barrier, and among attending neonatologists and neonatology nurse practitioners, there was decreased perception of the risk of diagnostic error impacting patient outcomes, relative to the perception among neonatology fellowship trainees. Future directions include addressing concerns over the perceived time investment required for a diagnostic time-out and increasing provider appreciation of the nature and impact of diagnostic error on patient outcomes.

CLINICS CARE POINTS

- The diagnostic process is dynamic and is inextricably influenced by the context and system in which it occurs.
- Diagnostic errors, including wrong, missed or delayed diagnoses, cause harm to patients.
- Diagnostic errors are often multi-factorial, but cognitive diagnostic errors either alone or in combination with systems-based errors, comprise the majority of diagnostic errors.
- In a busy critical care setting, there may be in an increased likelihood of poor diagnostic calibration (the degree of concordance between diagnostic confidence and accuracy), which may stem from bias-related overconfidence or cognitive burden-induced complacency wherein a provider underestimates the possibility or impact of a diagnostic error.
- A diagnostic time-out provides a quick, elective, and standardized template for changing diagnostic reasoning to an analytical process to address and counteract heuristic thinking.
- Diagnostic time-outs should be a multi-disciplinary activity, as collective knowledge and diverse input from varying team members improve diagnosis.
- Opportune scenarios for diagnostic time-outs include transitions of care and changes in patient status, as well as clinician intuition.
- Survey results among neonatology providers identify time constraints and feelings of discomfort as barriers to implementation of the diagnostic time-out. Ongoing work is needed to address these concerns and increase provider appreciation of the nature and impact of diagnostic error on patient outcomes.

DISCLOSURE

The authors have nothing to disclose.

REFERENCES

1. Committee on Diagnostic Error in Health Care, Board on Health Care Services, Institute of Medicine, The National Academies of Sciences, Engineering, and Medicine. In: Balogh EP, Miller BT, Ball JR, editors. Improving diagnosis in health care. Washington, DC: National Academies Press; 2015. Available at: http://www.nap.edu/catalog/21794. Accessed July 18, 2016.

2. Abbas Q, Memon F, Laghari P, et al. Potentially preventable mortality in the pediatric intensive care unit: findings from a retrospective mortality analysis. Cureus 2020;12(3):e7358.

3. Custer JW, Winters BD, Goode V, et al. Diagnostic errors in the pediatric and neonatal ICU: a systematic review. Pediatr Crit Care Med 2015;16(1):29–36.

4. Graber ML, Franklin N, Gordon R. Diagnostic error in internal medicine. Arch Intern Med 2005;165(13):1493–9.

5. Croskerry P. Bias: a normal operating characteristic of the diagnosing brain. Diagnosis 2014;1(1):23–7.

6. Ely JW, Graber ML, Croskerry P. Checklists to reduce diagnostic errors. Acad Med 2011;86(3):307–13.

7. Ely JW, Graber ML. Preventing diagnostic errors in primary care. Am Fam Physician 2016;94(6):426–32.

8. Sloman SA. The empirical case for two systems of reasoning. Psychol Bull 1996; 119(1):3.

9. Croskerry P. Diagnostic failure: a cognitive and affective approach. In: Henriksen K, Battles JB, Marks ES, et al, editors. Advances in patient safety: from research to implementation (volume 2: concepts and methodology). Advances in patient safety. Agency for Healthcare Research and Quality (US); 2005. Available at: http://www.ncbi.nlm.nih.gov/books/NBK20487/. Accessed August 1, 2021.

10. Patel VL, Buchman TG. Cognitive overload in the ICU. Available at: https://psnet.ahrq.gov/web-mm/cognitive-overload-icu. Accessed August 1, 2021.

11. Patel VL, Zhang J, Yoskowitz NA, et al. Translational cognition for decision support in critical care environments: a review. J Biomed Inform 2008;41(3):413–31.

12. Sweller J. Cognitive load theory, learning difficulty, and instructional design. Learn Instruction 1994;4(4):295–312.

13. Sutcliffe K, Wears R. Still not safe: patient safety and the middle-managing of American medicine. New York: Oxford University Press; 2019.

14. Croskerry P. From mindless to mindful practice–cognitive bias and clinical decision making. N Engl J Med 2013;368(26):2445–8.

15. Berner ES, Graber ML. Overconfidence as a cause of diagnostic error in medicine. Am J Med 2008;121(5 Suppl):S2–23.

16. Emil S. Surgical strategies in complex gastroschisis. Semin Pediatr Surg 2018; 27(5):309–15.

17. Suominen J, Rintala R. Medium and long-term outcomes of gastroschisis. Semin Pediatr Surg 2018;27(5):327–9.

18. Sibbald M, de Bruin ABH, Yu E, et al. Why verifying diagnostic decisions with a checklist can help: insights from eye tracking. Adv Health Sci Educ Theory Pract 2015;20(4):1053–60.

19. Trowbridge RL. Twelve tips for teaching avoidance of diagnostic errors. Med Teach 2008;30(5):496–500.

20. Huang GC, Kriegel G, Wheaton C, et al. Implementation of diagnostic pauses in the ambulatory setting. BMJ Qual Saf 2018;27(6):492–7.

21. Berkwitt A, Osborn R, Grossman M. Walking a tightrope: balancing the risk of diagnostic error in inpatient pediatrics. Hosp Pediatr 2016;6(9):566–8.

22. Marsicek SM, Odom B, Woodard A, et al. Time for a time-out: the value of a diagnostic time-out in prolonged fever and lymphadenopathy. Hosp Pediatr 2019; 9(2):139–41.

23. Royce CS, Hayes MM, Schwartzstein RM. Teaching critical thinking: a case for instruction in cognitive biases to reduce diagnostic errors and improve patient safety. Acad Med 2019;94(2):187–94.

24. West RF, Meserve RJ, Stanovich KE. Cognitive sophistication does not attenuate the bias blind spot. J Pers Soc Psychol 2012;103(3):506–19.

25. Holmboe ES, Durning SJ. Assessing clinical reasoning: moving from in vitro to in vivo. Diagnosis (Berl) 2014;1(1):111–7.

26. Dunlop M, Schwartzstein RM. Reducing diagnostic error in the intensive care unit. Engaging uncertainty when teaching clinical reasoning. ATS Scholar 2020; 1(4):364–71.

27. Oakes MC, Porto M, Chung JH. Advances in prenatal and perinatal diagnosis and management of gastroschisis. Semin Pediatr Surg 2018;27(5):289–99.

28. McDonald KM, Matesic B, Contopoulos-Ioannidis DG, et al. Patient safety strategies targeted at diagnostic errors: a systematic review. Ann Intern Med 2013; 158(5 Pt 2):381–9.

Subtypes and Mimics of Sepsis

John A. Kellum, MD, MCCM[a,b,]*, Cassandra L. Formeck, MD, MS[a,c,d],
Kate F. Kernan, MD[a,b,d], Hernando Gómez, MD[a,b], Joseph A. Carcillo, MD[a,b,d]

KEYWORDS

- Endotoxin • Endotoxemia • Polymyxin B • Blood purification
- Macrophage activation syndrome • Atypical hemolytic uremic syndrome

KEY POINTS

- Inflammation is central to many acute conditions, ranging from infection to sterile tissue injury to rheumatic diseases and to drug/toxin reactions. These conditions easily can be confused with one another.
- Sepsis is extremely heterogenous at both the clinical and molecular levels. Emerging evidence points to various subphenotypes with divergent pathophysiology.
- Macrophage activation syndrome is a life-threatening complication of systemic inflammatory disorders, most commonly systemic juvenile idiopathic arthritis, adult-onset Still disease, and systemic lupus erythematosus.
- Atypical hemolytic uremic syndrome is associated with genetic or acquired disorders that lead to dysregulation of the complement system and thrombotic microangiopathy, resulting in multiple organ failure.
- Endotoxemic shock occurs in approximately half of patients with septic shock and often is refractory to standard therapy. The source of endotoxin often is loss of gut barrier function.

INTRODUCTION

The "Third International Consensus Definitions for Sepsis and Septic Shock" define sepsis as life-threatening organ dysfunction caused by a dysregulated host response to infection.[1] Other causes of life-threatening organ dysfunction, however, can be present in patients with known or suspected infection. Some are sepsis mimics in that a

[a] Center for Critical Care Nephrology, University of Pittsburgh, Pittsburgh, PA 15213, USA; [b] Department of Critical Care Medicine, University of Pittsburgh School of Medicine, Pittsburgh, PA 15213, USA; [c] Division of Nephrology, Department of Pediatrics, University of Pittsburgh School of Medicine, Pittsburgh, PA 15213, USA; [d] UPMC Children's Hospital of Pittsburgh, Pittsburgh, PA 15224, USA
* Corresponding author. Center for Critical Care Nephrology, 3347 Forbes Avenue, Suite 220, Pittsburgh, PA 15213.
E-mail address: kellum@pitt.edu
Twitter: kellumja (J.A.K.)

Crit Care Clin 38 (2022) 195–211
https://doi.org/10.1016/j.ccc.2021.11.013   criticalcare.theclinics.com
0749-0704/22/© 2021 Elsevier Inc. All rights reserved.

patient does not have sepsis but has another syndrome that is mistaken for sepsis (eg, noninfectious febrile conditions, such as malignant hyperthermia and serotonin syndrome—see "Common presentations of rare drug reactions and atypical presentations of common drug reactions" in this issue). In other instances, a patient technically meets criteria for sepsis but has dysfunction that is not directly attributable to infection. Because the host response is not routinely measured directly and cannot easily determine the presence of a dysregulated state, it is a matter of conjecture as to the cause of organ dysfunction in a patient with infection. Consider the common scenario where a patient presents with fever, cough, and infiltrates on chest radiograph, a presentation most often consistent with pneumonia. If that patient then develops acute kidney injury (AKI), the combination of organ dysfunction and presumed infection meets criteria for sepsis. Suppose, however, that the patient has heart failure and an upper respiratory tract infection? Suppose the AKI is related to the heart failure or its treatment? These clinical uncertainties, in which the organ dysfunction may not be directly attributable to the host response to infection, happen regularly. In a study of 2029 patients admitted to a hospital with a clinical diagnosis of community-acquired pneumonia, a diagnosis of pneumonia subsequently was ruled out in 134 patients (6.6%).[2]

In addition to these sepsis mimics, there also are instances when patients indeed may have sepsis but have an unusual subtype that may be amenable only to therapy specific for that subtype. This review considers this latter group of rare and not-so-rare conditions that may be responsible for a disproportionally high number of deaths from sepsis. Importantly, existing and emerging therapies are available for these subtypes. Although controversial, these therapies offer potential benefit in some patients currently labeled as having typical sepsis.

PATHOPHYSIOLOGY OF SEPSIS

The pathophysiology of sepsis is complex and incompletely understood.[3] Sepsis currently is conceptualized as a result of an imbalance in the systemic inflammatory response that affects immune function, the neuroendocrine axis, and coagulation, ultimately resulting in organ injury. Inflammation plays a critical role in the pathogenesis of sepsis, beginning with—in response to invasive pathogens—an initial release of cytokines, damage-associated molecular patterns (DAMPs), and pathogen-associated molecular patterns (PAMPs) (**Table 1**). PAMPs stimulate monocytes to release procoagulants and other mediators to activate platelets, neutrophils, and endothelial cells. DAMPs—comprising histones, chromosomal DNA, mitochondrial DNA, nucleosomes, and a variety of proteins—are released from neutrophils and activate inflammation and coagulation. Damaged endothelial cells further promote coagulation

Table 1	
Damage-associated and pathogen-associated molecular patterns	
Damage-associated Molecular Patterns	**Pathogen-associated Molecular Patterns**
• HMGB1	• Endotoxin
• Heat-shock proteins	• Flagellin
• Hyaluronan fragments	• Lipoteichoic acid (gram-positive bacteria)
• Uric acid	• Peptidoglycan
• Heparin sulfate	• Nucleic acid variants (viruses) for example,
• DNA	double-stranded RNA, unmethylated CpG motifs

Abbreviation: HMGB1, high mobility group box 1 protein.

through disruption of the glycocalyx and expression of von Willebrand factor. Shedding of the glycocalyx leads to exposure of E-selectin and other adhesion molecules, leading to adhesion of platelets and neutrophils, causing thrombus and fibrin formation.

Because inflammation is not specific to infection, inflammatory diseases most easily are confused with infection. This includes many rheumatic diseases as well as conditions associated with extensive tissue injury, such as polytrauma, burns, pancreatitis, and chemical pneumonitis. These conditions release various DAMPs into the circulation, engaging the molecular machinery that produces the same cardinal features of infection, including fever, increased capillary permeability, and activation of immune effector cells.

PAMPs produce the same proinflammatory effects as DAMPs. Endotoxin, the most important and well-characterized PAMP, is particularly well suited to causing systemic inflammation, activating the immune response through multiple pathways, including some shared by DAMPs. Responses to endotoxin vary throughout the animal kingdom, with mammals generally the most sensitive; humans are exquisitely sensitive to endotoxin compared with other mammals.[4] The gastrointestinal (GI) tract is an enormous reservoir for endotoxin—some estimates suggest that enough endotoxin is present inside the gut of a single human to kill an entire city if given intravenously.[5] For this reason, any condition that jeopardizes intestinal barrier function from inflammatory bowel disease to ischemic enteritis can produce endotoxemia. COVID-19 infection also is a cause of endotoxemia, presumably from the GI tract.[6]

Because inflammation on a systemic level is dangerous, endogenous mechanisms to regulate inflammation exist and are vital for survival. Both proinflammatory and anti-inflammatory cytokines are released, and engagement of complement and coagulation cascades have built-in braking mechanisms to ensure the system is controlled as much as possible. Sepsis is the most common form of dysregulated inflammation, but others also exist. This review considers 3 syndromes that can mimic sepsis or exist as subtypes of sepsis. These syndromes are macrophage activation syndrome (MAS), atypical hemolytic uremic syndrome (aHUS), and endotoxemic shock. Finally, the overlap between these syndromes and what recent studies using artificial intelligence reveal about subtypes of sepsis and how they might relate to these syndromes are examined.

EVIDENCE FOR PHENOTYPIC AND GENETIC VARIATION IN SEPSIS

Sepsis may cause a wide range of organ failures, both in terms of which organs are involved and the severity that is observed (**Fig. 1**). There is no clear connection between the severity of organ failure and the number of organs failing. For example, a patient may have severe, even refractory shock but remain on room air with only mild dysfunction of the kidneys and brain. Conversely, some patients develop severe AKI or acute respiratory distress syndrome (ARDS) but maintain appropriate hemodynamics. Hospital mortality does correlate with the number of organs affected as well as the severity, but enormous heterogeneity exists.

In adults, sepsis disproportionally affects older patients, many of whom may have underlying organ dysfunction. Classifying organ dysfunction in sepsis in the presence of underlying chronic disease is challenging: classification systems for sepsis-associated organ failure like the sepsis-related organ failure assessment (SOFA) conflate acute and chronic organ dysfunction.[7] For example, the score for a patient with chronic kidney disease, hepatic cirrhosis, and home oxygen therapy for chronic lung disease could start at 6 points or 8 points prior to assessing any acute illness-

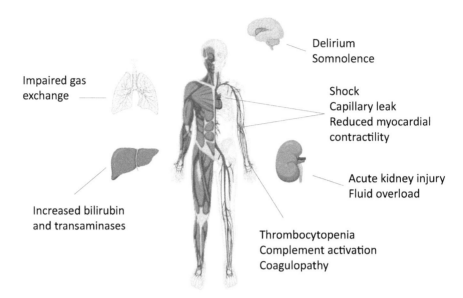

Delirium
Somnolence

Impaired gas exchange

Shock
Capillary leak
Reduced myocardial contractility

Acute kidney injury
Fluid overload

Increased bilirubin and transaminases

Thrombocytopenia
Complement activation
Coagulopathy

Fig. 1. The spectrum of organ failure seen in sepsis.

related features. Although many investigators are careful to exclude points for chronic disease, it often is difficult to know what was present prior to sepsis, especially if a patient has not had regular medical attention. To make matters worse, interventions for sepsis can add to organ dysfunction. For example, patients given large amounts of fluids for shock may develop respiratory failure and require mechanical ventilation. They also may require sedation to tolerate mechanical ventilation, and this may, in turn, worsen shock. Antibiotics and other medications can be nephrotoxic or lead to thrombocytopenia or liver dysfunction. Thus, in any given patient, some degree of organ dysfunction may be from the treatment of sepsis rather than the sepsis itself.

Some amount of phenotypic variation also may come from genetic differences. A Danish study showed a near 6-fold increase in the risk of death from infection before age 50 for adoptees whose biological parents also died from infection under 50 years of age.[8] Despite great variation in host responses, identifying genetic variants contributing to sepsis outcomes has proved challenging. Most genomic studies in sepsis have treated all patients as a single group, assuming shared genetic risk factors. They also have focused on correlations between common polymorphisms and sepsis outcome with limited functional studies to support associations.[9,10] Recently, the authors performed whole-exome sequencing (WES) on a small number of adults with sepsis[11] taken from a large cohort enrolled in the Protocolized Care for Early Septic Shock (ProCESS) trial.[12] The hypothesis was that certain genetic variants implicated in the pathogenesis of MAS and aHUS, as well as conditions like cryopyrin-associated periodic syndromes (CAPS) and familial Mediterranean fever, might be more common in patients with sepsis manifesting extreme inflammation. Using serum ferritin greater than 7000 ng/mL as a screen, the authors performed WES on 6 patients. All 6 exhibited 1 or more gene variants associated with these conditions (**Table 2**).

Although all the variants associated with MAS and aHUS reported in this study have been classified as pathogenic or likely pathogenic, they may or may not have been causal. Moreover, even if genetic variation played a role in the extreme phenotypes exhibited in these cases, the application of immunomodulatory therapies to septic

Table 2
Potentially pathologic variants identified in patients with septic shock

Subject	Gene	Variant	Amino Acid Change	Disease	Minor Allele Frequency[a]	Putative Therapy
1	C3	c.1407G>C NM_000064.2	p.Glu469Asp	aHUS	0.00394	Eculizumab
	UNC13D	c.1579C>T NM_199242.2	p.Arg527Trp	HLH	0.00523	IL1-RA
2	CD46	c.1058C>T NM_172359.2	p.Ala353Val	aHUS	0.01532	Eculizumab
	CFHR5	c.832G>A NM_030787	p.Gly278Ser	aHUS	0.00729	
3	UNC13D	c.2782C>T NM199242.2	p.Arg928Cys	HLH	0.02986	IL1RA
4	NLRP3	c.2113C>A NM_004895.4	p.Gln705Lys	CAPS	0.0495	IL1RA
	MEFV	c.250G>A NM_000243.2	p.Glu84Lys	FMF	0.00012	IL1RA
5	UNC13D	c.2983G>C NM_199242.2	p.Ala995Pro	HLH	0.00096	IL1RA
		c.2542A>C. NM_199242.2	p.Ile848Leu		0.00090	
6	CD46	c.1058C>T NM_172359.2	p.Ala353Val	aHUS	0.01532	Eculizumab
	MEFV	c.2084A>G NM_000243.2	p.Lys695Arg	FMF	0.00550	IL1RA

Previously reported pathogenic variants identified during WES analysis of sepsis patients with extreme hyperferritinemia. Numbers 1 to 6 indicate individual study subjects, whereas rows represent identified variants. Columns indicate genes with variants identified, specific variant, and genetic disorder associated with them.

Abbreviations: FMF, familial Mediterranean fever; HLH, hemophagocytic lymphohistiocytosis.

[a] Putative targeted therapies have been suggested based on the identification of these variants in other clinical contexts.

Adapted from Kernan, K.F., Ghaloul-Gonzalez, L., Shakoory, B. et al. Adults with septic shock and extreme hyperferritinemia exhibit pathogenic immune variation. Genes Immun 20, 520–526 (2019). https://doi.org/10.1038/s41435-018-0030-3; with permission.

individuals with these variants is of unclear benefit or harm. These findings provide evidence, however, that screening select sepsis patients can identify unappreciated heritable disease and could facilitate genome-driven precision medicine in the treatment of sepsis.

MACROPHAGE ACTIVATION SYNDROME

MAS is life-threatening complication of systemic inflammatory disorders, most commonly systemic juvenile idiopathic arthritis (sJIA), adult-onset Still disease, and systemic lupus erythematosus. Clinical and laboratory features of MAS include sustained fever, hyperferritinemia, pancytopenia, fibrinolytic coagulopathy, and liver dysfunction.[13] Thus, MAS looks much like sepsis, especially in cases where pancytopenia is absent or when only thrombocytopenia manifests. Typically, an underlying history of rheumatic disease makes a diagnosis easier, but MAS easily can be confused with sepsis. To make matters worse, certain infections can lead to MAS, notably Epstein-Barr virus (EBV), and, more recently recognized, severe cases of COVID-19.[14] The initial reports of cytokine storm in COVID-19 prompted many of the trials testing immune-modulating therapies for affected patients. Given that sepsis often is bacterial culture–negative, patients who develop clinical features of sepsis rarely have a diagnosis of sepsis challenged or affirmatively disproved. If a patient gets better on antibiotics, confirmation bias about the cause of the disease is succumbed to. Likewise, if a patient does not improve, confirmation bias leads to assuming that the sepsis was refractory to therapy, rather than sepsis not being the cause of the patient's illness.

A definitive diagnosis of MAS can be elusive, although careful physical examination and directed laboratory evaluation can establish a diagnosis. Cardinal features of MAS include persistently high fevers, hepatosplenomegaly, hyperferritinemia, pancytopenia, increased liver enzymes, increased fibrinogen, and hypertriglyceridemia (**Table 3**). Bone marrow biopsy that reveals macrophage hemophagocytosis also is suggestive, especially if there increased CD163 staining. To calculate the probability of MAS from these findings, an HScore has been developed,[15,16] and on-line calculators are available (such as at mdcalc.com).

Pathogenesis and Pathophysiology of Macrophage Activation Syndrome

Several recent reviews have characterized the pathogenesis of MAS in detail.[17,18] The prototype disease is familial hemophagocytic lymphohistiocytosis (fHLH), a constellation of rare autosomal recessive immune disorders resulting from homozygous deficiency in cytolytic pathway proteins.[19] In fHLH, defects in natural killer (NK) cell and cytotoxic T-cell function result in uncontrolled expansion of macrophages and T cells,[19,20] which leads to unregulated hypersecretion of cytokines, resulting in hematologic alterations and organ damage (**Fig. 2**).[21] The term *cytokine storm* often is used in this context but it is important to appreciate that the strikingly high levels of

Table 3
Clinical feature of typical sepsis versus macrophage activation syndrome and atypical hemolytic uremic syndrome

Characteristic	Sepsis	Macrophage Activation Syndrome	Atypical Hemolytic Uremic Syndrome
Fever	++	+++	+
Hepatomegaly, splenomegaly lymphadenopathy	±	+++	−
Encephalopathy	++	++	+++
ARDS	++	−	−
AKI	++	±	+++
ESR	↑↑	↓	↑↑
White blood cell count	↑↑	↓	↑
Increased AST	±	++	−
DIC	±	++	−
Thrombocytopenia	±	++	+++
Hypertriglyceridemia	−	++	−
Increased lactate dehydrogenase	−	+	+++
Increased ferritin	±	+++	±

Abbreviations: AST, aspartate aminotransferase; ESR, erythrocyte sedimentation rate.

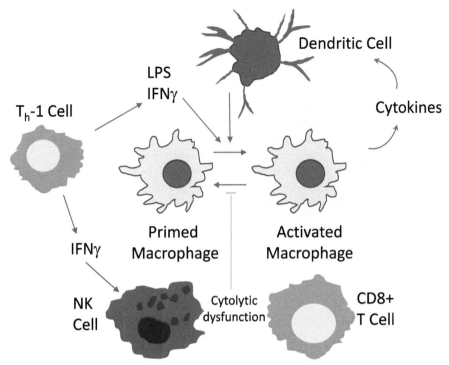

Fig. 2. Pathogenesis of MAS. IFNγ, interferon gamma; T_h-1, type 1 helper T cells.

cytokines reported in many studies of fHLH pale in comparison to what can be seen in typical cases of sepsis. For example, Henter and colleagues[22] reported levels of interleukin (IL)-6 between 25 pg/mL and 130 pg/mL in the plasma of children with active fHLH; other studies have reported only modest elevations in IL-6 and tumor necrosis factor levels (226 pg/mL and 24 pg/mL, respectively) in patients with clinically defined MAS in the setting of COVID-19.[23] Meanwhile, patients with bacterial sepsis may have levels of these cytokines many times higher.[24] Expression of cytokines in the periphery, however, may belie the degree of cytokine activation in the tissue (eg, liver), leading to local organ damage.[25] In addition, the efficacy of certain anticytokine therapies (discussed later) strongly argues for an important role of cytokines in the pathobiology of MAS. Whether the defects in NK-cell and T-cell cytolytic function in MAS are acquired or are related to genetic susceptibility is unknown. MAS and fHLH may share some of the same genetics. For example, the same biallelic pathogenic variants in the *UNC13D* gene reported in fHLH have been identified in some patients with MAS in the setting of sJIA.[26] Genetic polymorphisms in the interferon regulatory factor 5 (*IRF5*) gene also have been found to be risk factors for MAS.[27] In other patients, however, no such cytolytic dysfunction or genetic linkages have been found.

Management of Macrophage Activation Syndrome

Definitive clinical trials for MAS are lacking and, therefore, treatment largely is empiric. Historically, high-dose corticosteroids and/or cyclosporine have been used, and in extreme cases etoposide.[18] Plasma exchange also has been tried with variable results. With recent development of specific anticytokine therapies, many more potential treatments for MAS exist (**Table 4**). Definitive evidence as to which of these agents is

Table 4
Potential immune-modulating therapies for macrophage activation syndrome

Agents	Target	Mechanism
Available agent		
Anakinra, canakinumab	IL-1	Receptor antagonist
Tocilizumab	IL-6	Anti–IL-6R monoclonal Ab
Abatacept	CD28	CTLA4-Ig
Tofacitinib	JAK1/2	JAK inhibitor
Theoretic/investigational		
	IL-18	IL-18 binding protein
	IL-10	Recombinant IL-10 protein
	IL-33	Anti–IL-33R monoclonal Ab
	IFN-γ	Anti–IFN-γ monoclonal Ab

Abbreviations: Ab, antibody; CTLA4, cytotoxic T-lymphocyte–associated protein 4; IFN-γ, interferon gamma; Ig, immunoglobulin; JAK, Janus kinase; R, receptor.

Adapted from Crayne CB, Albeituni S, Nichols KE, Cron RQ. The Immunology of Macrophage Activation Syndrome. Front Immunol. 2019;10:119. Published 2019 Feb 1. https://doi.org/10.3389/fimmu.2019.00119; with permission.

most effective, however, still is lacking. COVID-19 has afforded an opportunity to test various immune-modulating drugs in the setting of infection-triggered inflammation, and some cases of COVID-19 resemble MAS. The RECOVERY trial randomized patients with COVID-19 to receive tocilizumab and used C-reactive protein (CRP) levels above 15.0 mg/dL as an indication of severe inflammation rather than MAS itself,[28] showing a mortality benefit, whereas a majority of other trials were either neutral or suggested harm. A recent follow-up analysis of the CORIMUNO-TOCI-1 trial[29] found a statistical interaction with CRP, such that patients with levels above 15.0 mg/dL experienced a large benefit in terms of 90-day mortality (9% with tocilizumab vs 35% with usual care; hazard ratio 0.18; 95% CI, 0.04–0.89) whereas no benefit was observed when CRP was below this threshold. Other immune-modulating therapies are being actively tested in COVID-19; whether the use of CRP for patient selection will prove useful is unknown.

Sepsis with Macrophage Activation Syndrome Features

An infectious trigger often is detected in sJIA patients with MAS, and EBV is the most common causative agent.[18] Even in patients without underlying rheumatic disease, however, there is a key question as to whether MAS could be triggered by sepsis in a small number of patients with particularly aggressive disease.[30] Prompt recognition and increasing compliance to best practices have reduced in-hospital mortality from sepsis for most patients over the past decade.[31–33] Some patients appear to be refractory to standard therapy, however, and some experts have hypothesized that MAS or a MAS-like condition might complicate some cases. One line of evidence in support of this hypothesis comes from a study by Shakoory and colleagues,[34] in which a post hoc analysis was performed on a randomized clinical trial investigating the effect of anakinra on mortality in sepsis. The investigators hypothesized that anakinra would improve survival in the subset of patients with sepsis who also presented with features of MAS, defined by concomitant hepatobiliary dysfunction (HBD) and disseminated intravascular coagulation (DIC). The investigators demonstrated that compared with placebo, anakinra resulted in a 50% relative risk reduction in mortality only in the subset of patients with features of MAS (approximately 6%) whereas the drug had no effect on the remaining patients.[35] The clinical phenotype of HBD plus DIC as a screen for MAS has the advantage that it is simple and objective and has been used as a more practical strategy for identifying patients with features of MAS during sepsis that may respond to anakinra.[11,35,36,37]

ATYPICAL HEMOLYTIC UREMIC SYNDROME

Hemolytic uremic syndrome (HUS) is characterized by hemolysis and renal failure. Typical HUS is caused by strains of bacteria (mainly *Escherichia coli*) producing Shiga toxins (STEC-HUS),[38] whereas an atypical form (aHUS) is associated with genetic or acquired disorders leading to dysregulation of the complement system.[39,40] Unlike typical HUS, aHUS occurs in the absence of Shiga toxin–producing bacterial infection and may be triggered by atypical infectious, drug, or environmental exposures, leading to microangiopathy, thrombocytopenia, and AKI. Cases of HUS can be familial or sporadic, and it is estimated that between 40% and 60% of affected patients harbor a rare variant that constitutes a genetic risk for disease.[41] More than 120 variants affecting various complement components and regulators have been described to date, accounting for 50% to 60% of cases.[42] Importantly, aHUS is thought to be an extremely rare disease, affecting fewer than 1 in 1 million adults and 3.5 per million children.[43] As a result, the disease rarely is considered, especially in patients with plausible alternate explanations for AKI, thrombocytopenia, and multiorgan failure, such as sepsis. The authors have discovered that more than 20% of patients in their center with sepsis and AKI develop severe thrombocytopenia (<50,000/μL) during their hospital course and yet only approximately 1% are diagnosed with aHUS or thrombotic thrombocytopenic purpura (TTP). As discussed previously, the authors also have identified genetic variation in some adults with septic shock known to be consistent with aHUS.[11]

Elsewhere in this issue, aHUS is discussed in detail, along with other forms of thrombotic microangiopathy in the context of uncommon causes of AKI—see Formeck and colleagues. Like MAS, aHUS is a disease of multiorgan failure that can be triggered by infection. Thus, it is difficult to distinguish from sepsis, a disorder that commonly causes AKI and thrombocytopenia (see **Table 3**). aHUS, however, causes thrombotic microangiopathy distinct from DIC and TTP. With DIC, coagulopathy also is present and the international normalized ratio (INR) usually is increased above 1.5. aHUS should be suspected in patients with sepsis and AKI when thrombocytopenia is unexplained by DIC, especially when there is evidence of hemolysis (eg, increased lactate dehydrogenase). Evidence of microvascular hemolysis on peripheral blood smears (eg, schistocytes) can be helpful but may be absent or episodic. aHUS can be distinguished from TTP on the basis of a disintegrin and metalloproteinase with a thrombospondin type 1 motif, member 13 (ADAMTS13) enzyme activity measurement.

ENDOTOXEMIC SHOCK

Endotoxin, also known as lipopolysaccharide (LPS), is a stabilizing molecule in the outer membrane of the cell wall of gram-negative bacteria. Endotoxin is highly immunostimulatory in mammals, especially humans, despite the fact that enormous quantities of it are carried around in the intestines—more than a million times the lethal dose if given intravenously.[5] Endotoxin can trigger all of the cardinal feature of sepsis on its own and likely is a modulating factor during the syndrome. This, in part, likely explains why the molecule and particular types of gram-negative bacteria have dominated sepsis experimental models and drug development for decades. Humans are especially sensitive to endotoxin, more so than any of their cousins in the animal kingdom.[4]

This exquisite sensitivity leads to a variety of responses, including activation of immune cells, which produce inflammatory proteins (eg, cytokines) that also are cytotoxic and whose actions result in the release of various DAMPs (see **Table 1**). This process ensures that even if the endotoxin exposure is transient, there will be a robust immune response lasting for some time.

In 1993, a laboratory technician self-administered 1 mg of Salmonella endotoxin, dissolved in sterile water, intravenously, in an attempt to treat a recently diagnosed tumor.[44] The patient presented 2.5 hours later in profound shock. Although the patient ultimately recovered, over the course of the next 72 hours, all the cardinal features of sepsis developed, including fever, tachycardia, increased cardiac output, leukocytosis with up to 45% immature neutrophils, thrombocytopenia with evidence of DIC, AKI, elevated hepatic transaminases, and mild hypoxemia requiring supplemental oxygen. Remarkably, the serum lactate concentration was only 2.0 mmol/L. The patient received a 100-mg dose of HA-1A antibody (Centoxin, Centocor, Malvern, Pennsylvania), a human IgM antibody for the lipid A domain of endotoxin, 23 hours after the endotoxin injection. The patient ultimately made a complete recovery and appeared to resolve the illness rather rapidly. Although fever remained for 60 hours and vasopressors were required for almost as long, sustained organ failure did not occur. The inflammatory response was attenuated substantially from its peak already at 24 hours after endotoxin injection, although it was still very abnormal and subsequent testing was not performed. The discrete, nonsustained nature of the exposure, perhaps helped by the HA-1A antibody, resulted in a relatively mild case of sepsis. The patient, however, developed rather severe shock, receiving 2 vasopressors and more than 15 L of resuscitation fluid. It is intriguing to speculate whether a different predisposition or a more sustained exposure would have resulted in a different outcome.

Endotoxin as a Trigger for Macrophage Activation Syndrome and Atypical Hemolytic Uremic Syndrome

Endotoxin is a potent activator of macrophages (see **Fig. 2**) and is the classic stimulus used in vitro. The patient, described previously, with self-administered endotoxemic shock had a serum IL-6 concentration of 263,510 pg/mL measured 6.8 hours after the injection.[44] Compared with the so-called cytokine storm reported in many patients with MAS, this is several orders of magnitude higher. Could ongoing exposure to endotoxin produce an MAS picture? Although persistent exposure to low doses of endotoxin induces a phenomenon known as endotoxin tolerance,[45] continuous infusions of high doses are required to induce sepsis in nonhuman primates[4] and a more sustained exposure to endotoxin might be expected to lead to irreversible organ failure in humans.

Endotoxin also is a potent activator of complement and is capable of activating both the classical and alternative complement pathways.[46] aHUS is a disorder of complement activation and it known that endotoxin can trigger aHUS in susceptible hosts. Typical HUS is caused by Shiga toxin, and, although it originates from some of the same species of bacteria, Shiga toxin and endotoxin are quite distinct. The patient described previously certainly had complement activation, although it was rapidly brought under control. It is plausible that sustained endotoxemia might provoke aHUS, even in humans without a genetic predisposition, because approximately 40% of cases have no known genetic association.[42]

Sources of Endotoxin in Sepsis

Although endotoxin is ubiquitous in the environment, in the soil, in food, and on skin,[5] endotoxemia rarely comes from such sources. Gram-negative infections may result in endotoxemia and antibiotics may release it as they kill bacteria. Each person carries, however, a massive reservoir of endotoxin in the intestines. Estimates of the amount of endotoxin present in GI tracts are as high as 10 g to 50 g.[5]

In the GI tract, the chemical barrier of the mucosal layer and the cellular immune system maintains a symbiotic relationship with commensal bacteria.[47] Tight junction proteins are required for the maintenance of epithelial barrier integrity. The intracellular signaling transduction system and several extracellular stimuli, including cytokines, small GTPases, and post-translational modifications, dynamically modulate the tight junction protein complexes. An imbalance in these regulators leads to compromised barrier integrity and is linked with pathologic conditions.[47] Bacterial products, chiefly endotoxin, can cross the dysfunctional barrier and result in endotoxemia.

Humans and other mammals tend to be most sensitive to endotoxin from commensal gram-negative bacteria—organisms that constitutively live on or inside the host. These organisms have 6 acyl chains on the lipid A portion of the molecule (hexa-acylated lipid A) and these forms of endotoxin are most immunostimulatory in mammals, whereas LPS with fewer acyl chains is less so. Endotoxin with hexa-acylated lipid A is found in mainly bacteria that live in the lung and gut mucosa of mammalian hosts, such as commensal *Enterobacteriaceae* (eg, *Escherichia coli*, *Klebsiella*, and *Salmonella*).[4]

Management of Endotoxemia

Efforts to neutralize endotoxin began in the 1970s and accelerated as the molecular structure of endotoxin was characterized.[48] Various antibodies to endotoxin have been studied, including the HA-1A antibody used in the case discussed previously. Clinical trials testing these therapies have been discouraging. Few studies, however, have examined the effect of these treatments in patients with detectable endotoxemia.[49,50] An analysis of HA-1A found that this monoclonal antibody reduced mortality among 27 patients with detectable endotoxemia but not for 55 patients without detectable endotoxemia.[50] In general, however, results in the endotoxemia-positive subgroups of patients have not been positive.[51] The reasons for the disconnect between strong preclinical data, biologic rationale, and negative trials have been pondered in multiple reviews.[48] Potential explanations include problems with the agents themselves, study populations, and timing of therapy.

An alternative strategy to pharmacologic neutralization of endotoxin is removal of the molecule using hemoperfusion. Polymyxins are a group of cyclic cationic polypeptide antibiotics that have well characterized endotoxin binding. Although toxicity limits the clinical use of polymyxin B as an antibiotic, polymyxin B can be bound to a hemoperfusion column, and circulating endotoxin can be removed effectively through exposure to immobilized polymyxin B without the systemic toxicity. This method has been available in Japan since 1994 and received CE mark approval in Europe in 1998. More than 100,000 patients have been treated in more than a dozen countries.[52] Analyses of clinical data from a national Japanese database using propensity matching and other techniques has demonstrated benefit in the range of 3% to 7% absolute risk reduction for hospital mortality.[53,54] No clinical trials have been adequately powered to find an effect size in this range. The 2 largest trials to date, the ABDOMIX trial in France[55] and the EUPHRATES trial in the United States,[56] did not find a survival benefit for polymyxin B hemoperfusion. The EUPHRATES trial, however, was significantly different in design compared with other trials. Midway through the trial, enrollment was restricted to patients with multiple organ dysfunction score (MODS) of 9 or less (MODS range, 0–24, with 24 the worst possible score),[57] and the MODS group with a greater than 9 score became the primary analysis. This change was prompted by evidence that any benefit appeared to be limited to patients with greater organ dysfunction. A similar conclusion recently was reached by Fujimori and colleagues[54] in an analysis of more than 4000 patients from Japan. In this analysis, the therapy was most effective for patients with more organ failure.

Another significant difference between the EUPHRATES trial and other studies was the use of the endotoxin activity assay (EAA). EAA is an immunoassay that uses anti–lipid A monoclonal antibody and whole blood. Endotoxin in the blood sample binds with the antibody, and this antibody-antigen complex stimulates neutrophils that also are in the sample. Reactive oxygen species produced by neutrophils then are measured by the luminol chemiluminescence reaction. Basal and maximally stimulated samples are measured in parallel as negative and positive controls, and endotoxin activity in the sample is expressed as a relative value (EAA level).[58] A level of 0.60 or higher is considered the threshold for high endotoxin activity and is associated with increased intensive care unit (ICU) mortality.[59] Enrollment into the EUPHRATES trial was restricted to patients with septic shock who were found to have EAA 0.60 or higher.

Overall, the EUPHRATES trial showed that even in the per protocol analysis restricted to patients with a MODS greater than 9, 28-day mortality was 33% with hemoperfusion versus 36.4% with sham, a difference that was not statistically significant.[56] The EA, however, cannot quantify circulating endotoxin precisely when EAA levels are 0.90 or greater and values in this range may not represent treatable levels. A reanalysis of the EUPHRATES trial data revealed that 17% of patients had EAA greater than or equal to 0.90. When these patients are removed, 28-day mortality was 26.1% for polymyxin B hemoperfusion versus 36.8% for sham (risk difference 10.7%; odds ratio 0.52, 95% CI, 0.27–0.99; $P = .047$).[60] These findings prompted the design of an ongoing trial in the United States.

SEPSIS AND ARTIFICIAL INTELLIGENCE

Sepsis is a heterogeneous syndrome; identification of distinct clinical phenotypes could allow for more precise therapy and improve care. Machine learning is a branch of artificial intelligence based on the notion that systems can learn from data, identify patterns, and make decisions without human intervention. If the input data are comprehensive, the results can be considered unbiased, and discovery using these approaches can complement more directed hypothesis testing and help generate new hypotheses. Seymour and colleagues[61] used machine learning and simulation to derive clusters of clinical characteristics (ie, phenotypes) from patients meeting the Sepsis-3 criteria[1] within 6 hours of hospital presentation. k-Means clustering was applied to all clinical and laboratory variables in the electronic health records (29 in all) from 16,552 patients and then validated in a second database (n = 31,160) and in prospective cohorts from observational studies and randomized controlled trials (n = 5320). Optimal fit was obtained with 4 derived phenotypes (α, β, γ, and δ) and host-response biomarkers (eg, cytokines); organ failure patterns and survival varied considerably across phenotypes (**Table 5**). Although all phenotypes included some dysfunction across organs, kidney, liver, and coagulation abnormalities tended to cluster in 1 phenotype (δ phenotype), and pulmonary involvement tended to be greatest in the γ phenotype. The δ phenotype was present in 10% to 15% of patients across data sets and was associated with a dramatically higher mortality rate (32% in-hospital mortality compared with 2% for the α phenotype.

Table 5
Characteristics of sepsis phenotypes identified by artificial intelligence

Characteristic	Total	Phenotype			
		α	β	γ	δ
Proportion of patients		33%	27%	27%	13%
Increased cytokines		+	+	++	+++
Coagulopathy		+	+	+	++
Liver dysfunction		+	+	+	++
AKI		+	++	+	+++
Days of mechanical ventilation, median (IQR)	5 (2–10)	4 (2–9)	4 (2–9)	6 (3–13)	4 (2–9)
Days of vasopressors, median (IQR)	3 (2–5)	2 (2–4)	3 (2–4)	3 (2–5)	3 (2–5)
Admitted to ICU	45%	25%	32%	63%	85%
In-hospital mortality	10%	2%	5%	15%	32%

Abbreviation: IQR, interquartile range.
   Data from Seymour CW, Kennedy JN, Wang S, et al. Derivation, Validation, and Potential Treatment Implications of Novel Clinical Phenotypes for Sepsis. JAMA. 2019;321(20):2003-2017. https://doi.org/10.1001/jama.2019.5791.

Given the distributions of organ failures and hyperinflammation seen in the δ phenotype and the associated mortality, it is likely that patients with sepsis who develop MAS and/or aHUS-like conditions would be included mainly in this phenotype. It is equally tempting to posit that endotoxemia may be a driver of this phenotype in many patients. Because endotoxin is not routinely quantified and because MAS and aHUS often are missed, further research is needed to confirm or refute the hypothesis that these conditions are driving the δ phenotype.

SUMMARY

Inflammation is central to many acute conditions across the spectrum, from infection to sterile tissue injury to rheumatic diseases and to drug/toxin reactions. The molecular basis for this nonspecific response involves various receptors and immune effector cells and has been elucidated, at least in part, in recent years. Sepsis is a heterogenous and imprecise syndrome that likely includes multiple phenotypes, some of which may be amenable to specific therapies. Progress in developing new therapies for sepsis almost certainly will require focusing on specific subsets of patients. Furthermore, careful evaluation of patients for sepsis mimics and for treatable diseases manifesting within the clinical classification of sepsis is key to improving care. Because sepsis is a common condition, it is easy to overlook unusual causes of organ failure and to succumb to confirmation bias about the nature of a patient's illness. Careful attention to past medical and family histories and specific use of an array of diagnostic testing and subspecialty input can help identify potentially treatable diseases masquerading as typical sepsis. The increasing use of artificial intelligence to sift through patterns of clinical characteristics also may help advance research into this complex area.

CLINICS CARE POINTS

- Sepsis can be missed in patients with underlying chronic organ dysfunction and always should be considered in any patient with infection, regardless of prior medical history.

- Sepsis also be may over-diagnosed: up to 10% of patients initially diagnosed with sepsis have an alternate diagnosis.
- aHUS should be considered when thrombocytopenia and intravascular hemolysis present along with AKI.
- A sepsis phenotype that includes liver dysfunction and DIC may occur in up to 10% of patients with sepsis. The condition appears to have features in common with MAS, including extremely high ferritin and poor survival.
- Endotoxin activity greater than 0.6 identifies a subset of sepsis patients with increased ICU mortality.

DISCLOSURE

J.A. Kellum discloses grant support and consulting fees from Astute Medical/Bio-Merieux and Baxter and currently is a full-time employee of Spectral Medical. H. Gómez discloses grant support and consulting fees from BioMerieux. All other authors declare no conflicts of interest.

REFERENCES

1. Singer M, Deutschman CS, Seymour CW, et al. The third international consensus definitions for sepsis and septic shock (Sepsis-3). JAMA 2016;315(8):801–10.
2. Kellum JA, Kong L, Fink MP, et al. Understanding the inflammatory cytokine response in pneumonia and sepsis: results of the genetic and inflammatory markers of sepsis (GenIMS) study. Arch Intern Med 2007;167(15):1655–63.
3. Angus DC, van der Poll T. Severe sepsis and septic shock. N Engl J Med 2013; 369(9):840–51.
4. Brinkworth JF, Valizadegan N. Sepsis and the evolution of human increased sensitivity to lipopolysaccharide. Evol Anthropol 2021;30(2):141–57.
5. Wassenaar TM, Zimmermann K. Lipopolysaccharides in food, food supplements, and probiotics: should we be worried? Eur J Microbiol Immunol (Bp) 2018; 8(3):63–9.
6. Sirivongrangson P, Kulvichit W, Payungporn S, et al. Endotoxemia and circulating bacteriome in severe COVID-19 patients. Intensive Care Med Exp 2020;8(1):72.
7. Vincent JL, Moreno R, Takala J, et al. The SOFA (Sepsis-related organ failure assessment) score to describe organ dysfunction/failure. On behalf of the working group on sepsis-related problems of the European society of intensive care medicine. Intensive Care Med 1996;22(7):707–10.
8. Sorensen TI, Nielsen GG, Andersen PK, et al. Genetic and environmental influences on premature death in adult adoptees. N Engl J Med 1988;318(12): 727–32.
9. Rautanen A, Mills TC, Gordon AC, et al. Genome-wide association study of survival from sepsis due to pneumonia: an observational cohort study. Lancet Respir Med 2015;3(1):53–60.
10. Scherag A, Schoneweck F, Kesselmeier M, et al. Genetic factors of the disease course after sepsis: a genome-wide study for 28Day mortality. EBioMedicine 2016;12:239–46.
11. Kernan KF, Ghaloul-Gonzalez L, Shakoory B, et al. Adults with septic shock and extreme hyperferritinemia exhibit pathogenic immune variation. Genes Immun 2019;20(6):520–6.

12. Yealy DM, Kellum JA, Huang DT, et al. A randomized trial of protocol-based care for early septic shock. N Engl J Med 2014;370(18):1683–93.
13. Crayne CB, Albeituni S, Nichols KE, et al. The immunology of macrophage activation syndrome. Front Immunol 2019;10:119.
14. Otsuka R, Seino KI. Macrophage activation syndrome and COVID-19. Inflamm Regen 2020;40:19.
15. Fardet L, Galicier L, Lambotte O, et al. Development and validation of the HScore, a score for the diagnosis of reactive hemophagocytic syndrome. Arthritis Rheumatol 2014;66(9):2613–20.
16. Debaugnies F, Mahadeb B, Ferster A, et al. Performances of the H-score for diagnosis of hemophagocytic lymphohistiocytosis in adult and pediatric patients. Am J Clin Pathol 2016;145(6):862–70.
17. Schulert GS, Grom AA. Pathogenesis of macrophage activation syndrome and potential for cytokine- directed therapies. Annu Rev Med 2015;66(1):145–59.
18. Ravelli A, Davi S, Minoia F, et al. Macrophage activation syndrome. Hematol Oncol Clin North Am 2015;29(5):927–41.
19. Henter JI, Horne A, Arico M, et al. HLH-2004: diagnostic and therapeutic guidelines for hemophagocytic lymphohistiocytosis. Pediatr Blood Cancer 2007;48(2):124–31.
20. Sullivan KE, Delaat CA, Douglas SD, et al. Defective natural killer cell function in patients with hemophagocytic lymphohistiocytosis and in first degree relatives. Pediatr Res 1998;44(4):465–8.
21. Janka G, zur Stadt U. Familial and acquired hemophagocytic lymphohistiocytosis. Hematology Am Soc Hematol Educ Program 2005;82–8.
22. Henter JI, Elinder G, Soder O, et al. Hypercytokinemia in familial hemophagocytic lymphohistiocytosis. Blood 1991;78(11):2918–22.
23. Lolachi S, Morin S, Coen M, et al. Macrophage activation syndrome as an unusual presentation of paucisymptomatic severe acute respiratory syndrome coronavirus 2 infection: a case report. Medicine 2020;99(32):e21570.
24. Kellum JA, Pike F, Yealy DM, et al. Relationship between alternative resuscitation strategies, host response and injury biomarkers, and outcome in septic shock: analysis of the protocol-based care for early septic shock study. Crit Care Med 2017;45(3):438–45.
25. Billiau AD, Roskams T, Van Damme-Lombaerts R, et al. Macrophage activation syndrome: characteristic findings on liver biopsy illustrating the key role of activated, IFN-gamma-producing lymphocytes and IL-6- and TNF-alpha-producing macrophages. Blood 2005;105(4):1648–51.
26. Hazen MM, Woodward AL, Hofmann I, et al. Mutations of the hemophagocytic lymphohistiocytosis-associated gene UNC13D in a patient with systemic juvenile idiopathic arthritis. Arthritis Rheum 2008;58(2):567–70.
27. Yanagimachi M, Goto H, Miyamae T, et al. Association of IRF5 polymorphisms with susceptibility to hemophagocytic lymphohistiocytosis in children. J Clin Immunol 2011;31(6):946–51.
28. RECOVERY Collaborative Group, Horby PW, Pessoa-Amorim G, et al. Tocilizumab in patients admitted to hospital with COVID-19 (RECOVERY): preliminary results of a randomised, controlled, open-label, platform trial. Lancet 2021;397(10285):1637–45.
29. Mariette X, Hermine O, Tharaux PL, et al. Effectiveness of tocilizumab in patients hospitalized with COVID-19: a follow-up of the CORIMUNO-TOCI-1 randomized clinical trial. JAMA Intern Med 2021;181(9):1241–3.

30. Carcillo JA, Shakoory B, Castillo L. Secondary hemophagocytic lymphohistiocytosis, macrophage activation syndrome, and hyperferritinemic sepsis-induced multiple-organ dysfunction syndrome in the pediatric ICU. In: Mastropietro C, Valentine K, editors. Pediatric critical care. Cham: Springer; 2019.

31. Ferrer R, Artigas A, Levy MM, et al. Improvement in process of care and outcome after a multicenter severe sepsis educational program in Spain. JAMA 2008; 299(19):2294–303.

32. Kaukonen KM, Bailey M, Suzuki S, et al. Mortality related to severe sepsis and septic shock among critically ill patients in Australia and New Zealand, 2000-2012. JAMA 2014;311(13):1308–16.

33. Levy MM, Rhodes A, Phillips GS, et al. Surviving Sepsis Campaign: association between performance metrics and outcomes in a 7.5-year study. Crit Care Med 2015;43(1):3–12.

34. Opal SM, Fisher CJ Jr, Dhainaut JF, et al. Confirmatory interleukin-1 receptor antagonist trial in severe sepsis: a phase III, randomized, double-blind, placebo-controlled, multicenter trial. The Interleukin-1 Receptor Antagonist Sepsis Investigator Group. Crit Care Med 1997;25(7):1115–24.

35. Shakoory B, Carcillo JA, Chatham WW, et al. Interleukin-1 receptor blockade is associated with reduced mortality in sepsis patients with features of macrophage activation syndrome: reanalysis of a prior phase III trial. Crit Care Med 2016; 44(2):275–81.

36. Carcillo JA, Halstead ES, Hall MW, et al. Three hypothetical inflammation pathobiology phenotypes and pediatric sepsis-induced multiple organ failure outcome. Pediatr Crit Care Med 2017;18(6):513–23.

37. Kyriazopoulou E, Leventogiannis K, Norrby-Teglund A, et al. Macrophage activation-like syndrome: an immunological entity associated with rapid progression to death in sepsis. BMC Med 2017;15(1):172.

38. Tarr PI, Gordon CA, Chandler WL. Shiga-toxin-producing Escherichia coli and haemolytic uraemic syndrome. Lancet 2005;365(9464):1073–86.

39. Noris M, Remuzzi G. Atypical hemolytic-uremic syndrome. N Engl J Med 2009; 361(17):1676–87.

40. Kavanagh D, Goodship T. Genetics and complement in atypical HUS. Pediatr Nephrol 2010;25(12):2431–42.

41. Osborne AJ, Breno M, Borsa NG, et al. Statistical validation of rare complement variants provides insights into the molecular basis of atypical hemolytic uremic syndrome and C3 Glomerulopathy. J Immunol 2018;200(7):2464–78.

42. Noris M, Mescia F, Remuzzi G. STEC-HUS, atypical HUS and TTP are all diseases of complement activation. Nat Rev Nephrol 2012;8(11):622–33.

43. Zimmerhackl LB, Besbas N, Jungraithmayr T, et al. Epidemiology, clinical presentation, and pathophysiology of atypical and recurrent hemolytic uremic syndrome. Semin Thromb Hemost 2006;32(2):113–20.

44. Taveira da Silva AM, Kaulbach HC, Chuidian FS, et al. Brief report: shock and multiple-organ dysfunction after self-administration of Salmonella endotoxin. N Engl J Med 1993;328(20):1457–60.

45. Beeson PB. Development of tolerance to typhoid bacterial pyrogen and its abolition by reticulo-endothelial blockade. Proc Soc Exp Biol Med 1946;61:248–50.

46. Fine DP. Activation of the classic and alternate complement pathways by endotoxin. J Immunol 1974;112(2):763–9.

47. Chelakkot C, Ghim J, Ryu SH. Mechanisms regulating intestinal barrier integrity and its pathological implications. Exp Mol Med 2018;50(8):1–9.

48. Hurley JC. Towards clinical applications of anti-endotoxin antibodies; a re-appraisal of the disconnect. Toxins (Basel) 2013;5(12):2589–620.
49. Behre G, Schedel I, Nentwig B, et al. Endotoxin concentration in neutropenic patients with suspected gram-negative sepsis: correlation with clinical outcome and determination of anti-endotoxin core antibodies during therapy with polyclonal immunoglobulin M-enriched immunoglobulins. Antimicrob Agents Chemother 1992;36(10):2139–46.
50. Wortel CH, von der Mohlen MA, van Deventer SJ, et al. Effectiveness of a human monoclonal anti-endotoxin antibody (HA-1A) in gram-negative sepsis: relationship to endotoxin and cytokine levels. J Infect Dis 1992;166(6):1367–74.
51. Opal SM, Laterre PF, Francois B, et al. Effect of eritoran, an antagonist of MD2-TLR4, on mortality in patients with severe sepsis: the ACCESS randomized trial. JAMA 2013;309(11):1154–62.
52. Shimizu T, Miyake T, Tani M. History and current status of polymyxin B-immobilized fiber column for treatment of severe sepsis and septic shock. Ann Gastroenterol Surg 2017;1(2):105–13.
53. Fujimori K, Tarasawa K, Fushimi K. Effects of polymyxin B hemoperfusion on septic shock patients requiring noradrenaline: analysis of a nationwide administrative database in Japan. Blood Purif 2021;50(4–5):560–5.
54. Fujimori K, Tarasawa K, Fushimi K. Effectiveness of polymyxin B hemoperfusion for sepsis depends on the baseline SOFA score: a nationwide observational study. Ann Intensive Care 2021;11(1):141.
55. Payen DM, Guilhot J, Launey Y, et al. Early use of polymyxin B hemoperfusion in patients with septic shock due to peritonitis: a multicenter randomized control trial. Intensive Care Med 2015;41(6):975–84.
56. Dellinger RP, Bagshaw SM, Antonelli M, et al. Effect of targeted polymyxin B hemoperfusion on 28-day mortality in patients with septic shock and elevated endotoxin level: the EUPHRATES randomized clinical trial. JAMA 2018;320(14):1455–63.
57. Carcillo JA, Kellum JA. Is there a role for plasmapheresis/plasma exchange therapy in septic shock, MODS, and thrombocytopenia-associated multiple organ failure? We still do not know–but perhaps we are closer. Intensive Care Med 2002;28(10):1373–5.
58. Ikeda T, Ikeda K, Suda S, et al. Usefulness of the endotoxin activity assay as a biomarker to assess the severity of endotoxemia in critically ill patients. Innate Immun 2014;20(8):881–7.
59. Marshall JC, Foster D, Vincent JL, et al. Diagnostic and prognostic implications of endotoxemia in critical illness: results of the MEDIC study. J Infect Dis 2004;190(3):527–34.
60. Klein DJ, Foster D, Schorr CA, et al. The EUPHRATES trial (Evaluating the use of Polymyxin B Hemoperfusion in a randomized controlled trial of adults treated for Endotoxemia and Septic shock): study protocol for a randomized controlled trial. Trials 2014;15(1):218.
61. Seymour CW, Kennedy JN, Wang S, et al. Derivation, validation, and potential treatment implications of novel clinical phenotypes for sepsis. JAMA 2019;321(20):2003–17.

All that Wheezes is not Asthma or Bronchiolitis

Erica Y. Chou, MD[a], Barry J. Pelz, MD[b], Asriani M. Chiu, MD[b], Paula J. Soung, MD[a],*

KEYWORDS

- Wheezing • Asthma • Asthma mimics • Bronchiolitis • Respiratory distress
- Respiratory failure

KEY POINTS

- The differential diagnosis of wheezing is broad.
- While asthma and bronchiolitis are both very common, these entities tend to follow a typical time course with a predictable response to targeted therapies.
- Astute clinical attention and a high index of suspicion are helpful in guiding the treatment of patients with respiratory symptoms.

INTRODUCTION

A wheeze is a high-pitched, musical, adventitious lung sound resulting from air passing through a narrowed or obstructed airway from the level of the larynx to the small bronchi.[1] In young children under the age of 2, the most common cause of wheezing is bronchiolitis, a condition in which airway obstruction is due to inflammation and mucous production; in older children and adults, the most common cause is asthma, which is characterized by bronchoconstriction, airway inflammation, and mucous production. However, almost any disorder that leads to the narrowing or obstruction of the respiratory tract may cause wheezing or other transmitted respiratory sounds that may be misinterpreted as wheezing.[1,2]

Bronchiolitis is the leading cause of hospital admission for respiratory distress in infants and the most common lower respiratory tract infectious process in children younger than 2 years of age.[3,4] It is a clinical diagnosis wherein children present with congestion, cough, wheezing, progressively worsening tachypnea, increased work of breathing and respiratory distress, and sometimes progression to acute respiratory failure. Evidence-based guidelines suggest limiting workup such as chest

[a] Department of Pediatrics, Medical College of Wisconsin, 9000 West Wisconsin Avenue, Milwaukee, WI 53226, USA; [b] Department of Pediatrics (Allergy and Immunology) and Medicine, Medical College of Wisconsin, 9000 West Wisconsin Avenue, Milwaukee, WI 53226, USA
* Corresponding author. C560 Children's Corporate Center, PO Box 1997, Milwaukee, WI 53201-1997.
E-mail address: psoung@mcw.edu

Crit Care Clin 38 (2022) 213–229
https://doi.org/10.1016/j.ccc.2021.11.002
0749-0704/22/© 2021 Elsevier Inc. All rights reserved.
criticalcare.theclinics.com

radiographs and viral testing. Management is primarily supportive, as bronchodilators, steroids, and other treatments have not been shown to improve outcomes and are not routinely recommended.[5] As a result, patients are diagnosed clinically, and with few beneficial interventions, it is difficult to assess for a lack of response, which might then lead to an expanded differential diagnosis. Triggers for evaluating alternative diagnoses in an infant or toddler presenting with wheezing may include abrupt onset, fluctuating or recurrent degree of distress, persistent symptoms inconsistent with typical disease progression, and/or the presence of additional history or clinical symptoms inconsistent with bronchiolitis.

Asthma is the most common cause of wheezing and dyspnea in children and adults. It is a heterogeneous syndrome characterized by variable, reversible airway obstruction, and hyperreactivity, that includes several categories such as extrinsic (allergic), intrinsic (nonallergic), exercise-induced, drug-induced, and atypical asthma, among others.[1] There is a wide range of severity of asthma exacerbations, from successful management with bronchodilators and steroids in the outpatient setting, to severe status asthmaticus resulting in respiratory failure and requiring intubation. A paucity of wheeze in asthma may result from either improving or worsening severity of bronchoconstriction and airflow obstruction.[1] Because asthma can present with variable respiratory symptoms and severities, the presence or absence of wheezing can be easily attributed to asthma, although at times incorrectly.[6] Considerations for evaluating for alternative diagnoses may include new-onset wheezing in older children and adults, focal or predominantly inspiratory wheezing, monophonic breath sounds, poor response to conventional asthma treatments, as well as atypical chronicity or recurrence of symptoms.

ASTHMA AND BRONCHIOLITIS MIMICS: THE DIFFERENTIAL DIAGNOSIS OF WHEEZING

A careful history and physical examination are essential to elucidating the cause of wheezing. Clinicians should consider etiologies beyond bronchiolitis and asthma if

---

Box 1
Red flag indicators for expanding the differential diagnosis of wheezing

Clubbing of digits

Dysphagia, drooling, aphonia

Episodic/recurrent respiratory distress

Growth failure or weight loss

Hemoptysis

Heart murmur

Lethargy

Persistent hyperinflation or asymmetric inflation on imaging

Recurrent sinopulmonary infections

Refractory lung infiltrates on imaging

Tripoding (sitting up-leaning forward posture)

Sudden onset of respiratory distress

Weakness or focal neurologic deficits

red flag findings are present (**Box 1**). The differential for wheezing can be narrowed by the pathophysiology and localization of the lesion (**Table 1**). We will review a variety of case presentations that highlight the broad differential of wheezing and clues that increase the index of suspicion for an alternative diagnosis to asthma or bronchiolitis.

Extrathoracic Upper Airway

Respiratory symptoms from extrathoracic upper airway sources often present with stridor and higher pitched inspiratory sounds and respond poorly to bronchodilators. While abnormal breath sounds are usually localized to the upper airway, they can also be transmitted throughout the lung fields making them difficult to distinguish from wheezing.[6]

Case: The Paradox
A 22-year-old female with a history of asthma and gastroesophageal reflux disease presented to a local emergency department (ED) in respiratory distress after being exposed to cleaning chemicals at work. She had a history of strong odors and fragrances triggering acute respiratory symptoms which were treated as recurrent asthma exacerbations with multiple ED visits and intensive care unit (ICU) admissions over a 2-year period. On arrival to the ED, she was in acute respiratory distress, unable to speak in full sentences, with pulse oximetry of 95% on room air (RA). She was given albuterol-ipratropium nebulizer treatments and intravenous steroids with minimal improvement. Her physical examination was pertinent for good aeration throughout all lung fields with no stridor and no wheezing, but visible increased work of breathing. She was transferred to the ICU whereby she was placed on BiPAP with improvement.

Differential and Diagnosis. With a history of recurrent asthma exacerbations, the natural inclination was to diagnose and treat the patient for asthma. However, given a lack of response to bronchodilators, lack of wheezing on examination, and improvement with positive pressure, the focus instead turned to upper airway obstruction, including laryngospasm, laryngeal angioedema (which can be associated with acute anaphylaxis, angiotensin-converting enzyme inhibitor therapy, or hereditary angioedema), laryngeal or tracheal stenosis, vocal fold abnormalities (including vocal cord paresis or paradoxic vocal cord motion), or excessive dynamic airway collapse (including laryngomalacia or tracheomalacia).

   She underwent direct laryngoscopy with videostroboscopy and had evidence of paradoxic vocal fold motion with abnormal adduction of the true vocal folds during inspiration, consistent with vocal cord dysfunction (VCD). She worked extensively with speech-language pathologists, with significant improvement in her VCD symptoms.

Discussion and Clinical Pearls. VCD, also known as intermittent laryngeal obstruction (ILO) or paradoxic vocal fold motion abnormality (PVFMA), is a condition whereby the vocal cords and larynx inappropriately narrow in response to external stimuli, from irritants such as fragrances or chemicals, exercise, and even strong emotions. During a symptomatic episode, inappropriate vocal fold adduction can occur during inspiration, expiration, or both.[7] While an important mimicker of asthma, VCD can be seen concomitantly with asthma in over 50% of patients, with positive methacholine challenge testing in up to 70% of VCD cases.[8]

   While both asthma and VCD can cause dyspnea, especially with exposure to irritants or exercise, VCD does not typically respond to bronchodilators or steroids. Most patients will complain of difficulty getting air "in" versus "out" which can be a significant distinguishing factor compared with asthma or lower respiratory tract

Table 1
Causes of wheezing by anatomic location

Extrathoracic Upper Airway	Intrathoracic Airways	Parenchymal/Interstitial
Anaphylaxis	*Upper Airway*	Allergic bronchopulmonary
Aspiration	Airway compression	aspergillosis
Epiglottitis	(mediastinal mass or	Hypersensitivity pneumonitis
Foreign body aspiration	lymph nodes)	Immunodeficiency disorders
Gastroesophageal reflux	Foreign body aspiration	Infections (bacterial, viral,
Goiter	Intrathoracic goiter	atypical or fungal
Hemangioma	Tracheal tumor or mass	pneumonia; parasitic,
Laryngeal cleft	Tracheal papillomatosis	turberculosis)
Laryngeal edema or stenosis	Tracheomalacia	Inhalation injury (including [a]
Laryngeal tumor or mass	Tracheal stenosis	EVALI)
Laryngomalacia	Vascular compression (ring	[c]Interstitial lung disease (ILD)
Papillomatosis	or sling)	Gastric aspiration
Retropharyngeal abscess	*Lower Airway*	Pulmonary cysts
Subglottic stenosis	Asthma	Pulmonary edema ([b]ARDS,
Tonsillar hypertrophy	Acute chest syndrome	cardiac)
Tracheoesophageal fistula	Bronchiolitis	Pulmonary embolism
Vocal cord dysfunction	Bronchospasm (anaphylaxis,	Pulmonary hemosiderosis
Vocal cord paralysis	postviral, drug induced)	Pulmonary sequestration
	Bronchopulmonary dysplasia	Sarcoidosis
	Bronchiectasis	Vasculitis
	Bronchial cysts, tumors, or	
	mass	
	Bronchial stenosis	
	Bronchomalacia	
	Bronchiolitis obliterans	
	Chronic obstructive	
	pulmonary disease	
	Cardiovascular anomalies	
	(cardiac asthma)	
	Carcinoid syndrome	
	Cystic fibrosis	
	Dyskinetic (immotile) cilia	
	syndrome	
	Inhalational injury	
	Lymphangiectasia	
	Neuromuscular weakness	
	(secretion clearance)	
	Plastic bronchitis syndrome	
	α_1-Antitrypsin deficiency	

[a] EVALI = Electronic cigarette (e-cigarette) or vaping product use-associated lung injury.
[b] ARDS = acute respiratory distress syndrome.
[c] ILD = includes a broad group of idiopathic, acquired, rheumatoid, infectious, immune-related, storage, and malignant related disease processes in addition to those included separately (hypersensitivity pneumonitis, pulmonary hemosiderosis, sarcoidosis, vasculitis).

obstruction. Patients are more likely to have anxiety or another associated mental health condition, and a history of childhood abuse is noted in many patients with VCD. Pulmonary function testing may be normal or show flattening of the inspiratory loop.[9] The diagnosis is made with laryngoscopy visualizing abnormal vocal cord adduction with bronchoprovocation with the inducer, or a substitute like methacholine or mannitol. Additionally, laryngoscopy is useful to exclude other causes of static and dynamic upper airway obstruction.[9] Long-term treatment of VCD is a multidisciplinary approach that includes identifying and avoiding inducers, and treatment with speech-language pathologists. Respiratory retraining including the use of lower abdominal breathing and coordination of timing between respiration and phonation has also been shown to help, as has whole body and upper neck and shoulder relaxation. Psychotherapy may also be part of the broad treatment plan.

Case: Achilles Heel
A 15-year-old previously healthy female adolescent presented with difficulty breathing in the setting of 2 weeks of rhinorrhea, congestion, and cough. She had been diagnosed with sinusitis and treated with antibiotics during this course. She presented with 3 days of increased difficulty breathing and a hoarse voice. In the ED, she had a respiratory rate of 40 and oxygen saturation of 81% on RA, requiring 4 liters per minute (LPM) oxygen. Chest and neck radiographs were normal. She was given racemic epinephrine, albuterol nebulizer treatments, and dexamethasone and was admitted for further monitoring.

On admission, physical examination was notable for dysphonia, inability to cough or clear secretions, and respiratory distress with coarse transmitted breath sounds and diminished aeration throughout both lung fields. On neurologic examination, she had mild bilateral ptosis, peripheral extremity weakness involving the upper and lower extremities with 3/5 hand grip strength and decreased patellar and Achilles reflexes.

Further history revealed symptoms of generalized weakness, numbness, and tingling in her extremities, and slight drooping of her right eye noted over the 2 days prior to admission.

Differential and Diagnosis. Acute respiratory distress is common in young children with upper respiratory symptoms; however, symptoms of airway obstruction in a previously healthy adolescent are atypical. While the primary presenting complaint was respiratory in nature, a detailed history and physical examination uncovered neurologic findings including lack of phonation and other findings of cranial nerve palsies, in addition to subtle peripheral weakness and neuropathy. Otolaryngology was consulted and urgently performed a bedside scope confirming bilateral vocal cord paresis with aspiration of secretions. The patient had rapid escalation to respiratory failure requiring intubation. The differential diagnosis included Guillain-Barré syndrome, multiple sclerosis, neuromyelitis optica, acute disseminated encephalomyelitis, myasthenia gravis, Lyme disease, and neurosarcoidosis.[10] MRIs of the brain and spine were normal and lumbar puncture with cerebrospinal fluid (CSF) studies were negative for albumin-cytologic dissociation or inflammation. Given the examination findings of cranial nerves palsies, upper extremity weakness, and decreased reflexes in the lower extremities, neurology diagnosed her clinically with Miller Fisher syndrome or the pharyngeal-cervical-brachial overlap variant of Guillain–Barré syndrome (GBS). She was treated with intravenous immunoglobulin leading to clinical improvement and extubation with near resolution of her neurologic deficits. Electromyography demonstrated polyneuropathy. Antibody testing returned positive for anti-GQ1b and anti-GD1b antibodies, supporting the diagnosis of a GBS variant.

Discussion and Clinical Pearls. GBS describes a heterogeneous group of disorders, including the variant Miller Fisher syndrome (MFS) and other GBS subtypes.[10] MFS is characterized by external ophthalmoplegia, ataxia, and muscle weakness with areflexia. The pharyngeal–cervical–brachial variant of GBS is characterized by acute weakness of the oropharyngeal, neck, and shoulder muscles with swallowing dysfunction and may overlap with MFS.[11,12] These GBS variants are uncommon in children but are more likely to present with respiratory symptoms, such as cough, stridor, wheezing, and respiratory distress early in the course of symptoms.[13] Variants with cranial nerve involvement may present more acutely from a respiratory standpoint than GBS with ascending weakness. Shared clinical features include a history of antecedent infection (usually upper respiratory infection or diarrhea symptoms) in more than 90% of patients, typically a monophasic disease course, and symmetric cranial or limb weakness.[10] Diagnosis may be supported by CSF albumin-cytological dissociation, abnormal nerve conduction studies, or the identification of antiganglioside antibodies, but these studies should not be relied on to make the clinical diagnosis, particularly if doing so delays treatment. When acute neurologic deficits are associated with respiratory distress, emergent evaluation is needed. Early diagnosis of GBS and its variants is important to guide appropriate treatment with immunotherapy. Uncovering other acute neurologic diagnoses on the differential is of equal urgency.

Intrathoracic Airway

While extrathoracic airway obstruction tends to be exacerbated by the effect of atmospheric pressure compressing the trachea during inspiration, intrathoracic airways are subject to dynamic airway collapse during expiration, resulting in more prominent expiratory wheezing with narrowing or obstruction. Fixed obstructions may result in biphasic wheezing.

Case: Mass Effect

A 9-year-old previously healthy female presented with persistent cough for 4 weeks, and 5 days of increased work of breathing. She had no previous diagnosis of asthma but had been prescribed albuterol by urgent care without relief. On the day of admission, she was struggling to catch her breath and talk in complete sentences. She was brought to the ED, where she was hypoxic to 88% on RA, tachycardic to the 180s, and tachypneic to the 40s. Examination was notable for poor air movement, prolonged expiration, and wheezing. She received continuous albuterol and intravenous magnesium. She became combative and confused, at which time intravenous (IV) epinephrine was given for severe respiratory distress. Chest radiograph showed hyperinflation and perihilar bronchovascular lung markings without focal pneumonia. Arterial blood gas showed a pH of 7.29 and Pco_2 of 46.6. She was admitted to the ICU on an 8 LPM nonrebreather oxygen mask. Symptoms initially improved with albuterol and IV steroids, but then she had multiple recurrent episodes of significant respiratory distress with desaturations, sometimes waking her from sleep anxious, where she would state "I can't breathe" and required positive pressure via bag-mask until calm.

Differential and Diagnosis. History of prolonged cough with associated acute respiratory distress along with documented wheezing on examination may be consistent with uncontrolled asthma. Given features of episodic and recurrent distress, desaturations, and concerns for anxiety or agitation, the differential was expanded to include foreign body, anatomic abnormality, and VCD. As mentioned previously, VCD should be considered in children and adults with recurrent episodic dyspnea and wheezing refractory to bronchodilators; however, oximetry and blood gas exchange are usually unaffected; if present, such findings warrant broader evaluation.[14,15] Tracheal or bronchial airway lesions involving external compression or internal narrowing may mimic symptoms of airway obstruction caused by asthma and should be on the differential diagnosis in patients with poor response to conventional asthma treatment.[16]

Otolaryngology performed a bronchoscopy which demonstrated a flesh-colored mass originating from the anterior tracheal wall 15 cm above the carina, nearly occluding the distal trachea. Computed tomography (CT) imaging of the neck and chest demonstrated a mildly enhancing lesion in the distal left anterolateral trachea associated with at least 50% narrowing of the tracheal lumen, with prominent paratracheal and supraclavicular adenopathy (**Fig. 1**). She underwent biopsy and endoscopic debulking of the mass which revealed anaplastic large cell lymphoma.

Discussion and Clinical Pearls. Tumors of the trachea or respiratory system are rare in the pediatric age group. Tracheal lesions almost always present with symptoms of airway obstruction such as cough, dyspnea, wheezing, stridor, or repeat pulmonary infections; and due to slow growth of the tumors, the respiratory symptoms are mistaken for symptoms of asthma.[17] Delay in diagnosis is common, with greater than 50% of airway masses being initially misdiagnosed and managed as asthma.[18] Children present with new-onset progressive symptoms that can be life threatening given that lesions often obstruct more than 50% of the airway lumen at diagnosis.[19,20] If patients are not responding to conventional treatments, it is important to consider airway evaluation. Tracheal bronchogenic cysts, thymic cysts or masses, and benign and malignant tumors involving the trachea or anterior mediastinum have been reported with acute respiratory presentations mimicking wheezing from infants to young adults.[17,19,21–25] Similarly, adults may present with new-onset wheezing and respiratory symptoms with bronchotracheal tumors or mediastinal masses causing extrinsic tracheal compression secondary to lesions such as goiter, squamous cell carcinoma, and lymphoma.[26,27] Timely diagnosis of tracheal masses requires a high index of suspicion and conducting definitive evaluation by bronchoscopy.[18]

Case: A Kernel of Truth

A 14-month-old male toddler with 2 days of cough, congestion, and tactile fevers presented to the ED with acute onset of increased work of breathing and tachypnea. He was given steroids, continuous albuterol, and intravenous magnesium for presumed reactive airway disease and was admitted to the acute care floor. After admission, his respiratory status worsened despite receiving scheduled albuterol, hypertonic

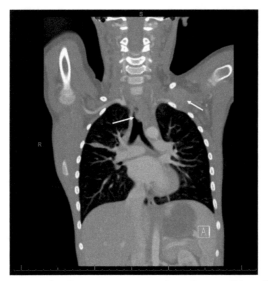

Fig. 1. Computed tomography demonstrating anaplastic large cell lymphoma of the distal left anterolateral trachea (*arrow*) with associated paratracheal and supraclavicular adenopathy.

saline, and positive expiratory pressure treatments. He was transferred to the ICU whereby he was placed on high-flow nasal cannula and heliox. Over several days, he was gradually weaned off oxygen, but he continued to have tachypnea, retractions, and significant inspiratory and expiratory wheezing bilaterally.

Differential and Diagnosis. Respiratory distress in the setting of cough, congestion, and fever suggests an infectious etiology. Viral respiratory infections may cause wheezing through inflammation and mucous secretion, as in bronchiolitis, or through induced bronchospasm.[28] This patient had symptoms that persisted longer than expected for a typical viral respiratory infection and did not respond to bronchodilator treatments. Atypical pneumonias should be considered, as wheeze can be a prominent feature and slow to resolve,[29] especially without treatment with a macrolide antibiotic.[30] Although *Mycoplasma* and *Chlamydia pneumoniae* are more common in children older than 3 years,[31,32] both were tested for in this patient and were negative. Cardiac asthma was considered but was lower on the differential diagnosis as he did not have a murmur, abnormal heart sounds, signs of fluid overload such as hepatomegaly or edema on examination, had a normal heart size on chest radiograph, and had been growing well before admission.

The patient had serial chest radiographs which showed peribronchial markings bilaterally, with shifting right upper lobe and left lower lobe atelectasis. Given the patient's persistent symptoms, pulmonology performed a bronchoscopy and found a popcorn kernel lodged in each mainstem bronchus. The foreign bodies were removed leading to rapid resolution of respiratory symptoms. In reviewing the history with his parents, they denied any history of choking, but an aunt did admit to feeding him popcorn before the onset of his symptoms.

Discussion and Clinical Pearls. Foreign body aspiration (FBA) occurs commonly in children between 1 to 3 years of age,[33] likely due to the introduction of solids and the oral exploratory behavior of toddlers.[34] Foods are the most frequently aspirated items, followed by other organic and nonorganic materials, such as small pieces of plastic from toys.[35] Clinical symptoms depend on the type, location, and size of foreign body. The objects may become lodged at any point in the bronchial tree, with variable degrees of obstruction. Symptoms may include cough, stridor, wheezing, shortness of breath, or respiratory failure in severe cases. Although there is a "clinical triad" of FBA (persistent cough, localized wheezing, and localized decreased breath sounds), few patients present with the complete triad, making it a specific, but not sensitive marker of FBA.[36] Sometimes the child or parent can remember a coughing or choking event preceding the onset of wheezing, which should increase the degree of suspicion for FBA.[36] Chest radiograph is frequently obtained to evaluate for foreign body despite most aspirated objects being radiolucent. A high percentage of children with FBA have normal chest radiographs, although localized air trapping and atelectasis may be seen (**Fig. 2**). Bronchoscopy is the definitive diagnostic procedure and treatment for foreign bodies in children.[34] Having a high degree of suspicion for FBA is important to avoid delay of diagnosis and management.

Case: Change of Heart

A 65-year-old male with a history of hypertension, diabetes, and asthma/COPD syndrome (ACOS) presented with 1 to 2 weeks of worsening cough and dyspnea on exertion, which acutely woke him from sleep before presentation. He used his albuterol rescue inhaler without improvement and presented to the ED whereby he was in respiratory distress with hypoxemia of 88% on room air and was subsequently admitted. He admitted to not using his asthma controller medications consistently, and he was a current smoker. Vitals were also pertinent for an elevated blood pressure of 180/100 mm Hg. On examination, he had difficulty speaking in complete sentences, wheezing on auscultation, decreased breath sounds at the bases, and tachycardia without any obvious murmurs. He did not have elevated jugular vein distention or any lower extremity edema. Basic laboratories including complete blood count with differential, serum electrolytes, liver function tests, and troponins were unremarkable. Chest radiograph showed increased interstitial markings; and a 12-lead EKG showed sinus tachycardia with nonspecific ST and T wave changes. He was given supplemental oxygen, albuterol nebulizer treatments, and intravenous steroids without improvement. Brain natriuretic peptide (BNP) was elevated at 500 pg/mL (normal <100 pg/mL, >400 pg/mL likely heart failure). An echocardiogram showed decreased ejection fraction. When he began to improve after starting diuretics, he also admitted to not using his antihypertensives consistently.

Differential and Diagnosis. Dyspnea on exertion and nocturnal dyspnea can be a common symptom with both pulmonary and cardiac causes and may be difficult to distinguish, especially if the patient has both cardiac disease and chronic obstructive lung disease, including asthma or COPD. The differential diagnosis includes pneumonia and pulmonary embolism, depending on the acuity of the presentation. Even in a patient with no known heart disease, reviewing the history and medication list may help identify cardiac risk factors. Severe hypertension, renal failure, or severe anemia may present with acute cardiac failure. In the pediatric population, common causes for low cardiac output or fluid overload include congenital heart defects. Many congenital heart defects manifest in infancy with cyanosis, tachypnea, wheezing, or difficulty feeding. Acute myocarditis and cardiomyopathy should also be considered in infants and older children as well as previously healthy young adults presenting with symptoms of chest pain, dyspnea, or respiratory distress.[37]

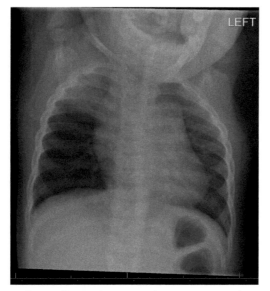

Fig. 2. Chest radiograph revealing atelectasis and air trapping in foreign body aspiration. Note the absence of a radiopaque foreign body.

Discussion and Clinical Pearls. Cardiac asthma may be more of a diagnostic challenge in patients that have mild or even compensated heart failure, especially if they also have coexisting obstructive lung disease. In this case, the patient did not have any known cardiac disease, but uncontrolled hypertension likely led to left ventricular hypertrophy and decreased ejection fraction. Given the lack of response to bronchodilators and steroids, obtaining the BNP was important in determining the correct diagnosis and subsequent treatment. Pulmonary function testing with bronchoprovocation testing, as well as echocardiography, may help differentiate cardiac and bronchial asthma.[38]

The wheezing of cardiac asthma is caused by compression of the intrathoracic airways by interstitial edema, as well as internal narrowing of the bronchial airways by vascular engorgement and airway remodeling, in addition to possible reflex bronchoconstriction, all of which may mimic acute asthma or even bronchiolitis in an infant.[38,39] In adult patients, the typical rales of heart failure may not be heard due to overall reduction in breath sounds in the setting of chronic obstructive lung disease. Murmurs, gallops, decreased heart sounds, or cardiomegaly on chest radiography are clues to cardiac asthma. However, these cardiac examination findings may be obscured by the pulmonary manifestations of cardiac asthma. A thorough history and examination for other findings of volume overload, including jugular venous distension, hepatomegaly, or peripheral edema, and an index of suspicion to explore nonpulmonary causes of respiratory distress, are required even in the absence of suggestive examination findings.[40]

Lung Interstitium–Parenchyma

Disorders leading to parenchymal inflammation may cause a variety of symptoms including cough, shortness of breath, chest tightness, and wheeze. Respiratory distress associated with transmitted respiratory sounds or even the absence of wheezes may be misconstrued as asthma with these associated symptoms. The differential for interstitial lung involvement is broad making additional historical cues essential in determining appropriate evaluation and management.

Case: A Hot Trend

A 17-year-old unimmunized male presented with 6 days of fever, myalgia, and sharp anterior chest pain triggered by coughing and inspiration. He was tachycardic to the 120s, tachypneic to the 30s, and hypoxemic to 85% on room air, which improved to greater than 90% on 2 LPM. On examination, he appeared in distress, with nasal flaring and accessory muscle use. He was taking shallow breaths and breath sounds were diminished. Laboratories showed elevated inflammatory markers. Chest radiograph showed diffuse coarse and hazy bilateral interstitial opacities (**Fig. 3**A). He had a CT angiogram which showed no evidence of pulmonary embolism, but extensive nodular ground-glass opacities were seen throughout both lungs (see **Fig. 3**B). He was admitted to the acute care floor, then transferred to the ICU for worsening tachypnea, hypoxemia to the 50s, and respiratory distress that progressed to failure, requiring intubation for several days.

Social history was significant for vaping and smoking marijuana, and frequenting public steam rooms at the local YMCA.

Differential and Diagnosis. Unimmunized status, fever, cough, respiratory distress, elevated inflammatory markers, and imaging findings of bilateral interstitial ground-glass opacities raised concern for lower respiratory tract infection. The patient had an extensive infectious workup, including assays for histoplasmosis, blastomycosis,

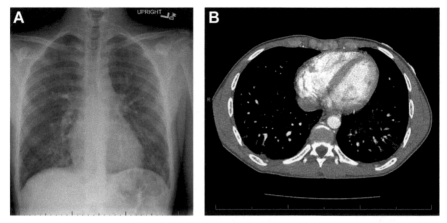

Fig. 3. Imaging findings in electronic cigarette (e-cigarette) or vaping product use-associated lung injury (EVALI). (*A*) Chest radiograph showing diffuse coarse and hazy bilateral interstitial opacities. (*B*) Computed tomography demonstrating extensive nodular ground-glass opacities throughout both lungs.

tick-borne illnesses, and legionella, all of which were negative. He was empirically given broad-spectrum antibiotics without improvement.

Differential diagnosis also included hypersensitivity pneumonitis (HP). HP is caused by the inhalation of an antigen to which the patient is sensitized and hyperresponsive, and often presents with fever, chills, cough, and shortness of breath.[41] Chest CT typically shows fine nodular opacities and widespread ground-glass opacities, and bronchoalveolar lavage (BAL) has a significantly elevated percentage of lymphocytes in HP.[42] Pulmonology was consulted and performed a bronchoscopy and BAL in our patient, which showed 60% neutrophils, only 5% lymphocytes, 1% eosinophils, and—notably—20% alveolar macrophages and a small-to-moderate amount of lipid-laden macrophages.

Given these BAL findings, in combination with the patient's history, signs and symptoms, other diagnostic findings, as well as lack of an identified infectious etiology and failure to improve on antibiotics, he was diagnosed with inhalational pneumonitis, specifically electronic cigarette (e-cigarette) or vaping product use-associated lung injury (EVALI). He was started on IV methylprednisolone with improvement clinically and radiographically. He was extubated and weaned to room air before discharge. Steroids were transitioned to oral prednisone with a 2-week taper.

Discussion and Clinical Pearls. EVALI is a relatively new condition, first reported in 2019. EVALI has been primarily described in teenagers and adults, with 37% of patients between 18 to 24 years old.[43] Symptoms of EVALI include constitutional symptoms, such as fever, night sweats, and fatigue; GI symptoms, including abdominal pain, nausea, vomiting, diarrhea, and weight loss; and respiratory symptoms, including cough, shortness of breath, and chest pain.[44] While wheezing is less commonly noted as a presenting symptom of EVALI, wheezing has been associated with e-cigarette use.[45,46] Tachycardia, tachypnea, and hypoxemia are frequently seen at the time of presentation, with up to one-third ultimately requiring intubation and mechanical ventilation.[44] Laboratory studies in EVALI can show leukocytosis and elevated inflammatory markers. BAL can show a predominance of macrophages, including lipid-laden macrophages, although it is unclear whether they are a marker of

EVALI or of vaping.[47] CT imaging predominantly shows peripheral or perilobular patchy bilateral ground-glass opacities or consolidation with subpleural sparing.[48] The mainstay of treatment of EVALI is systemic corticosteroids, although regimens are variable in the dose and length of treatment.

Solvents in e-cigarettes, including Vitamin E acetate and aromatic/volatile hydrocarbons can cause damage to the respiratory epithelium when inhaled and heated in e-cigarette products. These trigger inflammatory lung responses believed to be the cause of EVALI.[49] A thorough environmental exposure history and social history for use of e-cigarettes or vaping products is key for adolescents and young adults presenting with respiratory distress.

Case: Vessel Disease
A 10-year-old male with a history of chronic cough presented with 5 days of gradually worsening cough along with new respiratory distress and fatigue. The patient's cough began 14 months prior and was described as nonproductive occurring throughout the day and occasionally overnight. He had numerous visits to his pediatrician and a pediatric pulmonologist. His CXR showed mildly hyperinflated lungs bilaterally with slightly increased peribronchial markings. His spirometry revealed mild obstruction (FEV1 89% predicted, FVC 116% predicted, and FEV1/FVC ratio of 56% predicted). He was treated with inhaled corticosteroids, intranasal steroids, antihistamines, and a proton pump inhibitor, all of which did not alleviate the cough. In the 5 days leading up to his current presentation, he reported a worsening cough that became more frequent and more intense, worsening nasal congestion, significant fatigue, and anorexia. His initial examination revealed a tired appearing male in mild respiratory distress with relatively decreased oxygen saturations of 90% on room air, accessory muscle use, and inspiratory and expiratory wheezes in all lung fields with prolonged inspiratory to expiratory phases. There were occasional crackles noted peripherally. Repeat spirometry revealed a significant decrease in lung function with severe obstruction (FEV1 44% predicted, FVC 61% predicted, and FEV1/FVC ratio of 65% predicted). He was admitted to the hospital and treated with 2 LPM supplemental oxygen by nasal cannula and oral corticosteroids. Due to his prolonged course of symptoms, rapid decline in lung function, and his lack of response to various conventional medications, a broad investigation of other potential causes was initiated with multidisciplinary involvement including pulmonary, rheumatology, hematology, infectious disease, and allergy-immunology specialists. Findings were notable for chest radiograph with symmetric hyperinflation and increased peribronchial cuffing, peripheral white blood cell count of 13,600, an absolute peripheral eosinophil count of 2030, and a total IgE level of 1364 with a total IgG of 1290.

Differential and Diagnosis. While cough and respiratory symptoms are extremely common in children—and specifically in children with asthma—significant eosinophilia (more than 1500 cells per microliter) and elevated IgE levels (more than 500) are not typically seen in asthma. These findings raise concern for a more systemic and inflammatory process such as allergic bronchopulmonary aspergillosis (ABPA), parasitic infection, hypereosinophilic syndrome, or vasculitis. As such, the patient underwent additional workup which included parasite evaluation, antineutrophil cytoplasmic antibody (ANCA) testing, troponin and echocardiogram to evaluate for cardiac involvement of eosinophilic inflammation, bone marrow biopsy, and ABPA testing, all of which were negative. The patient had CT imaging of the sinuses and the lungs which revealed soft tissue densities throughout the paranasal sinuses and nasal cavities and circumferential wall thickening along the lobar, segmental, and subsegmental bronchi throughout both lungs with ground-glass and linear opacities in both lungs. He underwent nasal endoscopy with biopsies and bronchoscopy with BAL. The BAL fluid had 47% eosinophils, and sinus biopsy revealed eosinophils accumulating in extravascular areas. Given these findings, the diagnosis of eosinophilic granulomatosis with polyangiitis (EGPA) was strongly suspected. As EGPA can lead to peripheral neuropathy (including symptoms of pain, numbness, and/or weakness), nerve conduction studies were performed and were normal. Following a prolonged course of oral corticosteroid treatment, the patient was started on high-dose mepolizumab and has clinically done well.

Discussion and Clinical Pearls. EGPA (formerly called Churg–Strauss Syndrome) is a multisystem disorder characterized by asthma, rhinosinusitis, and peripheral eosinophilia. The disorder involves vasculitic inflammation of the small and medium-sized arteries and is characterized by eosinophilic infiltration with or without vasculitis in various affected tissues (including the skin, nerves, kidneys, gastrointestinal tract, or respiratory tract). Asthma is one of the cardinal features of EGPA, found in more than 90% of patients with EGPA.[50] Asthma in EGPA is often poorly controlled with inhaled corticosteroids and usually complicated by frequent and/or severe asthma exacerbations.

While both asthma and allergic rhinitis can lead to bronchoconstriction, nasal congestion, and rhinorrhea, these conditions do not typically result in high levels of peripheral eosinophilia or the other organ system involvement that can be seen in EGPA. Perhaps more importantly, asthma and allergic rhinitis tend to respond well to many of the immediate and readily available targeted therapies, including bronchodilators, antihistamines, inhaled and systemic steroids. Lack of response to typical medications as well as the continued escalation of symptoms led to a broader workup, leading to a diagnosis, and long-term therapeutic plan.

Case: Immunity Matters
A 17-year-old female adolescent with a history of recurrent viral upper respiratory infections presented with 7 days of shortness of breath, productive cough, fever, and chills. She was seen in the ED with examination findings of scattered crackles and wheezing. She was treated with an albuterol inhaler and a 5-day course of azithromycin with no improvement, after which she returned to the ED with persistent and worsening symptoms. A CT scan of the chest showed extensive multifocal nodular opacities in both lungs, ground-glass attenuation, traction bronchiectasis, mediastinal lymphadenopathy, and splenomegaly. She was hospitalized for intravenous antibiotics and oxygen supplementation. Of note, this treatment course marked her third documented pneumonia in the preceding 2 years, and she had additionally received multiple courses of antibiotics for sinusitis in the past.

She was referred to allergy and immunology whereby additional evaluation revealed panhypogammaglobulinemia with an IgG 129 mg/dL (reference range 508–1080), IgA 16 (52–232), and IgM 4 (36–226). She had low antibody responses to *Haemophilus influenzae*, *Tetanus*, and *Streptococcus pneumoniae*, and did not significantly respond after repeat vaccination. Lymphocyte enumeration by flow cytometry revealed moderate lymphopenia, with low B cells, low CD8 T cells, and a skewed ratio of memory to naïve T cells with an increased number of activated T cells. HIV and Hepatitis C testing were both negative by polymerase chain reaction.

Differential and Diagnosis. The combination of markedly reduced serum IgG along with low levels of IgA and/or IgM, poor response to immunizations, and an absence of any other defined immunodeficiency are hallmarks of common variable immunodeficiency (CVID). The differential for hypogammaglobulinemia is broad and includes both secondary and primary causes. Notable secondary causes include medications including glucocorticoids, antiseizure medications, and immunosuppressants. In young children, primary causes of hypogammaglobulinemia, including X-linked agammaglobulinemia, must be carefully excluded.

Specific to the acute on chronic respiratory complaints, the patient's lung disease and recurrent pneumonia raise concerns for cystic fibrosis, primary ciliary dyskinesia, and interstitial lung disease, all of which must be carefully excluded, depending on the clinical scenario. Additionally, there is a broad spectrum of pulmonary manifestations in primary immunodeficiencies, raising concern for the myriad of infectious, structural (e.g., bronchiectasis), malignant, and inflammatory abnormalities that can occur within primary immunodeficiencies. One of these is granulomatous and lymphocytic interstitial lung disease (GLILD) which affects a subset of patients with CVID. GLILD typically presents with dyspnea on exertion and a new or altered cough, which may mimic asthma. Some patients are asymptomatic but have characteristic findings on chest imaging, leading to the diagnosis. Other pulmonary diseases that should be considered include organizing pneumonia and bronchial-associated lymphoid tissue (BALT) lymphoma.

This patient was ultimately diagnosed with CVID. She underwent a video-assisted thoracoscopic surgery (VATS) with biopsy that was highly suspicious for GLILD. She was started on gammaglobulin replacement therapy for CVID and treatment with rituximab and azathioprine for GLILD with clinical improvement.[51,52]

Discussion and Clinical Pearls. CVID is the most common primary immunodeficiency affecting both children and adults.[53] Approximately 20% of patients with CVID are diagnosed before 20 years of age, while the majority is diagnosed between 20 and 45 years of age.[54,55] CVID should be considered in any patient with recurrent bacterial sinopulmonary infections. Many patients with CVID also have evidence of immune dysregulation, which can lead to chronic lung disease, gastrointestinal disease, hematologic disease, and/or malignancy. CVID is an important consideration in patients presenting with pulmonary complaints, especially if there is a history of additional infections or immune involvement (such as thrombocytopenia or thymoma). Other conditions that lead to recurrent pulmonary infections such as cystic fibrosis and primary ciliary dyskinesia should also be excluded.

SUMMARY

Wheezing is a symptom, not a diagnosis. Assessment of patients with wheezing can be diagnostically challenging when considering the vast array of focal and systemic disorders that may cause narrowing or obstruction of the airways, bronchial secretions or wall edema, parenchymal inflammation, as well as respiratory weakness that may contribute to this symptom.[1,2] All that wheezes is not asthma or bronchiolitis, and establishing an accurate diagnosis requires attention to the patient's history, physical examination, and response to therapy,[27] as well as having a high index of suspicion for alternative diagnoses.

CLINICS CARE POINTS

- A thorough history and examination may reveal diagnostic clues for the source of wheezing and aid in accurate diagnosis.

- Acuity and chronicity of symptoms, attempts to localize examination findings to an anatomic location, as well as the age of the patient, may lend direction to differential diagnoses to be considered.
- If there is a poor response to the routine therapeutic management of wheezing, a high index of suspicion for alternative diagnoses is required.

DISCLOSURE

The authors have no conflicts of interest to disclose.

REFERENCES

1. Gong H. Wheezing and asthma. In: Walker HK, Hall WD, Hurst JW, editors. Clinical methods: the history, physical, and Laboratory examinations. 3rd edition. Butterworths; 1990. Available at: http://www.ncbi.nlm.nih.gov/books/NBK358/. Accessed July 12, 2021.
2. Patel PH, Mirabile VS, Sharma S. Wheezing. In: StatPearls. Treasure Island (FL): StatPearls Publishing; 2021. Available at: http://www.ncbi.nlm.nih.gov/books/NBK482454/. Accessed June 7, 2021.
3. Hall CB, Weinberg GA, Iwane MK, et al. The burden of respiratory syncytial virus infection in young children. N Engl J Med 2009;360(6):588–98.
4. Erickson EN, Bhakta RT, Mendez MD. Pediatric bronchiolitis. In: StatPearls. Treasure Island (FL): StatPearls Publishing; 2021. Available at: http://www.ncbi.nlm.nih.gov/books/NBK519506/. Accessed July 12, 2021.
5. Clinical Practice Guideline. The diagnosis, management, and Prevention of bronchiolitis | American Academy of pediatrics. Available at: https://pediatrics.aappublications.org/content/134/5/e1474. Accessed July 19, 2021.
6. Weinberger M, Abu-Hasan M. Pseudo-asthma: when cough, wheezing, and dyspnea are not asthma. Pediatrics 2007;120(4):855–64.
7. Dunn NM, Katial RK, Hoyte FCL. Vocal cord dysfunction: a review. Asthma Res Pract 2015;1(1):9.
8. Perkins MPJ, Morris LMJ. Vocal cord dysfunction induced by methacholine challenge testing. Chest 2002;122(6):1988–93.
9. Fretzayas A, Moustaki M, Loukou I, et al. Differentiating vocal cord dysfunction from asthma. J Asthma Allergy 2017;10:277–83.
10. Wakerley BR, Yuki N. Mimics and chameleons in Guillain-Barré and Miller Fisher syndromes. Pract Neurol 2015;15(2):90–9.
11. Lametery E, Dubois-Teklali F, Millet A, et al. [Pharyngeal-cervical-brachial syndrome: a rare form of Guillain-Barré syndrome with severe acute bulbar palsy]. Arch Pediatr Organe Off Soc Francaise Pediatr 2016;23(2):176–9.
12. Lyu R-K, Chen S-T. Acute multiple cranial neuropathy: a variant of Guillain-Barré syndrome? Muscle Nerve 2004;30(4):433–6.
13. Uysalol M, Tatlı B, Uzel N, et al. A rare form of Guillan Barre syndrome: a child diagnosed with anti-GD1a and anti-GD1b positive pharyngeal-cervical-brachial variant. Balk Med J 2013;30(3):337–41.
14. Sharma A. Respiratory distress. In: Nelson pediatric symptom-based diagnosis. Philadelphia: Elsevier; 2018. p. 39–60.e1.
15. Noyes BE, Kemp JS. Vocal cord dysfunction in children. Paediatr Respir Rev 2007;8(2):155–63.

16. Paraskakis E, Froudarakis M, Tsalkidou EA, et al. An eight-year-old girl with tracheal mass treated as a difficult asthma case. *J Asthma* Published Online September 2020;29:1–5.
17. Baghai-Wadji M, Sianati M, Nikpour H, et al. Pleomorphic adenoma of the trachea in an 8-year-old boy: a case report. J Pediatr Surg 2006;41(8):e23–6.
18. Desai DP, Holinger LD, Gonzalez-Crussi F. Tracheal Neoplasms in children. Ann Otol Rhinol Laryngol 1998;107(9):790–6.
19. Romão RLP, de Barros F, Maksoud Filho JG, et al. Malignant tumor of the trachea in children: diagnostic pitfalls and surgical management. J Pediatr Surg 2009;44(11):e1–4.
20. Gjonaj ST, Lowenthal DB, Dozor AJ, et al. Pneumonias, asthma, Pneumothorax, and respiratory arrest caused by a tracheal mass. Pediatrics 1997;99(4):604–5.
21. Stewart B, Cochran A, Iglesia K, et al. Unusual case of stridor and wheeze in an infant: tracheal bronchogenic cyst. Pediatr Pulmonol 2002;34(4):320–3. https://doi.org/10.1002/ppul.10129.
22. Youngson GG, Ein SH, Geddie WR, et al. Infected thymic cyst: an unusual cause of respiratory distress in a child. Pediatr Pulmonol 1987;3(4):276–9. https://doi.org/10.1002/ppul.1950030414.
23. Javia L, Harris MA, Fuller S. Rings, slings, and other tracheal disorders in the neonate. Semin Fetal Neonatal Med 2016;21(4):277–84.
24. Welsh JH, Maxson T, Jaksic T, et al. Tracheobronchial mucoepidermoid carcinoma in childhood and adolescence: case report and review of the literature. Int J Pediatr Otorhinolaryngol 1998;45(3):265–73.
25. Yester MA, Ajizian SJ. Atypical presentation of a mediastinal mass in an adolescent: Critical care considerations. Pediatr Crit Care Med 2010;11(4):e44.
26. Cengiz K, Aykin A, Demirci A, et al. Intrathoracic goiter with hyperthyroidism, tracheal compression, superior vena cava syndrome, and horner's syndrome. Chest 1990;97(4):1005–6.
27. Krieger BP. When wheezing may not mean asthma. Other common and uncommon causes to consider. Postgrad Med 2002;112(2):101–2, 105-108, 111.
28. Tan WC. Viruses in asthma exacerbations. Curr Opin Intern Med 2005;4(2):178–83.
29. Laitinen LA, Miettinen AK, Kuosma E, et al. Lung function impairment following mycoplasmal and other acute pneumonias. Eur Respir J 1992;5(6):670–4.
30. Esposito S, Blasi F, Arosio C, et al. Importance of acute Mycoplasma pneumoniae and Chlamydia pneumoniae infections in children with wheezing. Eur Respir J 2000;16(6):1142–6.
31. Shim JY. Current perspectives on atypical pneumonia in children. Clin Exp Pediatr 2020;63(12):469–76.
32. Lieberman D, Lieberman D, Printz S, et al. Atypical Pathogen infection in adults with acute exacerbation of bronchial asthma. Am J Respir Crit Care Med 2003;167(3):406–10.
33. Oğuz F, Çıtak A, Ünüvar E, et al. Airway foreign bodies in childhood. Int J Pediatr Otorhinolaryngol 2000;52(1):11–6.
34. Lima JAB, Fischer GB. Foreign body aspiration in children. Paediatr Respir Rev 2002;3(4):303–7.
35. Rothmann BF, Boeckman CR. Foreign bodies in the larynx and tracheobronchial tree in children: a review of 225 cases. Ann Otol Rhinol Laryngol 1980;89(5):434–6.
36. Midulla F, Guidi R, Barbato A, et al. Foreign body aspiration in children. Pediatr Int 2005;47(6):663–8.
37. Sertogullarindan B, Ozbay B, Gumrukcuoglu HA, et al. A case of viral myocarditis presenting with acute asthma attack. J Clin Med Res 2012;4(3):224–6. https://doi.org/10.4021/jocmr823w.

38. Tanabe T, Rozycki HJ, Kanoh S, et al. Cardiac asthma: new insights into an old disease. Expert Rev Respir Med 2012;6(6):705–14.
39. Jorge S, Becquemin M-H, Delerme S, et al. Cardiac asthma in elderly patients: incidence, clinical presentation and outcome. BMC Cardiovasc Disord 2007; 7(1):16.
40. Carter K, Moskowitz W. Cardiac asthma: old disease, new considerations. Clin Pulm Med 2014;21(4):173–80.
41. Spagnolo P, Rossi G, Cavazza A, et al. Hypersensitivity pneumonitis: a comprehensive review. J Investig Allergol Clin Immunol 2015;25(4):237–50.
42. Ratjen F, Costabel U, Griese M, et al. Bronchoalveolar lavage fluid findings in children with hypersensitivity pneumonitis. Eur Respir J 2003;21(1):144–8.
43. Outbreak of lung injury associated with the use of E-cigarette, or vaping, products. Centers for disease control and prevention. 2020. Available at: https://www.cdc.gov/tobacco/basic_information/e-cigarettes/severe-lung-disease.html. Accessed July 8, 2021.
44. Layden JE, Ghinai I, Pray I, et al. Pulmonary illness related to E-cigarette use in Illinois and Wisconsin — final report. N Engl J Med 2020;382(10):903–16.
45. Vardavas CI, Anagnostopoulos N, Kougias M, et al. Short-term pulmonary effects of using an electronic cigarette: Impact on respiratory flow Resistance, Impedance, and Exhaled Nitric Oxide. CHEST 2012;141(6):1400–6.
46. Li D, Sundar IK, McIntosh S, et al. Association of smoking and electronic cigarette use with wheezing and related respiratory symptoms in adults: cross-sectional results from the Population Assessment of Tobacco and Health (PATH) study, wave 2. Tob Control 2020;29(2):140–7.
47. Aberegg SK, Cirulis MM, Maddock SD, et al. Clinical, bronchoscopic, and imaging findings of e-cigarette, or vaping, product use–associated lung injury among patients treated at an Academic medical Center. JAMA Netw Open 2020;3(11): e2019176.
48. Thakrar PD, Boyd KP, Swanson CP, et al. E-cigarette, or vaping, product use-associated lung injury in adolescents: a review of imaging features. Pediatr Radiol 2020;50(3):338–44.
49. Blount BC, Karwowski MP, Shields PG, et al. Vitamin E acetate in bronchoalveolar-lavage fluid associated with EVALI. N Engl J Med 2020;382(8):697–705.
50. Comarmond C, Pagnoux C, Khellaf M, et al. Eosinophilic granulomatosis with polyangiitis (Churg-Strauss): clinical characteristics and long-term followup of the 383 patients enrolled in the French Vasculitis Study Group cohort. Arthritis Rheum 2013;65(1):270–81.
51. Verbsky JW, Hintermeyer MK, Simpson PM, et al. Rituximab and antimetabolite treatment of granulomatous and lymphocytic interstitial lung disease in common variable immunodeficiency. J Allergy Clin Immunol 2021;147(2):704–12.e17.
52. Chase NM, Verbsky JW, Hintermeyer MK, et al. Use of combination chemotherapy for treatment of granulomatous and lymphocytic interstitial lung disease (GLILD) in patients with common variable immunodeficiency (CVID). J Clin Immunol 2013;33(1):30–9.
53. Sullivan KE, Puck JM, Notarangelo LD, et al. USIDNET: a strategy to build a community of clinical immunologists. J Clin Immunol 2014;34(4):428–35.
54. Cunningham-Rundles C, Bodian C. Common variable immunodeficiency: clinical and immunological features of 248 patients. Clin Immunol 1999;92(1):34–48.
55. Resnick ES, Moshier EL, Godbold JH, et al. Morbidity and mortality in common variable immune deficiency over 4 decades. Blood 2012;119(7):1650–7.

Recognition and Management Considerations of Cardiac Channelopathies in the Intensive Care Unit

Anoop Kumar Singh, MB BCh

KEYWORDS

- Long QT Syndrome • Brugada syndrome
- Catecholaminergic polymorphic ventricular tachycardia • Sudden cardiac arrest
- Critical care

KEY POINTS

- There are many medical decisions that can potentially incite ventricular tachycardia in patients with long QT syndrome, Brugada syndrome, and catecholaminergic polymorphic ventricular tachycardia.
- A basic understanding of implantable cardioverter-defibrillators is essential in managing patients with channelopathies.
- A previously healthy patient presenting with a sudden cardiac arrest requires an extensive diagnostic evaluation to determine the underlying condition.
- Electrical storm in patients with a cardiac channelopathy requires some modifications to the advanced cardiac life support protocol taking into account the use of disease-specific medications and avoidance of other drugs.
- All of the aforementioned should be ideally done in conjunction with a specialist facile in the management of sudden cardiac arrest conditions.

INTRODUCTION

Cardiac output is the product of heart rate by stroke volume. In turn, the underpinning of both cardiac rate and stroke volume is the electrical system of the heart that sets the pace and coordinates a synchronized contraction from the atrial and ventricular chambers. The impact of cardiac arrhythmias runs the gamut from minor to malignant problems. This article focuses specifically on genetic arrhythmia syndromes (ie, channelopathies) that may present with a life-threatening tachyarrhythmia.

Medical College of Wisconsi, 9000 West Wisconsin Avenue, MS 713, Milwaukee, WI 53226, USA
E-mail address: asingh@chw.org

Crit Care Clin 38 (2022) 231–242
https://doi.org/10.1016/j.ccc.2021.11.014
0749-0704/22/© 2021 Elsevier Inc. All rights reserved.

criticalcare.theclinics.com

BACKGROUND
Cellular Electrophysiology

The cycling of sodium, calcium, and potassium into and out of cardiac myocytes is regulated by ion channels. The cardiac action potential starts with the cell holding a negative membrane potential, which, when triggered, initiates depolarization by a rapid influx of sodium ions into the cell.[1] After cellular repolarization the cell's path back to a negative membrane potential is delayed by calcium influx. This plateau phase in the action potential is critical for multiple reasons including the release of intracellular calcium for muscular contraction (excitation-contraction coupling)[2] and the prevention of immediate cardiac restimulation (tetany). As the plateau phase ends, there is an unopposed efflux of potassium from the myocyte, which repolarizes the cell. A basic understanding of cardiac depolarization, plateau phase, and repolarization is critical to understanding the pathophysiology and management of inherited arrhythmia syndromes.

Cardiac Cycle

Although ion channels dictate the cellular events, it is the interconnected nature of cardiac myocytes that results in global cardiac conduction and contraction. Cardiac myocytes work as a functional syncytium with 2 units: the atrial and ventricular syncytia. The annulus fibrosis electrically separates the atria from the ventricles. The coordination of myocytes depends on an organized electrical signal to orchestrate atrial and then ventricular contraction.

Electrocardiogram (ECG): an ECG transcribes the electrical events of the cardiac cycle. In sinus rhythm, the sinoatrial node initiates a propagation wave through the atria that results in a P-wave on the ECG. Because the annulus fibrosis prevents further transmission to the ventricles, the only path for electrical wavefront is through the atrioventricular node (AVN). The delay at the AVN is represented on the ECG by an isoelectric period (the PR segment). Once the AVN conducts to the penetrating bundle of His (the only normal electrical connection through the annulus fibrosis), ventricular depolarization happens rapidly and symmetrically via the bundle branches and Purkinje fibers, resulting in the normal, narrow QRS on the ECG. The conclusion of this cycle is the T-wave that represents ventricular repolarization. The ECG is the fundamental tool for defining a malignant arrhythmia as the cause for a cardiac arrest.

Tachyarrhythmias: an increase in cardiac output brought about by tachycardia eventually reaches a threshold, and then at supraphysiologic rates there is a drop in cardiac output due to a decline in stroke volume. A disorganized electrical signal can result in pockets of myocardium contracting at different times, which can be symptomatic in the atria (ie, atrial fibrillation) and life threatening in the ventricles (ie, ventricular fibrillation [VF]). The abrupt drop in cardiac output during a cardiac arrest is most often a function of poor ventricular filling and uncoordinated ventricular contraction. The genetic arrhythmia conditions that will be discussed can all produce the similar endpoint of an unstable ventricular tachyarrhythmia.

THE MAJOR GENETIC ARRHYTHMIA SYNDROMES
Long QT Syndrome

Long QT Syndrome (LQTS) is the prototypical cardiac channelopathy. Pathogenic variants in genes coding for either potassium or sodium channel proteins are the main causes of congenital LQTS. This genetic abnormality prolongs ventricular repolarization, manifests on an ECG with a prolonged QT interval (**Fig. 1**), and creates a vulnerable situation for a triggered, polymorphic ventricular tachycardia (VT) ("torsade de

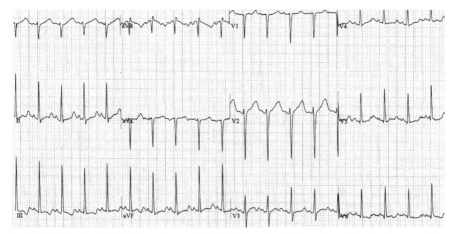

Fig. 1. Twelve-lead ECG of a patient with LQTS showing QT prolongation during exercise.

pointes"). The incidence of LQTS is estimated at 1:2000 live births.[3] There is no male or female predominance but the lifetime risk for an LQTS cardiac arrhythmia is higher in women than in men. The presentation of LQTS can occur at any age but is most commonly diagnosed during adolescence.[4] LQTS is primarily inherited in an autosomal dominant fashion, so familial screening is a key part of the workup for probands. Jervell and Lange-Nielsen syndrome, the autosomal recessive form of LQTS, is characterized by congenital deafness and malignant arrhythmias.

Most of the people with LQTS will be clinically asymptomatic with no physical examination findings of note. The clinical predisposition for polymorphic VT can be unmasked by triggering events such as exertion, being startled, use of specific drugs, hypokalemia, hypomagnesemia, and more. Short (ie, self-resolving within 30 seconds) arrhythmic episodes in LQTS generally present as syncope or a seizure.[5] Prolonged VT in LQTS results in cardiac arrest where emergent treatment is needed to prevent death.

For patients with a known diagnosis of LQTS a universal recommendation for prevention is avoidance of LQTS triggers. A comprehensive list of medications to avoid is regularly updated (crediblemeds.org),[6] including some types of antiarrhythmics, anticonvulsants, anesthetics, benzodiazepines, beta-agonists, antihistamines, antidepressants, and antibiotics. In addition, hypokalemia, hypomagnesemia, and hypocalcemia are all to be avoided for patients with LQTS. Finally, depending on the type of LQTS, there may be restrictions on the type and degree of exercise participation. From a medical standpoint β-blockers are a frequently used drug to prevent VT in LQTS. For patients at very high risk of a sudden cardiac arrest (based on their individual risk factors) or for those who have survived a cardiac arrest, advanced therapies are often used, such as an implantable cardioverter-defibrillator (ICD) or left cardiac sympathetic denervation.

The acute management for torsade de pointes involves prompt defibrillation. For patients with ongoing VT, intravenous magnesium sulfate helps to stabilize the dysrhythmia. In the acute setting use of an intravenous β-blocker and rapid correction of hypokalemia, hypocalcemia, and hypomagnesemia are helpful steps in preventing further VT.

Brugada Syndrome

The Brugada syndrome (BrS) is an inherited arrhythmia syndrome characterized by focal ECG changes and a predisposition to VF. Unlike LQTS, where a pathogenic gene variant is identified in ~80% of cases, patients with BrS have a pathogenic genetic variant identified only 25% of the time, with the vast majority being in genes coding for sodium channel proteins. The prevalence of the condition remains unclear but estimates range from 1:2000 to 1:5000 with a marked male predominance (estimated as 8 times greater in men than women).[7]

The mean age of presentation for BrS is approximately 40 years. The characteristic ECG finding ("Brugada pattern") is found in leads V1-V3 with j-point elevation greater than 2 mm, a coved ST segment, and inverted T wave (**Fig. 2**). Arrhythmic events happen most often during sleep but can also be triggered by fever or certain medications. Symptomatic patients present with syncope, seizures, and agonal respirations due to rapid, polymorphic VT or VF. If the ventricular arrhythmia sustains, sudden cardiac death will follow if not managed emergently. The acute management of VF with BrS requires immediate defibrillation. If the patient has ongoing ventricular arrhythmias then isoproterenol can provide some stabilization. The drug quinidine is particularly useful for patients with BrS, and a discussion with a cardiac rhythm specialist would be recommended to assist in the use of this medication.

For patients with BrS who have survived a malignant ventricular arrhythmia, the mainstay of treatment is ICD implantation. Because fever is a particular trigger for childhood presentations, temperature regulation is a preventative measure for this age group. Although not as extensive a list as in LQTS, there are specific medications to be avoided (www.brugadadrugs.org),[8] which could precipitate VF in patients with BrS.

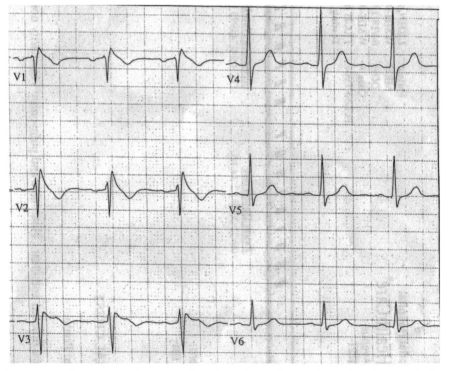

Fig. 2. Brugada pattern ECG showing focal j-point elevation and coved ST elevation in the right precordial leads.

Catecholaminergic Polymorphic Ventricular Tachycardia

Catecholaminergic polymorphic ventricular tachycardia (CPVT) is a channelopathy characterized by adrenergic-mediated VT. The underlying genetic problem causes abnormal calcium release from the sarcoplasmic reticulum. The commonest pathogenic CPVT variants are in the ryanodine receptor, specifically in *RYR2*, and this form of CPVT is inherited in autosomal dominant fashion. Pathogenic variants in both calsequestrin genes cause an autosomal recessive form of CPVT.[9] Many probands with CPVT have de novo variants, so the family history may be unremarkable in this condition.

The prevalence of CPVT is unknown but the condition is less common than LQTS or BrS, with some estimates at 1:10,000 births. The age of presentation tends to be younger in CPVT with a mean age at presentation of 8 years.[9] Symptoms, which classically occur with exertion or emotional stress, include palpitations, syncope, seizures, or sudden cardiac arrest. Unlike LQTS and BrS, patients with CPVT do not have a classic resting ECG pattern that would define the condition. The diagnosis is made by the history and often electrocardiographic monitoring during exercise. During a stress test the classic progression with increasing exertion would be as follows: normal rhythm, development of premature ventricular contraction (PVCs), bidirectional PVCs, bidirectional VT, and possibly, if the test is not stopped, VF. Finally, although VT is the hallmark dysrhythmia for CPVT, many patients can have supraventricular arrhythmias, particularly multifocal atrial tachycardia.

The management for CPVT includes minimizing exertional triggers, which entails a discussion between the provider and patient about their individualized risk of sudden cardiac arrest during sports. High-dose β-blockers are a standard therapy with consideration given for the addition of flecainide to prevent arrhythmias. Surgical left cardiac sympathetic denervation has a role in cases of CPVT with frequent, malignant arrhythmias.[10] The use of ICDs in CPVT is more challenging than its use for LQTS and BrS. Bidirectional VT in CPVT may be a perfusing rhythm (eg, the conscious patient is able to describe palpitations) and as such ICD discharges occur in an aware patient. Also worrisome is that ICD shocks may not convert bidirectional VT to sinus rhythm.[11] The combination of ICD shocks with an adrenergically mediated arrhythmia syndrome sets the stage for "electrical storm" (VT triggers an ICD shock that triggers an adrenaline surge that triggers VT again that leads to another ICD shock, and so forth). Thus, intravenous β-blockers are the critical medication in breaking the cycle of electrical storm in CPVT. It is less clear how effective verapamil is in the acute setting; however, there are case reports describing its efficacy for incessant VT with CPVT.[12]

CRITICAL CARE CONSIDERATIONS FOR A PATIENT WITH A CARDIAC CHANNELOPATHY
General Considerations

There are some stark differences in the management of the different arrhythmia syndromes discussed in this article. However, there are general points that are applicable to all patients with known genetic arrhythmias. The patient should be under continuous ECG monitoring capable of alarming for sustained and nonsustained arrhythmias. Depending on the specific situation a defibrillator may be bedside, but at a minimum the location of the nearest defibrillator with appropriate-sized pads should be discussed among the health care team.

If the patient or their family can provide a complete history then the medical provider should obtain pertinent information regarding the specific diagnosis, current medications, presence of a cardiac implanted electronic device (eg, ICD, pacemaker), and known arrhythmic triggers. A patient history of a sudden cardiac arrest or documented, unstable ventricular arrhythmia is important, as that finding not surprisingly increases the patient's risk for future arrhythmias.

In addition to the information that the patient and family can provide, it is high yield to communicate with the physician who manages the patient's arrhythmia condition. Their cardiologist/electrophysiologist should corroborate the arrhythmia diagnosis, provide information about pacemaker lower rate and/or ICD shock rate (when applicable), and serve as a consultant for decisions on best options for intensive care unit (ICU) management in light of the patient's genetic arrhythmia syndrome.

Basics of Implantable Cardioverter-Defibrillators

Knowledge of ICDs is important in managing a patient within the ICU setting. The basic components of all ICDs are a pulse generator (houses the circuitry, capacitor, and battery), a coil to complete the shock vector, and a sensing lead to detect the patient's rhythm. With the exception of subcutaneous ICDs, all ICDs have a minimum ability to pace the ventricle. For those with dual-chamber ICDs both atrial and ventricular pacing can be programmed if needed. The primary function of an ICD is to count the patient's heart rate. If the rate exceeds programmed thresholds and occurs for several seconds, the ICD will trigger a tachyarrhythmia intervention. For slower VTs, a rapid burst of ventricular pacing (antitachycardia pacing) can be used to attempt rhythm termination. If antitachycardia pacing fails or if the rate is too fast, the ICD will charge and deliver a biphasic shock to the patient. ICDs can deliver a sequence of multiple shocks (often up to 6 total) if rhythm reassessment shows continued tachycardia greater than the rate threshold.

A provider should be familiar with the limitations of an ICD. Although there is some capacity to distinguish supraventricular versus ventricular tachyarrhythmias, ICDs can deliver shocks for sinus tachycardia or supraventricular tachycardia if the rate exceeds the ICD rate limits. Also, patients can experience inappropriate shocks if an ICD "double counts" the rate by sensing both the QRS complex and the T wave for each beat. Placing a strong magnet over an ICD will disable its ability to detect and thus treat tachyarrhythmias. This magnet behavior of an ICD does not affect its ability to pace.

Disease-specific Considerations

LQTS: congenital LQTS is an important comorbidity to be considered during an ICU admission. Although many patients with LQTS will have never had a prior episode of VT, the circumstances leading to admission and subsequent management can place these patients at risk for their first, severe arrhythmic event. There are several ways that LQTS can affect ICU care. Some examples would include the following:

- Electrolyte depletion: a patient with hypovolemic shock may be at risk for ongoing potassium, calcium, or magnesium loss and should have these electrolytes regularly monitored and replaced if low.
- Hypothermia: although LQTS is not a contraindication to using targeted temperature management, the QT prolonging effects of hypothermia need to be considered during the process.
- Antibiotics: when feasible, a patient with atypical pneumonia would ideally receive an antibiotic alternative to macrolides due to their QT prolonging effect.

- Antiemetics: similarly, patients with a high need for antiemetic agents would need close QT monitoring, as many of these medications are on the drugs-to-avoid list for LQTS.
- Asthma: in patients with severe asthma exacerbations and LQTS, beta-agonist therapy is largely unavoidable but some adjunctive strategies include the use of magnesium sulfate and ipratropium bromide.
- Procedural sedation and anesthesia: when a patient requires sedation or anesthesia a review of LQTS drugs to avoid will list many of the commonly used drugs. Although there is no definitive safe protocol some drugs such as dexmedetomidine and sevoflurane are preferably avoided due to their higher potential for causing torsade de pointes.[13]

BrS: for BrS management the disease-specific considerations involve aggressive management of the arrhythmia triggers. In the ICU various situations pose a risk for patients with BrS.

- Sepsis: septic shock creates multiple problems, including relative hypovolemia and fever. Fever should be treated aggressively with antipyretics for patients with BrS, especially in younger patients in whom fever can precipitate VF. Although appropriate fluid resuscitation is not problematic, the use of alpha-agonist drugs (eg, norepinephrine, phenylephrine) to maintain vasomotor tone can trigger VF in patients with BrS.[14]
- Intracranial trauma: bradycardia and high vagal tone are seen after some brain injuries, and this slow heart rate increases the risk of VF for patients with BrS. Management of the underlying neurologic injury will help but isoproterenol should be available if needed for bradycardia-triggered tachyarrhythmias.
- Analgesia and anesthetics: although not nearly as extensive a list as seen for LQTS, there are still a handful of drugs to be avoided for BrS. For pain management bupivacaine is to be avoided because of its sodium channel blocking effect. Propofol, especially when given for a prolonged period, is contraindicated for patients with BrS.

CPVT: in the ICU the main impact of an underlying diagnosis of CPVT is avoiding adrenergic stimulation. So, when needed, appropriate pain management is important. If beta-agonist drugs are needed then consultation with an arrhythmia specialist is strongly encouraged for CPVT.

MANAGEMENT AND EVALUATION OF A PATIENT AFTER AN OUT-OF-HOSPITAL CARDIAC ARREST

The immediate management and workup of a patient who has suffered a sudden cardiac arrest is beyond the scope of this article. However, there are some specific points to be made about both the immediate management and subsequent workup. If the patient has a known cardiac condition then therapy can be tailored to their specific diagnosis. For a patient with no prior diagnosis the management is broader. The following sections discuss considerations for the patient with a recent cardiac arrest.

Prehospital Phase

Any data from the prehospital care may be useful to the ICU or perhaps later the cardiology team. If an automated external defibrillator or first-responder defibrillator was used to shock the patient, then rhythm strips from the device may be invaluable for later decision-making. The use of antiarrhythmic and inotropic medications in the field and the rhythm response to those interventions should be noted. The estimated "down time" for the patient until the return of spontaneous circulation may factor into the decision for temperature-based neuroprotection. Any bystander accounts of the cardiac arrest should be recorded, as it may be the only history available for the event. Finally, the age of the patient is a critical piece of information in the planning for ICU arrival. Coronary artery disease is the commonest underlying diagnosis for adults with out-of-hospital cardiac arrest,[15] but for a person younger than 35 years, strong consideration should be given to genetic cardiomyopathies and channelopathies.

At Presentation to the Intensive Care Unit

If the patient is relatively stable on arrival, a baseline ECG and echocardiogram would be useful initial tests. A Brugada pattern on the ECG could be seen soon after the cardiac arrest, and an echocardiogram could define structural heart anomalies as the undiagnosed condition. At the same time any details about the patient's history and antecedent events leading to the cardiac arrest may provide potential clues as to the underlying problem. A seemingly healthy teenager or young adult participating in sport at the time of their arrest should be strongly considered for either LQTS or CPVT (if their baseline echocardiogram ruled out structural heart disease). In addition to the standard medical history, there should be a detailed personal history with a focus on potential past cardiac events (eg, exertional syncope, seizures, near drowning event) and a family history looking for sudden, unexplained death at a young age.

If there is ongoing hemodynamic instability, advanced cardiac life support protocols should be followed, especially if the underlying cause for cardiac arrest is unknown. However, if ECG monitoring offers a clue for a cardiac channelopathy, this knowledge may prove useful to avoid provoking arrhythmias or electrical storm. In the case of LQTS, the ECG finding of T-wave alternans (**Fig. 3**) corresponds to marked QT prolongation. This degree of electrical instability may be a marker for future VT and should prompt immediate LQTS-specific management.

Standard advanced cardiac life support protocol when followed after sudden cardiac arrest should be monitored for any evidence that the treatment itself could be proarrhythmic for the patient. For example, amiodarone, which is a drug used for pulseless VT, prolongs the QT interval and may perpetuate torsade de pointes in a patient with LQTS. Epinephrine is frequently used to restore circulation and improve cardiac output. However, the drug could provoke increasing ventricular ectopy and then VT in a patient with underlying CPVT. And although β-blockers have an important role in the acute management of arrhythmias in patients with LQTS or CPVT, they are contraindicated in patients with BrS where the antagonistic drug (isoproterenol) is used in managing ongoing electrical storm.

Postarrest Workup

There are 2 broad reasons for identifying an inherited condition in a patient who has just suffered a cardiac arrest: (1) to assist in the acute and ongoing management for the patient and (2) to determine if first-degree relatives should be evaluated for the same condition. This workup should be done in conjunction with the cardiology service to ensure proper testing is ordered. The evaluation for structural heart disease may yield an obvious diagnosis. But if the patient is determined to have a structurally normal heart, then the genetic arrhythmia workup should be moved to the forefront of the differential diagnoses.

The initial ECG, although proving helpful for acute management, may be misleading with respect to the underlying diagnosis, as the QT interval is often prolonged

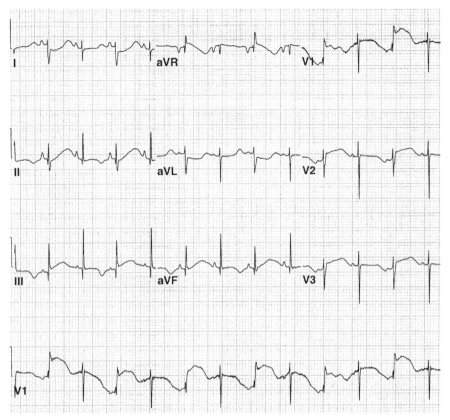

Fig. 3. Macroscopic T-wave alternans (seen best in lead III) in a patient with LQTS at risk for imminent torsade de pointes.

immediately after a cardiac arrest. Moreover, if the patient is being managed with therapeutic hypothermia the QT interval is likely iatrogenically prolonged. Thus, serial 12-lead ECGs over several days should be used looking for the "true QT interval" and also for the Brugada pattern in the right precordial leads to suggest BrS. Because CPVT has no classic baseline ECG finding, the patient's continuous, bedside ECG monitoring should be evaluated on a daily basis looking for clues such as increasing PVCs with tachycardia and bidirectional VT (**Fig. 4**).

Genetic testing for sudden cardiac arrest conditions is readily available through commercial laboratories. Although genetic testing may be a crucial part of the evaluation, the test requires a comprehensive discussion with the patient and/or family by specialists well versed in cardiomyopathies and channelopathies. This pretest discussion is critical for the later explanation of results. At present, most laboratories offer panel testing, which permits genetic assessment for multiple cardiomyopathy and channelopathy conditions. At a minimum, the ICU team managing the patient should have a blood sample drawn and held for the genetic arrhythmia team to decide on later testing.

In a worst-case scenario where a sudden cardiac arrest progresses to death, the medical team needs to encourage premortem and postmortem analysis for the underlying condition. The potential of an inherited condition places relatives at risk, and the

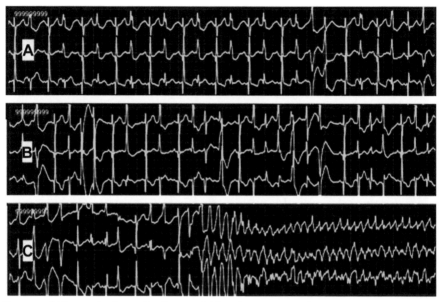

Fig. 4. Bedside monitoring strips from a child with a recent cardiac arrest. (*A*) Isolated PVCs noted. (*B*) Increasing agitation and tachycardia with resultant polymorphic ventricular ectopy and couplets. (*C*) Degeneration into sustained, polymorphic VT.

highest yield of cardiac and genetic testing would be with the patient who suffered a cardiac arrest. Thus a complete autopsy that includes consideration for genetic testing (if not performed pre-mortem) is a critical part of care.[16]

SUMMARY

People with cardiac channelopathies can present in childhood, adulthood, or be completely asymptomatic. However, the low likelihood of a severe cardiac event is increased for these patients during episodes of medical care as medications, fever, and electrolyte derangements may place them at high risk for provoked ventricular arrhythmias. Thus, a basic understanding of these conditions and the relevant electrophysiology is essential for ICU management. Disease-specific care, in conjunction with a cardiac rhythm specialist, is needed for a patient with a cardiac channelopathy when experiencing electrical storm. Finally, for a patient who has suffered a cardiac arrest, the ICU team plays a vital role in both the acute management and subsequent diagnostic evaluation.

CLINICS CARE POINTS

- For patients with long QT syndrome, avoidance of QT prolonging drugs and electrolyte derangements are key for ICU management.
- In Brugada syndrome key management issues include aggressively treating fever and avoiding drugs that cause sodium channel blockade.

- Catecholaminergic polymorphic ventricular tachycardia is managed with beta-blockers and flecainide while avoiding adrenergic drugs.
- ACLS-guided treatments should be monitored for response as amiodarone, epinephrine, and lidocaine can be proarrhythmic depending on the underlying channelopathy.

DISCLOSURE

The author has no commercial or financial conflicts of interest or funding sources.

REFERENCES

1. Nerbonne JM, Kass RS. Molecular physiology of cardiac repolarization. Physiol Rev 2005;85(4):1205–53.
2. Cooper PJ, Soeller C, Cannell MB. Excitation–contraction coupling in human heart failure examined by action potential clamp in rat cardiac myocytes. J Mol Cell Cardiol 2010;49(6):911–7.
3. Schwartz PJ, Stramba-Badiale M, Crotti L, et al. Prevalence of the congenital long-QT syndrome. Circulation 2009;120(18):1761–7.
4. Wilde AAM, Amin AS, Postema PG. Diagnosis, management and therapeutic strategies for congenital long QT syndrome. Heart 2021. https://doi.org/10.1136/heartjnl-2020-318259.
5. Priori SG, Wilde AA, Horie M, et al. Executive summary: HRS/EHRA/APHRS expert consensus statement on the diagnosis and management of patients with inherited primary arrhythmia syndromes. Heart Rhythm 2013;10(12): e85–108.
6. Woosley RL, Heise CW, Gallo T, Tate J, Woosley D and Romero KA, www.CredibleMeds.org, QTdrugs List, 12/14/2021, AZCERT, Inc. 1457 E. Desert Garden Dr., Tucson, AZ 85718
7. Brugada J, Campuzano O, Arbelo E, et al. Present status of brugada syndrome. J Am Coll Cardiol 2018;72(9):1046–59.
8. Postema PG, Wolpert C, Amin AS, et al. Drugs and Brugada syndrome patients: review of the literature, recommendations, and an up-to-date website (www.brugadadrugs.org). Heart Rhythm 2009;6(9):1335–41. https://doi.org/10.1016/j.hrthm.2009.07.002.
9. Pflaumer A, Davis AM. An update on the diagnosis and management of catecholaminergic polymorphic ventricular tachycardia. Heart Lung Circ 2019;28(3): 366–9.
10. Pflaumer A, Wilde AAM, Charafeddine F, et al. 50 Years of catecholaminergic polymorphic ventricular tachycardia (CPVT) – time to explore the dark side of the moon. Heart Lung Circ 2020;29(4):520–8.
11. Miyake CY, Webster G, Czosek RJ, et al. Efficacy of implantable cardioverter defibrillators in young patients with catecholaminergic polymorphic ventricular tachycardia: success depends on substrate. Circ Arrhythm Electrophysiol 2013;6(3):579–87.
12. Fagundes A, De Magalhaes LP, Russo M, et al. Pharmacological treatment of electrical storm in cathecolaminergic polymorphic ventricular tachycardia. Pacing Clin Electrophysiol 2010;33(3):e27–31.
13. O'Hare M, Maldonado Y, Munro J, et al. Perioperative management of patients with congenital or acquired disorders of the QT interval. Br J Anaesth 2018; 120(4):629–44.

14. Dendramis G, Brugada P. Intensive care and anesthetic management of patients with Brugada syndrome and COVID-19 infection. Pacing Clin Electrophysiol 2020;43(10):1184–9.
15. Virani SS, Alonso A, Benjamin EJ, et al. Heart disease and stroke statistics—2020 update: a report from the american heart association. Circulation 2020;141(9). https://doi.org/10.1161/CIR.0000000000000757.
16. Stiles MK, Wilde AAM, Abrams DJ, et al. 2020 APHRS/HRS expert consensus statement on the investigation of decedents with sudden unexplained death and patients with sudden cardiac arrest, and of their families. Heart Rhythm 2021;18(1):e1–50.

Undiagnosed and Rare Diseases in Critical Care
Severe Mucocutaneous Medication Reactions

Bridget E. Shields, MD[a],*, Karolyn A. Wanat, MD[b,c],
Yvonne E. Chiu, MD[b,d]

KEYWORDS

- Drug reaction with eosinophilia and systemic symptoms (DRESS)
- Drug-induced hypersensitivity syndrome (DIHS) • Stevens-Johnson syndrome (SJS)
- Toxic-epidermal necrolysis (TEN)
- Reactive infectious mucocutaneus eruption (RIME)
- Methotrexate-induced epidermal necrosis (MEN)

KEY POINTS

- Severe cutaneous adverse reactions (SCARs) result in significant patient morbidity and mortality.
- Early recognition of SCARs coupled with rapid culprit medication withdrawal can improve patient outcomes significantly.
- Despite similar clinical presentations across SCARs, distinct clinical and histologic features allow for distinction between entities as well as targeted management.

DRUG REACTION WITH EOSINOPHILIA AND SYSTEMIC SYMPTOMS/DRUG-INDUCED HYPERSENSITIVITY SYNDROME

Drug reaction with eosinophilia and systemic symptoms (DRESS), also referred to as drug-induced hypersensitivity syndrome, is a severe and potentially life-threatening medication hypersensitivity reaction. The overall population risk has been estimated at between 1 in 1000 to 10,000 drug exposures.[1,2] The proposed pathogenesis of DRESS includes genetic predisposition (pathogenic variants in specific HLA alleles or in genes encoding drug detoxification enzymes),[1,3,4] accumulation of drug metabolites,[3] and reactivation of viral infections.[4] A risk factor for the development of DRESS

[a] Department of Dermatology, University of Wisconsin, 1 South Park Street, Madison, WI 53703, USA; [b] Department of Dermatology, Medical College of Wisconsin, 8701 Watertown Plank Road, Milwaukee, WI 53226, USA; [c] Department of Pathology, Medical College of Wisconsin, 8701 Watertown Plank Road, Milwaukee, WI 53226, USA; [d] Department of Pediatrics, Medical College of Wisconsin, 8701 Watertown Plank Road, Milwaukee, WI 53226, USA
* Corresponding author.
E-mail address: bshields@dermatology.wisc.edu

Crit Care Clin 38 (2022) 243–269
https://doi.org/10.1016/j.ccc.2021.11.003
0749-0704/22/© 2021 Elsevier Inc. All rights reserved.
criticalcare.theclinics.com

is immunosuppression, specifically, decreased total B-lymphocyte counts and serum immunoglobulin levels at onset,[5] which may explain the frequent reactivation of herpesvirus infections in DRESS.[4] Human herpesvirus (HHV)-6, HHV-7, cytomegalovirus, and Epstein-Barr virus reactivation have been identified in many patients with DRESS with a proposed similar mechanism to that seen in viral reactivation of graft-versus-host disease (GVHD).[6,7] Prior studies have identified HHV-6 DNA (via polymerase chain reaction [PCR]) and mRNA (via in situ hybridization) in lesional skin of DRESS patients.[2,8]

Many medications have been implicated in the development of DRESS, most commonly anticonvulsant medications (specifically, aromatic antiepileptics), allopurinol, antimicrobial sulfonamides or dapsone, and other antibiotics (**Table 1**).[9] DRESS

Table 1
Medications frequently associated with drug reaction with eosinophilia and systemic symptoms/drug-induced hypersensitivity syndrome[4,9]

Anticonvulsants	Carbamazepine
	Lamotrigine
	Oxcarbazepine
	Phenobarbital
	Phenytoin
	Valproic acid
	Zonisamide
Antibiotics	Amoxicillin
	Ampicillin
	Cefotaxime
	Daptomycin
	Ethambutol
	Isoniazid
	Linezolid
	Metronidazole
	Minocycline
	Pyrazinamide
	Quinine
	Rifampin
	Streptomycin
	Vancomycin
Antivirals	Abacavir
	Nevirapine
	Zalcitabine
Antidepressants	Bupropion
	Fluoxetine
Antihypertensives	Amlodipine
	Captopril
Biologics	Efalizumab
	Imatinib
Sulfonamides	Dapsone
	Sulfadiazine
	Trimethoprim/sulfamethoxazole
	Sulfasalazine
Other	Allopurinol
	Celecoxib
	Ibuprofen
	Mexiletine
	Ranitidine
	Erythropoietin alfa

usually occurs 2 weeks to 6 weeks after initial medication exposure; however, symptoms may develop more rapidly upon re-exposure.[1,4] DRESS occurs in both adult and pediatric patients, and patients often have a febrile prodrome lasting days prior to development of the cutaneous eruption. Skin lesions may be pruritic and typically involve the face, neck, and upper extremities before generalizing. The cutaneous exanthem is classically morbilliform but can exhibit numerous morphologies, including pustules, vesicles, bullae, purpura, and targetoid lesions.[4,10] With time, the eruption evolves from pink to violaceous or purpuric erythema before desquamating.[4] Significant facial edema frequently is noted and is best observed in the periorbital and midfacial regions. Patients typically exhibit associated systemic symptoms, including fever, lymphadenopathy, and hematologic abnormalities. Multiorgan system involvement can occur and affects the pulmonary, renal, cardiac, gastrointestinal, neurologic, and endocrine systems. Some medications have been associated with a higher risk of specific internal organ involvement (**Table 2**).[4] Peripheral eosinophilia is thought to drive systemic manifestations because eosinophil granule proteins are toxic to many tissues.[1]

Anicteric hepatitis is common in DRESS and may present with hepatosplenomegaly. Studies have reported between 70% and 90% of patients exhibit elevated alanine aminotransferase.[10,11] Liver enzymes may remain elevated even after the culprit medication has been withdrawn, and normalization may lag behind other laboratory test results. Hepatic necrosis is the most common cause of mortality in DRESS and can result in coagulopathy, liver failure, and sepsis.[4]

Renal involvement in DRESS typically presents with proteinuria and hematuria as well as elevated creatinine and blood urea nitrogen levels. It is seen most frequently in those patients with preexisting kidney disease and in elderly patients.[12] Although most patients recover quickly with withdrawal of the offending medication, renal failure may result in rare cases of interstitial nephritis development. There is no current evidence to suggest that more aggressive systemic therapy prevents risk of development of interstitial nephritis.

Pulmonary manifestations of DRESS may include acute interstitial pneumonitis, lymphocytic interstitial pneumonia, pleuritis, and acute respiratory distress syndrome (ARDS).[11] The most commonly identified symptoms are shortness of breath and nonproductive cough.[4]

Myocarditis has been associated with DRESS and may present later in the disease course, sometimes months after the offending medication has been withdrawn.[13] Hypersensitivity myocarditis and acute necrotizing eosinophilic myocarditis (ANEM) have been described. Patients may present with dyspnea, tachycardia, chest pain, or hypotension, and electrocardiogram may reveal arrythmias, sinus tachycardia, conduction

Table 2
Medications with specific internal organ risk in drug reaction with eosinophilia and systemic symptoms/drug-induced hypersensitivity syndromes[4]

Medication	Organ System Involved
Allopurinol	Renal
Ampicillin	Cardiac
Carbamazepine	Renal
Dapsone	Hepatic and renal
Minocycline	Hepatic, pulmonary, cardiac
Phenytoin	Hepatic

delays, ST segment, or T-wave changes.[12] Decreased ejection fraction may be noted on echocardiogram, and cardiac enzymes (creatinine kinase and troponin I) may be elevated.[12] ANEM is associated with high mortality and is identified by echocardiography that reveals decompensated systolic function, biventricular cardiac failure, and pericardial effusion.[12,13]

DRESS has been associated with hemophagocytic syndrome (HLH), which should be suspected a few weeks after the onset of the cutaneous eruption. Presentation is associated classically with fever, jaundice, hepatosplenomegaly, and a hyperinflamed state on laboratory evaluation.[12]

Uncommonly, neurologic manifestations, such as delayed-onset encephalitis and meningitis, have been reported in patients with DRESS.[12] Symptoms at presentation have included muscle weakness, distorted speech, headache, seizure, or coma.[12] Similarly, gastroenteritis resulting in chronic enteropathy can occur in patients with DRESS.[4,12] Endocrine abnormalities often occur after recovery from the acute event and in a delayed fashion. Most commonly, the thyroid is affected, and chronic complications may include thyroiditis or sick euthyroid syndrome.[3] Antithyroid antibodies have been detected up to 1 year after resolution of acute DRESS syndrome.[4] For this reason, thyroid function screening is recommended for 2 years in patients who have suffered from DRESS syndrome.[3] Pancreatitis and type 1 diabetes mellitus also have been identified in patients with DRESS.

Currently, no consistently reproducible diagnostic criteria exist to make the diagnosis of DRESS. The European Registry of Severe Cutaneous Adverse Reaction (EuroSCAR) validation criteria and the Japanese Research Committee on Severe Cutaneous Adverse Reaction criteria have been proposed.[14] The histopathologic features in DRESS are nonspecific but most commonly described as a perivascular lymphocytic infiltrate in the papillary dermis with extravasated erythrocytes and eosinophils.[1,3,4,15] Atypical lymphocytes also may be seen.[4,15]

Treatment of DRESS includes immediate removal of the culprit medication and initiation of systemic corticosteroids.[16] Early recognition and administration of systemic corticosteroid therapy at a minimum dose of 1.0 mg/kg/d prednisone equivalent are recommended.[16] In patients who are unresponsive to or intolerant of oral corticosteroids, intravenous methylprednisolone may be used in pulsed fashion at 30 mg/kg, intravenous administration, for 3 days.[17] Slow corticosteroid taper over 3 months to 6 months often is required to prevent disease recurrence. Cyclosporine A (CsA) has been used successfully as a steroid-sparing agent to treat DRESS syndrome.[18] Although intravenous immunoglobulin (IVIG) at 1 g/kg for 2 days has been reported in the treatment of DRESS,[19,20] larger studies have found IVIG monotherapy to be insufficient in most cases.[21] Supportive therapies often are implemented and include fluid resuscitation, electrolyte stabilization, external temperature regulation, calorie replacement, and appropriate topical corticosteroids.[16] Patients may require care in an intensive care or burn unit setting, especially if they manifest significant exfoliative dermatitis.[16] The use of empiric antibiotics or anti-inflammatory therapies is not recommended routinely and actually may worsen DRESS in certain patients.[17] Organ-specific laboratory testing and imaging should be used to drive appropriate consultation from multidisciplinary specialists. **Fig. 1** proposes an algorithm for diagnosis, management, and treatment of DRESS syndrome, as described by Husain and colleagues.[16]

The differential diagnosis for DRESS is broad and can include exanthematous/morbilliform medication eruption, viral exanthem, erythema multiforme (EM), leukemia cutis, GVHD, and Stevens-Johnson syndrome (SJS) or toxic epidermal necrolysis (TEN). Mononucleosis may be considered due to clinical lymphadenopathy and/or

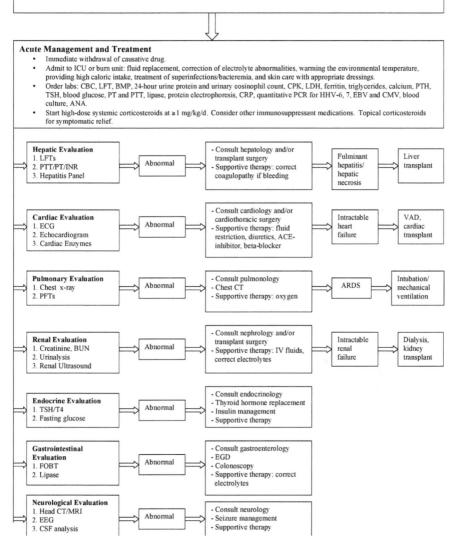

Fig. 1. Proposed evaluation and management of DRESS syndrome. ANA, anti-nuclear antibody; ARDS, acute respiratory distress syndrome; BMP, basic metabolic panel; BUN, blood urea nitrogen; CBC, complete blood count; CMV, cytomegalovirus; CPK, creatine phosphokinase; CRP, C-reactive protein; CSF, cerebrospinal fluid; CT, computed tomography; EBV, Epstein-Barr virus; ECG, electrocardiogram; EEG, electroencephalogram; EGD, esophagoduodenoscopy; FOBT, fecal occult blood test; ICU, intensive care unit; INR, international normalized ratio; J-SCAR, Japanese Research Committee on Severe Cutaneous Adverse Reaction; LDH, lactate dehydrogenase; LFT, liver function test; MRI, magnetic resonance imaging; PFT, pulmonary function test; PT, prothrombin time; PTT, partial thromboplastin time; T4, thyroxine; TSH, thyroid stimulating hormone; VAD, ventricular assist device. (*From* Husain Z, Reddy BY, Schwartz RA. DRESS syndrome: Part II. Management and therapeutics. J Am Acad Dermatol. 2013;68(5):709.e1-720. https://doi.org/10.1016/j.jaad.2013.01.032; with permission)

the presence of atypical lymphocytes on complete blood counts. DRESS should be considered an emergency, and assessment for internal organ involvement is of utmost importance. Management with consultative physicians, early supportive care, and initiation of pharmacologic therapy may decrease morbidity and mortality. Medications causative of DRESS should be placed on allergy lists, because re-exposure and rechallenge are contraindicated.

STEVENS-JOHNSON SYNDROME/TOXIC EPIDERMAL NECROLYSIS

SJS and TEN are life-threatening adverse cutaneous medication reactions associated with mortality rates as high as 30%.[22–24] SJS and TEN are reported to affect 1.6 to 9.2 patients per million annually in the United States.[25] SJS and TEN are characterized clinically by widespread mucocutaneous desquamation with full-thickness epidermal necrosis on histology.[26] SJS/TEN exist on a spectrum and are characterized by extent of epidermal detachment when disease is at its worst. Epidermal detachment of less than 10% body surface area (BSA) is seen in SJS, whereas between 10% and 30% BSA characterizes SJS/TEN overlap, and epidermal loss above 30% BSA a defines TEN.[27]

SJS/TEN can affect persons of all ages and occurs with increased incidence in adult patients with human immunodeficiency virus, malignancy, immunosuppression, and autoimmune disease.[26] SJS/TEN is triggered by a medication in upwards of 95% of cases[26]; however, infectious etiologies and idiopathic disease are described.[28] Some reported cases of infection-triggered SJS/TEN may be better classified as reactive infectious mucocutaneous eruption (RIME), discussed later. SJS/TEN usually occurs between 1 week and 8 weeks of medication ingestion with an average time to onset of 1 week to 2 weeks.[26] Previous exposure to a culprit medication can result in the more rapid onset of symptoms upon re-exposure. SJS/TEN can occur as the result of a dose adjustment or a change in medication formulation.

The exact pathogenesis of SJS/TEN remains unknown, but it is thought to be a hypersensitivity reaction that leads to CD8$^+$ cytotoxic T-cell–mediated apoptosis of keratinocytes facilitated by Fas ligand (FasL), tumor necrosis factor (TNF)-α, granulysin, perforin/granzyme B, and nitric oxide.[26] Major histocompatibility complex class I allotype may predispose specific populations to the development of SJS/TEN upon medication exposure as well as play an important role in disease pathogenesis.[26] Increased risk of SJS/TEN has been associated with HLA-A29, HLA-B12, and HLA-DR7 and exposure to sulfonamide[29]; HLA-A2, HLA-B12 with oxicam-type nonsteroidal anti-inflammatory drugs (NSAIDs)[29]; HLA-A*3101 and HLA-B*1502 with carbamazepine; HLA-B*5801 with allopurinol; and HLA-B*5701 with abacavir, among others.[26] This has led to routine HLA testing performed in patients of East Asian descent prior to carbamazepine initiation and in all patients before beginning abacavir.[26]

The most common causative agents of SJS/TEN include antiretrovirals, antiepileptic agents, sulfonamides, NSAIDs, and antibiotics, as outlined in **Table 3**.[23,26,30] In the largest retrospective chart review to date, the most common medication cause of SJS/TEN was trimethoprim/sulfamethoxazole.[31] The algorithm of drug causality for epidermal necrolysis (ALDEN) was developed from cases enrolled in the EuroSCAR, and it may be used as an objective scoring tool that allows for causality assessment in select cases.[32]

SJS/TEN typically begins with a prodromal fever, rhinorrhea, malaise, headache, and anorexia.[26] A morbilliform eruption may precede mucocutaneous sloughing and often is characterized by atypical targetoid macules that are dusky and nonblanching.[26] During the acute phase, flaccid bullae, erosions, and painful epidermal

Table 3
Medications causing drug-induced Stevens-Johnson syndrome/toxic epidermal necrolysis[23,26,29–31]

Medication Class	Medication
Antibiotics	Aminopenicillins
	β-Lactams
	Fluoroquinolones
	Sulfonamides
	Tetracyclines
	Trimethoprim/sulfamethoxazole
Anticonvulsants	Carbamazepine
	Lamotrigine
	Phenobarbital
	Phenytoin
Anti-inflammatories	NSAIDs
	Sulfasalazine
Antivirals	Abacavir
	Nevirapine
Other	Allopurinol
	Acetaminophen

denudation may result in sheets of wet cigar paper–like tissue loss.[26,33] Nikolsky and Asboe-Hansen signs are characteristically positive.[26] The process usually develops rapidly over 24 hours to 48 hours but also may evolve slowly over 2 weeks.[33] At least 2 mucosal surfaces are involved, and pharyngitis, dysphagia, photophobia, or dysuria may be reported early in the disease course. Appropriate subspecialists should be consulted for oral, ocular, and genital involvement to limit tissue damage and prevent scarring. SJS/TEN may result in acute, multiorgan system damage involving the kidneys, liver, lungs, and hematopoietic system.[26]

A diagnosis of SJS/TEN is made through clinical and histologic findings. Characteristic histopathology includes a subepidermal split with full-thickness epidermal necrosis, lymphocytic inflammation at the dermoepidermal junction, and CD8$^+$ T cells in the epidermis.[26] Endothelial apoptosis and CD4$^+$ T cells invariably are present in the dermis.[26,34] Frozen sections can be used to rapidly ascertain a diagnosis of SJS/TEN and reveal full-thickness epidermal necrosis. Although serum markers, such as FasL, perforin/granzyme B, granulysin, and soluble CD40 ligand, have been studied to assist in diagnosing SJS/TEN, larger studies are needed to clarify the utility of these assays.[26,34]

Because SJS/TEN portends significant morbidity and mortality, a series of tools for prognostic prediction has been developed. The Severity of Illness Score for Toxic Epidermal Necrolysis (SCORTEN) is the most broadly used prognostic tool and is outlined in **Table 4**.[26] Each prognostic factor is given a score of 1, and the number of positive criteria corresponds to mortality rates (0–1: 3.2%; 2: 12.1%; 3: 35.3%; 4: 58.3%; or 5 or greater: 90.0%).[27] The SCORTEN should be calculated on day 1 of hospitalization to maximize utility[26,34]; unfortunately, reports of overestimation and underestimation of SJS/TEN-related in-hospital mortality exist.[35,36] The ABCD-10 recently has been proposed as a novel mortality prediction model that utilizes age at admission (≥50 years) (1 point), epidermal detachment (>10% BSA) (1 point), serum bicarbonate (<20 mmol/L) (1 point), active malignancy (2 points), and dialysis (3 points) to predict

Table 4
Severity of illness score for toxic epidermal necrolysis[27]

Independent Prognostic Factors	Weight
Age (y) ≥40	1
Presence of malignancy (yes)	1
≥10% BSA detached	1
Tachycardia (≥120 bpm)	1
Serum bicarbonate (<20 mEq/L) (<20 mmol/L)	1
Serum glucose (>252 mg/dL) (>14 mmol/L)	1
Serum urea nitrogen (>28 mg/dL) (>10 mmol/L)	1

mortality.[35,36] Additional studies are needed to determine the generalizability of this new prognostic tool.

Treatment of SJS/TEN includes immediate discontinuation of the culprit medication, along with cessation of any non–life-sustaining medications.[34] Patients with SJS/TEN require significant supportive care, which should be completed in an intensive care setting or burn unit.[34] Attention should be focused on wound care, ocular care, oral care, urogenital care, fluid and electrolyte balance, airway management, stress ulcer prophylaxis, anticoagulation, and infection prevention and treatment.[25,34] There are no internationally accepted management guidelines for SJS/TEN. The Society of Dermatology Hospitalists recommends preservation of detached epidermis as a biologic dressing as well as limiting dressing changes, use of an air-fluidized bed, and nonadherent dressings (complete guidelines in **Table 5**).[25] Gentle cleansing with sterile water or dilute chlorhexidine may be completed with dressing changes followed by emollient application (petrolatum jelly is preferred) to minimize transcutaneous water loss and enhance barrier function.[25,37] Nonadherent, silver-impregnated dressings and absorptive dressings also can be considered.[25] Dressing changes should be completed with the assistance of oral and intravenous pain medication (ranging from acetaminophen to morphine or fentanyl).[25] Gabapentin and pregabalin have been used to limit opioid use and improve neuropathic pain.[38–40]

Fluid resuscitation with crystalloid is adapted from the care of burn patients and can be targeted to a urine output of 0.5 mL/kg/h to 1 mL/kg/h.[25,34,41,42] Evidence surrounding use of colloid fluids and albumin is lacking.[25] Patients with SJS/TEN have increased caloric needs, and ideal caloric intake should be between 30 kcal/kg and 35 kcal/kg.[43] Due to mucosal sloughing, a nasogastric tube may be required to provide enteral nutrition. Parenteral nutrition may be needed but has been associated with increased mortality,[44] as has hyperglycemia.[45] Complete recommendations are outlined in **Table 5**.

Pharmacologic therapies employed in the treatment of SJS/TEN include systemic corticosteroids, IVIG, CsA, TNF-α antagonists (with etanercept most supported by existing evidence), and traditional immunosuppressive medications.[46] There is a lack of randomized controlled trials (RCTs) to support the use of specific therapies; existing evidence is limited to retrospective observational studies. In a large retrospective cohort, more than 70% of patients received pharmacologic therapy versus supportive care alone (29.3%).[31] Most patients received corticosteroids (42.5%), IVIG (35.5%), or both (20.3%).[31] Stratified by therapy received, the standardized mortality ratio was lowest among those patients receiving both corticosteroids and IVIG.[31]

Re-epithelialization can take up to 4 weeks dependent on extent of initial cutaneous involvement.[47] Sepsis resulting in multiorgan failure has been reported as the most

Table 5
Society of Dermatology Hospitalists supportive care guidelines for the management of Stevens-Johnson syndrome and toxic epidermal necrosis in adults

Variable	Level of evidence[a]	Strength of recommendation[b]
Hospital setting and care team		
Management of patients with SJS/TEN requires a multidisciplinary team that may include dermatology, intensive care, pulmonology, ophthalmology, otorhinolaryngology, gynecology, urology, nephrology, plastic surgery, nutrition, nursing, psychology/psychiatry, and other fields.	4	D (GPP)
Dermatologists are experts in the disease state of SJS/TEN and should directly participate in the management of such patients.	4	D (GPP)
Staff should have specific training in the care of patients with SJS/TEN.	4	D (GPP)
Chronic conditions and comorbidities play a significant role in the mortality of patients with SJS/TEN and the need for specialized care, and hospital transfers should take into account these comorbidities.	3	C
Medical or burn intensive care unit settings of care for SJS/TEN patients are recommended.	2–/3	D
SJS/TEN patients must be cared for in a private room.	3	D
Patient rooms should be controlled for humidity.	4	D
Sterile sheets should be obtained and used for patient bedding, where available.	4	D
At least 1 nurse should take care of 1 patient with SJS/TEN (at least 1:1 ratio).	4	D
Wound care		
Determine % BSA of epidermal detachment (only skin that already is necrotic or detached or skin with positive Nikolsky sign).	3	D
Avoid unnecessary wound manipulation by limiting the number of dressing changes.	3	D
Use an air-fluidized bed to minimize friction.	3	D

(continued on next page)

Table 5
(continued)

Variable	Level of evidence[a]	Strength of recommendation[b]
Gently cleanse all areas with sterile water, normal saline, or dilute chlorhexidine (0.05%) solution with dressing changes.	4	D
The detached and detachable epidermis should be left in place as a biologic dressing.	4	D (GPP)
Lyse large or painful bullae for comfort only.	4	D (GPP)
Wound débridement of necrotic skin is not recommended.	4	D (GPP)
Apply topical emollients, such as petroleum jelly, on the entire epidermis.	3	D
Apply nonadherent sterile dressings to denuded skin.	3	D
Select nonadherent silver-impregnated primary dressings for optimal moisture retention and antibacterial properties.	2+/3	D
Apply secondary dressing to absorb exudate.	3	D
Ocular care		
Patients thought to have SJS/TEN should be examined by an ophthalmologist as part of the initial assessment.	4	D (GPP)
Patients should be examined at least every 24 h until it is clear there is no worsening, and, thereafter, the frequency of follow-up should be determined on a case-by case basis.	4	D (GPP)
Educate the appropriate staff regarding the need for immediate ophthalmologic evaluation of all SJS/TEN patients and the proper application of topical ocular medications (drops and ointments).	4	D (GPP)
The entire ocular surface—eyelid skin, eyelid margin, conjunctiva, and cornea—should be examined daily. The eyelids should be everted, and the eyes rotated to look for forniceal and tarsal conjunctival epithelial defects and early symblephara.	4	D (GPP)
Fluorescein staining should be done in all patients.	4	D
Resting eyelid position should be assessed for lagophthalmos.	4	D
Grade the ocular examination findings to facilitate medical decision making.	3	D

Recommendation		
Consider AMT during the initial evaluation of any patient thought to have SJS/TEN and at each follow-up examination during the acute phase.	1+/2+	B
Offer AMT to patients with moderate to severe conjunctival injection, significant conjunctival epithelial defects (especially the eyelid margin, tarsal conjunctiva, and fornices), significant corneal epithelial defects, or membranes or pseudomembranes.	1+/2+	B
AMT ideally is performed within 5 d of onset but may be offered later.	1+/2+	B
Amniotic membrane should cover the entire ocular surface.	1+/2+	B
Apply artificial tears every 1–2 h for any patient with any ocular surface inflammation.	4	D
Apply ophthalmic ointment to the eyelid margin every 2–24 h.	4	D
Eye drops containing preservatives should be avoided.	4	D
Apply a moisture chamber over the eyes for lagophthalmos. A facemask or moist occlusive dressing may be used for this purpose.	4	D
Rinse the eyes every 2–24 h with sterile saline.	4	D
Remove/lyse adherent debris and membranes daily.	4	D
Apply a topical anesthetic (eg, proparacaine or tetracaine) if needed.	4	D
Apply a corticosteroid-containing ointment to the eyelid margin and eyelashes at least once daily and a corticosteroid drop to the ocular surface at least twice daily for any patient with any ocular surface inflammation.	2–	D
If there is clinical suspicion of infectious conjunctivitis, obtain a bacterial (and consider a fungal) culture of the ocular surface and begin application of a topical broad-spectrum antibiotic (fourth-generation quinolone commonly used).	4	D
Avoid chloramphenicol drops and tetracycline-containing ointment because these have been associated with late complications, in particular dry eyes.	3	D
The mouth should be examined as part of the initial assessment of a patient with SJS/TEN.	4	D (GPP)
Daily oral examination is required during acute illness.	4	D (GPP)

(continued on next page)

Table 5
(continued)

Variable	Level of evidence[a]	Strength of recommendation[b]
Have a low threshold for HSV PCR, bacterial, and fungal cultures if infection is suspected.	4	D (GPP)
Petrolatum ointment should be applied on the lips immediately and then every 2 h throughout the acute illness.	3	D
Viscous lidocaine 2%, 15 mL per application, can be used every 3 h (and before cleanses) as an oral rinse to control pain.	3	D
Clean the mouth daily with warm saline mouthwashes or an oral sponge, sweeping the sponge gently in the labial and buccal sulci to reduce the risk of fibrotic scars and prevent buildup of hemorrhagic crust.	3	D
An antiseptic oral rinse should be used twice daily to reduce bacterial colonization of the mucosa.	3	D
A topical steroid (ultrapotent) ointment can be applied up to 4 times a day during the acute phase.	3	D
Consider diluted chlorhexidine digluconate mouthwash (2–3 times daily).	3	D
Consider the use of oral coating agents for pain reduction in patients with oral mucosal involvement.	4	D
Examine the urogenital tract as part of the initial assessment of a patient with SJS/TEN.	4	D (GPP)
Urogenital examination ideally should be performed by a gynecologist, urologist, or urogynecology specialist.	4	D (GPP)
Daily examination is required during the acute illness.	4	D (GPP)
If there is clinical suspicion for vaginal candidiasis in the setting of vaginal steroid use, consider obtaining a KOH and fungal culture and beginning treatment with antifungal medications.	4	D (GPP)
During the acute phase of the disease, the vulvar/urogenital skin/mucosa should be coated with an ointment and/or ointment gauze to help reduce pain, reduce adhesion formation, and facilitate healing.	3	D

An intravaginal device, such as a dilator/tampon/vaginal mold/roll of gauze covered in a lubricated condom, can be used to treat vaginal disease.	3	D
Intravaginal devices may be left in place for no longer than 24 h, at which time they should be replaced.	3	D
Even for virginal patients, use of a small mold or a condom-covered tampon should be encouraged if the patient is emotionally and physically comfortable with the regimen.	4	D
Patients uncomfortable with using an intravaginal device can apply medication twice daily with a vaginal applicator.	4	D
Topical anesthetics (eg, lidocaine 5% ointment) can be used at the vaginal introitus, once open sores have healed, to reduce discomfort with use of the vaginal dilators.	3	D
It is at the provider's discretion to use either a nonsteroidal ointment (eg, petrolatum jelly) with reapplication as frequently as necessary (2–4 times daily) to maintain barrier protection and/or consider 1–2 times daily application of a high-potency steroid ointment if active inflammation is observed, with the caveat that consideration for tapering of steroid use should be based on clinical improvement.	3	D
Consider the medication on the dilator can be changed to, or alternated with, estrogen cream to help promote healing of the vaginal mucosa.	4	D
Consider menstrual suppression to reduce discomfort and possibly to decrease the risk of vaginal adenosis.	3	D
Consider division of any fine (vaginal) adhesions to prevent the development of thick fibrous bands that could lead to problems inserting tampons and during sexual intercourse later in life.	3	D
Consider urinary catheters to decrease pain with urination, prevent urinary obstruction, and monitor fluid balance.	3	D
Evaluation and treatment of pain are priorities in the acute phase, especially during wound management.	4	D (GPP)
Pain should be evaluated every 4 h.	4	D (GPP)

(continued on next page)

Table 5
(continued)

Variable	Level of evidence[a]	Strength of recommendation[b]
A validated pain tool should be used to assess pain in all conscious patients at least once a day.	4	D (GPP)
If the score is mild, pain control with acetaminophen should be introduced.	3	D
If acetaminophen is not enough, oral synthetic opiates, such as tramadol, should be considered.	3	D
If the pain score is moderate to severe, then morphine or fentanyl should be delivered enterally, by PCA, or by infusion.	3	D
Procedures, such as dressing changes and bathing, may require additional pain control.	3	D
Consider adding low-dose ketamine infusions.	3	D
Consider adding gabapentin or pregabalin.	3	D
NSAIDs should be avoided due to renal or gastric injury.	3	D
Hand hygiene and other infection control measures should be strictly applied.	3	D (GPP)
Patients should be monitored carefully for signs of systemic infection, such as confusion, hypotension, reduced urine output, and reduced oxygen saturation.	3	D
Cutaneous infection may be accompanied by increase in skin pain.	3	D
Consider activation of HSV in eroded or vesicular areas that are slow to heal, particularly in genital and oral sites. Take viral swabs if herpes virus infection is suspected.	3	D
In patients with diarrhea who are immobile, consider a fecal management system to prevent fecal soiling of wounds.	3	D
Prophylactic antibiotic treatment is not recommended.	4	D
Administer systemic antibiotics only if there are clinical signs of infection. The choice of systemic antibiotic should be guided by local microbiologic resistance patterns.	3	D

Severe ENT involvement is significantly associated with pulmonary infection. ENT evaluation using nasal fiberoptic endoscopy should be suggested when dysphonia or dyspnea is present.	3	D
Fluid and electrolyte management		
Peripheral catheters preferred for vascular access with implantation in uninjured skin and fixed with nonadhesive dressings.	3	D
Change peripheral venous cannulas every 48 h if possible.	3	D
Monitor electrolytes and fluid balance daily.	4	D (GPP)
Consider invasive fluid balance monitoring with Foley catheter.	3	D
Fluid administration should be titrated to urine output (0.5–1 mL/kg/h).	3	D
Nutrition and stress ulcer prophylaxis		
Maintain adequate nutrition orally; use a nasogastric tube if necessary. Enteral feeding reduces stress ulcers and reduces bacterial translocation and enterogenic infection.	3	D
Supplement enteral nutrition with parenteral if intake via the enteral route is insufficient to meet caloric needs.	3	D
Avoid nasogastric tube placement if there is involvement of the nasopharyngeal mucosa.	3	D
Deliver daily caloric requirement of 30–35 kcal/kg.	3	D
Maintain close glycemic control.	3	D (GPP)
In patients receiving enteral nutrition, pharmacologic stress ulcer prophylaxis is not recommended.	4	D (GPP)
Pharmacologic stress ulcer prophylaxis with PPIs should be limited to patients at high risk for clinically important bleeding (respiratory failure, coagulopathy, liver disease, use of renal replacement therapy, 3 or more coexisting diseases).	4	D (GPP)
PPIs should be used over H_2 receptor antagonists (due to decrease in gastrointestinal bleeding events).	4	D (GPP)
Airway management		

(continued on next page)

Table 5
(continued)

Variable	Level of evidence[a]	Strength of recommendation[b]
The nose should be examined as part of the initial assessment of a patient with SJS/TEN.	4	D (GPP)
Daily nasal examinations are required during acute illness.	4	D (GPP)
Pulmonary care includes normal saline aerosols, bronchial aspiration, and postural drainage by turning the patient to different sides.	4	D
Severe ENT involvement is significantly associated with pulmonary infection. ENT evaluation using nasal fiberoptic endoscopy should be suggested when dysphonia or dyspnea is present.	3/4	D
Chest x-ray imaging and arterial blood gases should be obtained upon admission for baseline respiratory function assessment.	3/4	D
Patients with ongoing respiratory symptoms should be monitored closely with pulmonary function testing and high-resolution computed tomography scanning.	3	D
Fiberoptic bronchoscopy should be undertaken in patients with respiratory symptoms and hypoxia.	3	D
Bronchoscopy should be done by an experienced technician due to risk of post-instrumental endobronchial bleeding.	3	D
Consider intubation and early tracheostomy in patients with oral involvement and 1 of the following:	3	D
• Initial BSA 70% or more		
• Progression of BSA involved from DOH 1 to DOH 3 of >15%		
• Underlying neurologic diagnosis prevents airway protection		
• Documented airway involvement on direct laryngoscopy		
Ventilation strategies should mimic ARDS management guidelines (low tidal volume and early prone positioning).	4	D
Anticoagulation		

Immobile patients should receive low-molecular-weight heparin.	4	D (GPP)
For acutely ill patients at increased risk of thrombosis who are bleeding or at high risk for major bleeding, mechanical thromboprophylaxis with graduated compression stockings or intermittent pneumatic compression is recommended.	4	D (GPP)

Abbreviations: AMT, amniotic membrane transplantation; DOH, day of hospitalization; ENT, ear-nose-throat; GPP, good practice point; HSV, herpes simplex virus; KOH, potassium hydroxide preparation; PCA, patient-controlled analgesia; PPI, proton pump inhibitor.

Level of evidence:

1++: high-quality meta-analyses, systematic reviews of RCTs or RCTs with a very low risk of bias.

1+: well-conducted meta-analyses, systematic reviews of RCTs or RCTs with a low risk of bias.

1−: meta-analyses, systematic reviews of RCTs or RCTs with a high risk of bias.

2++: high-quality systematic reviews of case-control or cohort studies. High-quality case-control or cohort studies with a very low risk of confounding or bias and a high probability that the relationship is causal.

2+: well-conducted case-control or cohort studies with a low risk of confounding or bias and a moderate probability that the relationship is causal.

2−: case-control or cohort studies with a high risk of confounding or bias and a significant risk that the relationship is not causal.

3: nonanalytical studies (eg, case reports or case series).

4: expert opinion, formal consensus.

Grade of recommendations

A: at least 1 meta-analysis, systematic review or RCT rated as 1++, and directly applicable to the target population, or a systematic review of RCTs or a body of evidence consisting principally of studies rated as 1+, directly applicable to the target population and demonstrating overall consistency of results.

B: a body of evidence, including studies rated as 2++, directly applicable to the target population and demonstrating overall consistency of results, or extrapolated evidence from studies rated as 1++ or 1+.

C: a body of evidence, including studies rated as 2+, directly applicable to the target population and demonstrating overall consistency of results, or extrapolated evidence from studies rated as 2++.

D: evidence level 3 or 4 or extrapolated evidence from studies rated as 2+ formal consensus.

A GPP is a recommendation for best practice based on the experience of the guideline development group.

From Seminario-Vidal L, Kroshinsky D, Malachowski SJ, et al. Society of Dermatology Hospitalists supportive care guidelines for the management of Stevens-Johnson syndrome/toxic epidermal necrolysis in adults. J Am Acad Dermatol. 2020;82(6):1553–1567. https://doi.org/10.1016/j.jaad.2020.02.066; with permission.

common cause of death in patients with SJS/TEN.[25,48–50] The empiric use of antibiotics currently is not recommended; instead, therapy should be tailored to skin cultures.[51,52] The most common organisms causing blood stream infections in patients with SJS/TEN include *Pseudomonas aeruginosa*, *Staphylococcus aureus*, and *Enterobacteriaceae*.[48] Regular monitoring for infection during re-epithelialization stages, including bacterial swabs of concerning areas, can guide management.

Because mucosal involvement is invariably present in SJS/TEN, regular assessment of mucosal surfaces, application of topical therapies to decrease pain and prevent adhesions, and consultation with medical subspecialists (including ophthalmologists, urologists, gynecologists, otolaryngologists, and gastroenterologists) should be considered. These recommendations are outlined in full in **Table 5**.[25] Early consultation and preventative management may decrease the development of long-term sequelae of SJS/TEN, which can include dyspigmentation, alopecia, abnormal nail growth, dental abnormalities, tongue dysmotility, gingival inflammation, sicca syndrome, chronic conjunctivitis, symblepharon, mucosal scarring, esophageal stricture, bronchiolitis obliterans, chronic bronchitis, bronchiectasis, chronic obstructive pulmonary disease, genital adhesions, dyspareunia, and stenosis.[53,54] Depression, posttraumatic stress syndrome, and anxiety all have been reported following SJS/TEN.[54]

REACTIVE INFECTIOUS MUCOCUTANEOUS ERUPTION

RIME is a recently described mucocutaneous entity previously classified as EM, SJS, or TEN. RIME can be triggered by *Mycoplasma pneumoniae* (*MP*), termed *MP-induced rash and mucositis*, or by other respiratory infections.[55,56] RIME is a condition predominantly affecting children and adolescents, and cases occur more commonly in male patients than female patients.[55] RIME is characterized by prominent mucositis, generally with lesser cutaneous involvement than is seen in SJS/TEN. When present, targetoid, atypical targetoid, vesiculobullous, or morbilliform lesions may be present initially and evolve to epidermal detachment.[57] Oral involvement can include erosions, ulcerations, vesiculobullous lesions, and mucosal denudation.[57] Ocular lesions have been characterized by conjunctivitis, photophobia, and eyelid edema.[57] Urogenital, anal, and oroesophageal mucositis also have been reported.[57] Prodromal symptoms often occur in RIME and may include fever, cough, and malaise preceding the eruption by approximately 1 week.[57]

RIME is a clinical diagnosis but PCR from sputum, nasopharyngeal aspirates, or oropharyngeal swabs can detect MP DNA early in infection.[58] MP antigen detection on enzyme immunoassay detects IgM between 7 days and 10 days of infection.[58] Chest radiograph may demonstrate consolidations or interstitial infiltrates consistent with pneumonia. Most patients with RIME require hospitalization, and those with extensive cutaneous involvement may require management in an intensive care setting.[57] Given the often extensive mucositis in RIME, fluid resuscitation, nutritional support, and pain control are key to management. Most patients receive antibiotics and systemic corticosteroids with or without IVIG.[57] The use of CsA,[59] etanercept,[60] and plasmapheresis to treat RIME has been reported.[61] Acute complications of RIME may include hematemesis, epiglottitis, pneumomediastinum, pericardial effusion, and hepatitis.[57] Although most patients make a complete recovery, long-term sequelae of RIME include mucosal scarring, dyspigmentation, anxiety, and posttraumatic stress disorder.[57] Up to 18% of RIME cases are recurrent, resulting in significant morbidity due to repeated hospitalizations.[55] Unfortunately, no evidence exists to support preventative treatment.[55]

In pediatric patients presenting with SJS-like mucositis, RIME should be considered in the differential diagnosis, especially when no clear medication trigger exists. The pathogenesis of RIME remains unelucidated, making the development of treatment algorithms challenging.

STEVENS-JOHNSON SYNDROME AND TOXIC EPIDERMAL NECROLYSIS–LIKE LUPUS ERYTHEMATOSUS

Lupus erythematosus (LE) is an autoimmune disease that is diagnosed through a constellation of clinical, serologic, and histologic criteria. SJS/TEN-like LE is a rare but life-threatening presentation of cutaneous LE.[62] Approximate prevalence for SJS/TEN-like LE is 7 out of 10,000 patients,[62] and data regarding this entity are limited to case reports and case series. SJS/TEN-like LE is characterized by large sheets of epidermal detachment that can be indistinguishable from classic SJS/TEN. Cutaneous lesions typically begin in a photo-distributed fashion and progress to red and dusky patches that evolve to frank bullae, erosions, and desquamation.[62] Rarely, patients can develop blistering and epidermal loss overlying prior lesions of cutaneous LE. SJS/TEN-like LE can either be the presenting sign of systemic LE (SLE) or can occur years after an initial SLE diagnosis.[62] It is thought that SJS/TEN-like LE is triggered by excess ultraviolet light exposure resulting in cytotoxic T lymphocyte activation and autoantibody-mediated degeneration of the basal epidermis.[63,64] On histology, variable degrees of epidermal necrosis, subepidermal blistering, and vacuolar degeneration may be seen.[62] Perivascular lymphocytic inflammation and periadnexal lymphocytic inflammation often are reported, and direct immunofluorescence may reveal multiple immunoglobulins deposited in a granular pattern along the dermoepidermal junction.[62]

In SJS/TEN-like LE, drug hypersensitivity and infectious etiologies should be excluded. Clarifying a medication timeline is critical to making the diagnosis. It was previously suggested that patients with SJS/TEN-like LE had less mucosal involvement than those with SJS/TEN; however, a recent case series noted that more than half of the SJS/TEN-like LE patients included had severe mucosal erosions.[62] Acral and distal extremity involvement seemed to be identified in a higher proportion of patients with SJS/TEN-like LE, a finding that is less common in medication-induced SJS/TEN.[62] Patients invariably meet European Alliance of Associations for Rheumatology criteria, generally with strongly positive immunologic profiles, confirming an underlying SLE diagnosis. Most patients diagnosed with SJS/TEN-like SLE exhibit markers of active disease at presentation, including elevated erythrocyte sedimentation rate, low complement levels, hematologic abnormalities, and renal involvement.[62]

Currently, no standardized treatment of SJS/TEN-like LE exists. Patients often require hospitalization in an intensive care setting, where systemic corticosteroids (often high-dose, pulsed therapy) in combination with steroid-sparing immunosuppressives (azathioprine, cyclophosphamide, and mycophenolate mofetil) have been used.[63] The use of IVIG and plasmapheresis also has been reported.[65,66] Supportive care, including fluid resuscitation, barrier protection, and infection control, is recommended, because sepsis remains a risk in these patients.[62] SJS/TEN-like LE typically follows a disease course similar to that of SJS/TEN with delayed re-epithelialization (average of 11 days) after therapy initiation.[62] SJS/TEN-like LE should be considered in patients presenting with epidermal necrosis in the absence of clear medication or infectious trigger.

METHOTREXATE-INDUCED EPIDERMAL NECROSIS

Methotrexate (4-amino-10-methylfolic acid) (MTX) is a folic acid analog and antagonist used in the treatment of numerous inflammatory and malignant processes.[67,68] MTX is first-line treatment of rheumatoid arthritis, juvenile idiopathic arthritis, psoriatic arthritis, and psoriasis.[67,69] MTX-induced epidermal necrosis (MEN) is a rare cutaneous reaction that mimics SJS or TEN.[69] MEN is thought to be the result of direct drug toxicity to keratinocytes without an increase in inflammatory cytokines, as is seen in SJS/TEN.[69] MEN presents with severe and widespread epidermal detachment and mucosal erosions, resulting in significant morbidity and mortality.[69] Age greater than 60 years has been associated with increased odds of the development of MEN,[69] as have high initial doses (>10 mg per week) of MTX, chronic kidney disease (irreversible eGFR <60 mL/min), and delayed clearance of MTX.[69] MEN has been reported in pediatric patients receiving high-dose MTX for malignancy.[70,71]

Patients with MEN initially present with painful cutaneous erosions and mucosal ulcerations.[69] They often fail to exhibit the targetoid lesions that can be seen in SJS/TEN.[69] In a single controlled study of 24 patients with MEN, patients exhibited between 8% and 80% total body epidermal detachment.[69] On histopathology, MEN often exhibits an atrophic epidermis with dyskeratotic keratinocytes and vacuolar change, epidermal necrosis, and epidermal atypia, the latter distinguishing it from SJS/TEN.[69] A subset of patients who develop MEN also develop leukopenia and thrombocytopenia.[69] There are no current criteria to predict disease severity; however, poor prognostic indicators include severe renal disease and leukopenia.[69]

Treatment of MEN historically has been with leucovorin and granulocyte colony-stimulating factor.[69] Premedication with systemic corticosteroids, followed by folinic acid post-MTX infusion, has been described in pediatric patients.[70] Supportive care, including fluid resuscitation, infection prevention, and skin-directed therapies, is similar to that used in SJS/TEN. MEN should be considered in patients initiating MTX, especially at high doses and with potential for delayed drug clearance (due to decreased renal function or other medication interactions). Histopathology typically can distinguish SJS/TEN-like LE from SJS/TEN by dyskeratotic keratinocytes, vacuolar change, and epidermal atypia. Treatment of MEN should be in an intensive care setting with a focus on supportive care and leucovorin.

STEVENS-JOHNSON SYNDROME AND TOXIC EPIDERMAL NECROLYSIS–LIKE GRAFT-VERSUS-HOST DISEASE

GVHD develops when immunologically competent donor cells identify foreign antigens on recipient tissue, leading to attack of the host. GVHD occurs most frequently following allogeneic hematopoietic stem cell transplantation (HSCT); however, it can develop in the setting of solid organ transplantation, following transfusion of nonirradiated blood products into an immunocompromised host, or after autologous HSCT.[72] GVHD is a life-threatening immune response with mortality approaching 15%.[73] Cutaneous GVHD often is the earliest manifestation of disease and typically presents as a diffuse, morbilliform eruption with variable amounts of pruritus. Monomorphic, pink to dusky violaceous macules with fine overlying scale may be present and identifiable on acral sites, ears, neck, upper back, and scalp with a predilection for hair follicles. Mucosal ulcerations and erosions commonly are present.

GVHD is graded by cutaneous, hepatic, and gastrointestinal involvement and is staged by clinical and histologic severity (stage 1 involving <25% BSA, stage 2 involving 25% to 50% BSA, stage 3 involving greater than 50% BSA with generalized erythroderma, and stage 4 with generalized erythroderma with bullae and desquamation).[74] Stage 4 GVHD is associated with poor prognosis and high mortality[75] and can be exceedingly challenging to distinguish from SJS/TEN when extensive mucosal involvement is present.[76] Histologic overlap exists between TEN and GVHD, with both conditions exhibiting epidermal necrosis, subepidermal blistering, and pauci-inflammatory dermal infiltrate.[75] When present, vacuolar degeneration of basal keratinocytes and follicular involvement are supportive of GVHD.[75] In both conditions, a predominance of cytotoxic CD8[+] T lymphocytes are present.[75]

Treatment of GVHD is dependent on number and severity of organ systems involved and includes initial adjustment of preventative immunosuppressive therapies. Limited cutaneous disease may be treated with topical corticosteroids and calcineurin inhibitors. Oral corticosteroids are first-line therapy for more extensive cutaneous or multiorgan system disease.[72] There is no consensus on optimal corticosteroid dosing. Trials have evaluated high-dose and low-dose intravenous 6-methylprednisolone (10 mg/kg/d and 2 mg/kg/d, respectively) with comparable improvement in acute GVHD and relapse rates following therapy.[77] In less severe acute GVHD, lower doses of prednisone equivalent (1 mg/kg/d) have shown similar nonrelapse mortality and overall survival.[78] In patients with limited response to oral corticosteroids, a variety of second-line agents have been used and include mycophenolate mofetil, MTX, mammalian target of rapamycin inhibitors, Janus kinase inhibitors, rituximab, phototherapy, and extracorporeal photopheresis, among others.[72] No consensus exists on which therapies provide superior outcomes. Supportive care in an intensive care setting should include wound care, fluid resuscitation, and infection prevention.

DISCUSSION

Although many severe cutaneous adverse reactions (SCARs) may present similarly, physicians should be able to recognize SCARs and their mimicking conditions. Understanding disease time course and likely causative medications allows for rapid medication withdrawal and the initiation of early supportive care. Differences in clinical presentation, histopathologic findings, serologies, and long-term sequelae can ensure appropriate consultations and future monitoring.

CLINICS CARE POINTS

- DRESS occurs 2 weeks to 6 weeks after initial medication exposure; however, features may develop more rapidly upon medication re-exposure.
- Multiorgan system involvement can occur with DRESS and affects the pulmonary, renal, cardiac, gastrointestinal, neurologic, and endocrine systems.
- Treatment of DRESS includes removal of the culprit medication and initiation of systemic corticosteroids at a minimum dose of 1 mg/kg/d prednisone equivalent.
- SJS and TEN exist on a spectrum and are characterized by extent of epidermal detachment when disease is at its worst.
- Treatment of SJS/TEN includes immediate discontinuation of the culprit medication and cessation of non–life-sustaining medications.
- Patients with SJS/TEN require significant supportive care, which should be completed in an intensive care setting or burn unit.
- SJS/TEN mimics include RIME, SJS/TEN-like LE, MEN, and GVHD, and these diagnoses should be considered in any patient presenting with extensive mucocutaneous denudation.

DISCLOSURE

The authors have nothing to disclose.

REFERENCES

1. Bocquet H, Bagot M, Roujeau JC. Drug-induced pseudolymphoma and drug hypersensitivity syndrome (drug rash with eosinophilia and systemic symptoms: dress). Semin Cutan Med Surg 1996;15(4):250–7. https://doi.org/10.1016/s1085-5629(96)80038-1.

2. Chiou CC, Yang LC, Hung SI, et al. Clinicopathological features and prognosis of drug rash with eosinophilia and systemic symptoms: a study of 30 cases in Taiwan. J Eur Acad Dermatol Venereol 2008;22(9):1044–9. https://doi.org/10.1111/j.1468-3083.2008.02585.x.

3. Tas S, Simonart T. Drug rash with eosinophilia and systemic symptoms (DRESS syndrome). Acta Clin Belg 1999;54(4):197–200.

4. Husain Z, Reddy BY, Schwartz RA. DRESS syndrome: part I. Clinical perspectives. J Am Acad Dermatol 2013;68(5):693.e1–14. https://doi.org/10.1016/j.jaad.2013.01.033 [quiz 706–8].

5. Hirahara K, Kano Y, Mitsuyama Y, et al. Differences in immunological alterations and underlying viral infections in two well-defined severe drug eruptions. Clin Exp Dermatol 2010;35(8):863–8. https://doi.org/10.1111/j.1365-2230.2010.03820.x.

6. Natkunarajah J, Watson K, Diaz-Cano S, et al. Drug rash with eosinophilia and systemic symptoms and graft-versus-host disease developing sequentially in a patient. Clin Exp Dermatol 2009;34(2):199–201. https://doi.org/10.1111/j.1365-2230.2008.02823.x.

7. Kano Y, Hiraharas K, Sakuma K, et al. Several herpesviruses can reactivate in a severe drug-induced multiorgan reaction in the same sequential order as in graft-versus-host disease. Br J Dermatol 2006;155(2):301–6. https://doi.org/10.1111/j.1365-2133.2006.07238.x.

8. Fernando SL, Henderson CJ, O'Connor KS. Drug-induced hypersensitivity syndrome with superficial granulomatous dermatitis–a novel finding. Am J Dermatopathol 2009;31(6):611–3. https://doi.org/10.1097/DAD.0b013e3181a18d64.

9. Kardaun SH, Sekula P, Valeyrie-Allanore L, et al. Drug reaction with eosinophilia and systemic symptoms (DRESS): an original multisystem adverse drug reaction. Results from the prospective RegiSCAR study. Br J Dermatol 2013;169(5):1071–80. https://doi.org/10.1111/bjd.12501.

10. Ang CC, Wang YS, Yoosuff EL, et al. Retrospective analysis of drug-induced hypersensitivity syndrome: a study of 27 patients. J Am Acad Dermatol 2010;63(2):219–27. https://doi.org/10.1016/j.jaad.2009.08.050.

11. Kano Y, Shiohara T. The variable clinical picture of drug-induced hypersensitivity syndrome/drug rash with eosinophilia and systemic symptoms in relation to the eliciting drug. Immunol Allergy Clin North Am 2009;29(3):481–501. https://doi.org/10.1016/j.iac.2009.04.007.

12. Kano Y, Ishida T, Hirahara K, et al. Visceral involvements and long-term sequelae in drug-induced hypersensitivity syndrome. Med Clin North Am 2010;94(4):743–59. https://doi.org/10.1016/j.mcna.2010.03.004, xi.

13. Bourgeois GP, Cafardi JA, Groysman V, et al. Fulminant myocarditis as a late sequela of DRESS: two cases. J Am Acad Dermatol 2011;65(4):889–90. https://doi.org/10.1016/j.jaad.2010.12.013.

14. Kardaun SH, Sidoroff A, Valeyrie-Allanore L, et al. Variability in the clinical pattern of cutaneous side-effects of drugs with systemic symptoms: does a DRESS syndrome really exist? Br J Dermatol 2007;156(3):609–11. https://doi.org/10.1111/j.1365-2133.2006.07704.x.

15. Roujeau JC. Clinical heterogeneity of drug hypersensitivity. Toxicology 2005; 209(2):123–9. https://doi.org/10.1016/j.tox.2004.12.022.
16. Husain Z, Reddy BY, Schwartz RA. DRESS syndrome: part II. Management and therapeutics. J Am Acad Dermatol 2013;68(5):709.e1–9. https://doi.org/10.1016/j.jaad.2013.01.032 [quiz 718–20].
17. Shiohara T, Inaoka M, Kano Y. Drug-induced hypersensitivity syndrome (DIHS): a reaction induced by a complex interplay among herpesviruses and antiviral and antidrug immune responses. Allergol Int 2006;55(1):1–8. https://doi.org/10.2332/allergolint.55.1.
18. Nguyen E, Yanes D, Imadojemu S, et al. Evaluation of cyclosporine for the treatment of DRESS syndrome. JAMA Dermatol 2020;156(6):704–6. https://doi.org/10.1001/jamadermatol.2020.0048.
19. Scheuerman O, Nofech-Moses Y, Rachmel A, et al. Successful treatment of antiepileptic drug hypersensitivity syndrome with intravenous immune globulin. Pediatrics 2001;107(1):E14. https://doi.org/10.1542/peds.107.1.e14.
20. Fields KS, Petersen MJ, Chiao E, et al. Case reports: treatment of nevirapine-associated dress syndrome with intravenous immune globulin (IVIG). J Drugs Dermatol 2005;4(4):510–3.
21. Joly P, Janela B, Tetart F, et al. Poor benefit/risk balance of intravenous immunoglobulins in DRESS. Arch Dermatol 2012;148(4):543–4. https://doi.org/10.1001/archderm.148.4.dlt120002-c.
22. Dodiuk-Gad RP, Chung WH, Valeyrie-Allanore L, et al. Stevens-Johnson syndrome and toxic epidermal necrolysis: an update. Am J Clin Dermatol 2015; 16(6):475–93. https://doi.org/10.1007/s40257-015-0158-0.
23. Mockenhaupt M, Viboud C, Dunant A, et al. Stevens-Johnson syndrome and toxic epidermal necrolysis: assessment of medication risks with emphasis on recently marketed drugs. The EuroSCAR-study. J Invest Dermatol 2008;128(1):35–44. https://doi.org/10.1038/sj.jid.5701033.
24. Sekula P, Dunant A, Mockenhaupt M, et al. Comprehensive survival analysis of a cohort of patients with Stevens-Johnson syndrome and toxic epidermal necrolysis. J Invest Dermatol 2013;133(5):1197–204. https://doi.org/10.1038/jid.2012.510.
25. Seminario-Vidal L, Kroshinsky D, Malachowski SJ, et al. Society of dermatology hospitalists supportive care guidelines for the management of Stevens-Johnson syndrome/toxic epidermal necrolysis in adults. J Am Acad Dermatol 2020; 82(6):1553–67. https://doi.org/10.1016/j.jaad.2020.02.066.
26. Schwartz RA, McDonough PH, Lee BW. Toxic epidermal necrolysis: Part I. Introduction, history, classification, clinical features, systemic manifestations, etiology, and immunopathogenesis. J Am Acad Dermatol 2013;69(2):173.e1–13. https://doi.org/10.1016/j.jaad.2013.05.003 [quiz 185–6].
27. Bastuji-Garin S, Rzany B, Stern RS, et al. Clinical classification of cases of toxic epidermal necrolysis, Stevens-Johnson syndrome, and erythema multiforme. Arch Dermatol 1993;129(1):92–6.
28. Chaby G, Ingen-Housz-Oro S, De Prost N, et al. Idiopathic Stevens-Johnson syndrome and toxic epidermal necrolysis: prevalence and patients' characteristics. J Am Acad Dermatol 2019;80(5):1453–5. https://doi.org/10.1016/j.jaad.2018.10.058.
29. Roujeau JC, Huynh TN, Bracq C, et al. Genetic susceptibility to toxic epidermal necrolysis. Arch Dermatol 1987;123(9):1171–3.

30. Roujeau JC, Kelly JP, Naldi L, et al. Medication use and the risk of Stevens-Johnson syndrome or toxic epidermal necrolysis. N Engl J Med 1995;333(24):1600–7. https://doi.org/10.1056/NEJM199512143332404.

31. Micheletti RG, Chiesa-Fuxench Z, Noe MH, et al. Stevens-johnson syndrome/toxic epidermal necrolysis: a multicenter retrospective study of 377 adult patients from the United States. J Invest Dermatol 2018;138(11):2315–21. https://doi.org/10.1016/j.jid.2018.04.027.

32. Sassolas B, Haddad C, Mockenhaupt M, et al. ALDEN, an algorithm for assessment of drug causality in Stevens-Johnson Syndrome and toxic epidermal necrolysis: comparison with case-control analysis. Clin Pharmacol Ther 2010;88(1):60–8. https://doi.org/10.1038/clpt.2009.252.

33. Revuz J, Penso D, Roujeau JC, et al. Toxic epidermal necrolysis. Clinical findings and prognosis factors in 87 patients. Arch Dermatol 1987;123(9):1160–5. https://doi.org/10.1001/archderm.123.9.1160.

34. Schwartz RA, McDonough PH, Lee BW. Toxic epidermal necrolysis: part II. Prognosis, sequelae, diagnosis, differential diagnosis, prevention, and treatment. J Am Acad Dermatol 2013;69(2):187.e1–16. https://doi.org/10.1016/j.jaad.2013.05.002 [quiz 203–4].

35. Noe MH, Hubbard RA, Micheletti RG. The ABCD-10 risk prediction model for in-hospital mortality among patients with stevens-johnson syndrome/toxic epidermal necrolysis-reply. JAMA Dermatol 2019;155(9):1088–9. https://doi.org/10.1001/jamadermatol.2019.0998.

36. Noe MH, Rosenbach M, Hubbard RA, et al. Development and validation of a risk prediction model for in-hospital mortality among patients with stevens-johnson syndrome/toxic epidermal necrolysis-ABCD-10. JAMA Dermatol 2019;155(4):448–54. https://doi.org/10.1001/jamadermatol.2018.5605.

37. Creamer D, Walsh SA, Dziewulski P, et al. U.K. guidelines for the management of Stevens-Johnson syndrome/toxic epidermal necrolysis in adults 2016. Br J Dermatol 2016;174(6):1194–227. https://doi.org/10.1111/bjd.14530.

38. Gray P, Kirby J, Smith MT, et al. Pregabalin in severe burn injury pain: a double-blind, randomised placebo-controlled trial. Pain 2011;152(6):1279–88. https://doi.org/10.1016/j.pain.2011.01.055.

39. Jones LM, Uribe AA, Coffey R, et al. Pregabalin in the reduction of pain and opioid consumption after burn injuries: a preliminary, randomized, double-blind, placebo-controlled study. Medicine (Baltimore) 2019;98(18):e15343. https://doi.org/10.1097/MD.0000000000015343.

40. Kaul I, Amin A, Rosenberg M, et al. Use of gabapentin and pregabalin for pruritus and neuropathic pain associated with major burn injury: a retrospective chart review. Burns 2018;44(2):414–22. https://doi.org/10.1016/j.burns.2017.07.018.

41. McCullough M, Burg M, Lin E, et al. Steven johnson syndrome and toxic epidermal necrolysis in a burn unit: a 15-year experience. Burns 2017;43(1):200–5. https://doi.org/10.1016/j.burns.2016.07.026.

42. Schneider JA, Cohen PR. Prognosis and management of Stevens-Johnson syndrome and toxic epidermal necrolysis. J Am Acad Dermatol 2017;77(4):e117. https://doi.org/10.1016/j.jaad.2017.05.057.

43. Gupta LK, Martin AM, Agarwal N, et al. Guidelines for the management of Stevens-Johnson syndrome/toxic epidermal necrolysis: an Indian perspective. Indian J Dermatol Venereol Leprol 2016;82(6):603–25. https://doi.org/10.4103/0378-6323.191134.

44. Palmieri TL, Greenhalgh DG, Saffle JR, et al. A multicenter review of toxic epidermal necrolysis treated in U.S. burn centers at the end of the twentieth

century. J Burn Care Rehabil 2002;23(2):87–96. https://doi.org/10.1097/00004630-200203000-00004.

45. Chave TA, Mortimer NJ, Sladden MJ, et al. Toxic epidermal necrolysis: current evidence, practical management and future directions. Br J Dermatol 2005;153(2): 241–53. https://doi.org/10.1111/j.1365-2133.2005.06721.x.

46. Lerch M, Mainetti C, Terziroli Beretta-Piccoli B, et al. Current perspectives on stevens-johnson syndrome and toxic epidermal necrolysis. Clin Rev Allergy Immunol 2018;54(1):147–76. https://doi.org/10.1007/s12016-017-8654-z.

47. Kamada N, Yoneyama K, Togawa Y, et al. Toxic epidermal necrolysis with severe hyperbilirubinemia: complete re-epithelialization after bilirubin reduction therapies. J Dermatol 2010;37(6):534–6. https://doi.org/10.1111/j.1346-8138.2009. 00770.x.

48. de Prost N, Ingen-Housz-Oro S, Duong TA, et al. Bacteremia in Stevens-Johnson syndrome and toxic epidermal necrolysis: epidemiology, risk factors, and predictive value of skin cultures. Medicine (Baltimore) 2010;89(1):28–36. https://doi.org/10.1097/MD.0b013e3181ca4290.

49. Kim HI, Kim SW, Park GY, et al. Causes and treatment outcomes of Stevens-Johnson syndrome and toxic epidermal necrolysis in 82 adult patients. Korean J Intern Med 2012;27(2):203–10. https://doi.org/10.3904/kjim.2012.27.2.203.

50. Rajaratnam R, Mann C, Balasubramaniam P, et al. Toxic epidermal necrolysis: retrospective analysis of 21 consecutive cases managed at a tertiary centre. Clin Exp Dermatol 2010;35(8):853–62. https://doi.org/10.1111/j.1365-2230.2010. 03826.x.

51. Schulz JT, Sheridan RL, Ryan CM, et al. A 10-year experience with toxic epidermal necrolysis. J Burn Care Rehabil 2000;21(3):199–204. https://doi.org/10.1097/00004630-200021030-00004.

52. Struck MF, Hilbert P, Mockenhaupt M, et al. Severe cutaneous adverse reactions: emergency approach to non-burn epidermolytic syndromes. Intensive Care Med 2010;36(1):22–32. https://doi.org/10.1007/s00134-009-1659-1.

53. Wang LL, Noe MH, Micheletti RG. Long-term sequelae from Stevens-Johnson syndrome/toxic epidermal necrolysis in a large retrospective cohort. J Am Acad Dermatol 2021;84(3):784–6. https://doi.org/10.1016/j.jaad.2020.04.020.

54. Hoffman M, Chansky PB, Bashyam AR, et al. Long-term physical and psychological outcomes of stevens-johnson syndrome/toxic epidermal necrolysis. JAMA Dermatol 2021;157(6):712–5. https://doi.org/10.1001/jamadermatol.2021.1136.

55. Liakos W, Xu A, Finelt N. Clinical features of recurrent Mycoplasma pneumoniae-induced rash and mucositis. Pediatr Dermatol 2021;38(1):154–8. https://doi.org/10.1111/pde.14472.

56. Gámez-González LB, Peña-Varela C, Ramírez-López JM, et al. Adenoviral-induced rash and mucositis: expanding the spectrum of reactive infectious mucocutaneous eruption. Pediatr Dermatol 2021;38(1):306–8. https://doi.org/10.1111/pde.14419.

57. Canavan TN, Mathes EF, Frieden I, et al. Mycoplasma pneumoniae-induced rash and mucositis as a syndrome distinct from Stevens-Johnson syndrome and erythema multiforme: a systematic review. J Am Acad Dermatol 2015;72(2):239–45. https://doi.org/10.1016/j.jaad.2014.06.026.

58. Waites KB, Xiao L, Liu Y, et al. Mycoplasma pneumoniae from the respiratory tract and beyond. Clin Microbiol Rev 2017;30(3):747–809. https://doi.org/10.1128/CMR.00114-16.

59. Li HO, Colantonio S, Ramien ML. Treatment of. J Cutan Med Surg 2019;23(6): 608–12. https://doi.org/10.1177/1203475419874444.

60. Miller MM, Kamath S, Hughes M, et al. Evaluation of etanercept for treatment of reactive infectious mucocutaneous eruption. JAMA Dermatol 2021;157(2):230–2. https://doi.org/10.1001/jamadermatol.2020.5166.

61. Calvano RA, Scacchi MF, Sojo MM, et al. [Toxic epidermal necrolysis associated with acute infection by Mycoplasma pneumoniae]. Arch Argent Pediatr 2013; 111(1):e24–7. https://doi.org/10.5546/aap.2013.e24.

62. Tankunakorn J, Sawatwarakul S, Vachiramon V, et al. Stevens-johnson syndrome and toxic epidermal necrolysis-like lupus erythematosus. J Clin Rheumatol 2019; 25(5):224–31. https://doi.org/10.1097/RHU.0000000000000830.

63. Yildirim Cetin G, Sayar H, Ozkan F, et al. A case of toxic epidermal necrolysis-like skin lesions with systemic lupus erythematosus and review of the literature. Lupus 2013;22(8):839–46. https://doi.org/10.1177/0961203313492242.

64. Hau E, Vignon Pennamen MD, Battistella M, et al. Neutrophilic skin lesions in autoimmune connective tissue diseases: nine cases and a literature review. Medicine (Baltimore) 2014;93(29):e346. https://doi.org/10.1097/MD.0000000000000346.

65. Simsek I, Cinar M, Erdem H, et al. Efficacy of plasmapheresis in the treatment of refractory toxic epidermal necrolysis-like acute cutaneous lupus erythematosus. Lupus 2008;17(6):605–6. https://doi.org/10.1177/0961203308089341.

66. Baker MG, Cresce ND, Ameri M, et al. Systemic lupus erythematosus presenting as Stevens-Johnson syndrome/toxic epidermal necrolysis. J Clin Rheumatol 2014;20(3):167–71. https://doi.org/10.1097/RHU.0000000000000088.

67. Bedoui Y, Guillot X, Sélambarom J, et al. Methotrexate an old drug with new tricks. Int J Mol Sci 2019;20(20):5023. https://doi.org/10.3390/ijms20205023.

68. Chan ES, Cronstein BN. Methotrexate–how does it really work? Nat Rev Rheumatol 2010;6(3):175–8. https://doi.org/10.1038/nrrheum.2010.5.

69. Chen TJ, Chung WH, Chen CB, et al. Methotrexate-induced epidermal necrosis: a case series of 24 patients. J Am Acad Dermatol 2017;77(2):247–55.e2. https://doi.org/10.1016/j.jaad.2017.02.021.

70. Ravi M, Ridpath A, Audino AN, et al. High-dose methotrexate-induced epidermal necrosis in two pediatric patients. Pediatr Dermatol 2021;38(3):659–63. https://doi.org/10.1111/pde.14591.

71. Tomás-Velázquez A, Rodríguez-Garijo N, Moreno-Artero E, et al. Methotrexate-induced epidermal necrosis in a child with osteosarcoma. J Dtsch Dermatol Ges 2020;18(9):1028–30. https://doi.org/10.1111/ddg.14176.

72. Ramachandran V, Kolli SS, Strowd LC. Review of graft-versus-host disease. Dermatol Clin 2019;37(4):569–82. https://doi.org/10.1016/j.det.2019.05.014.

73. Jagasia M, Arora M, Flowers ME, et al. Risk factors for acute GVHD and survival after hematopoietic cell transplantation. Blood 2012;119(1):296–307. https://doi.org/10.1182/blood-2011-06-364265.

74. Strong Rodrigues K, Oliveira-Ribeiro C, de Abreu Fiuza Gomes S, et al. Cutaneous graft-versus-host disease: diagnosis and treatment. Am J Clin Dermatol 2018;19(1):33–50. https://doi.org/10.1007/s40257-017-0306-9.

75. Naik H, Lockwood S, Saavedra A. A pilot study comparing histological and immunophenotypic patterns in stage 4 skin graft vs host disease from toxic epidermal necrolysis. J Cutan Pathol 2017;44(10):857–60. https://doi.org/10.1111/cup.12986.

76. Chen A, Chao K, Rodriguez L, et al. Toxic epidermal necrolysis versus cutaneous graft-versus-host disease in a hematopoietic stem cell transplant recipient: the role of elafin. Leuk Lymphoma 2018;59(9):2261–3. https://doi.org/10.1080/10428194.2017.1422867.

77. Van Lint MT, Uderzo C, Locasciulli A, et al. Early treatment of acute graft-versus-host disease with high- or low-dose 6-methylprednisolone: a multicenter randomized trial from the Italian Group for Bone Marrow Transplantation. Blood 1998; 92(7):2288–93.
78. Mielcarek M, Furlong T, Storer BE, et al. Effectiveness and safety of lower dose prednisone for initial treatment of acute graft-versus-host disease: a randomized controlled trial. Haematologica 2015;100(6):842–8. https://doi.org/10.3324/haematol.2014.118471.

Uncommon Causes of Rhabdomyolysis

Matthew Harmelink, MD

KEYWORDS

- Rhabdomyolysis • Myoglobin • Creatine kinase • HyperCKemia

KEY POINTS

- Rhabdomyolysis is a complex end-stage process caused by either direct myocyte trauma or energy insufficiency.
- The complications of rhabdomyolysis are diffuse, resulting in complex cases in which the rhabdomyolysis can be the primary driver of systemic injury or merely a symptom of a more systemic process.
- There are diverse causes of rhabdomyolysis, and a broad differential diagnosis is needed to uncover the underlying cause.

INTRODUCTION

Rhabdomyolysis is a relatively common disease that involves the pathologic process of muscle breakdown. Initially caused by either energy depletion or direct myocyte injury, both inciting problems can result in increased calcium release and myocyte breakdown.[1] Most patients with rhabdomyolysis will not require intensive care and can be managed either as an outpatient or in an acute care setting. In the critical care patient, depending on sedation and the presence of other systemic diseases, a secondary rhabdomyolysis can easily be missed. Additionally, the differentiation between rhabdomyolysis and hyperCKemia is essential in understanding the appropriate treatment and diagnostic methods. Although the most common causes of rhabdomyolysis—infectious, exercise-induced, and traumatic—are typically readily identified, there are many uncommon triggers or underlying disorders that can predispose to rhabdomyolysis.[2,3] A framework for understanding rhabdomyolysis and for approaching the diagnostic evaluation of uncommon causes will be provided.

DEFINITIONS AND GENERAL FEATURES

Rhabdomyolysis is a final terminal pathway that results in skeletal myocyte necrosis, sarcolemma membrane permeability, and release of toxic intracellular contents into

Department of Neurology, Medical College of Wisconsin, CCC Suite 540, 5000 W. Wisconsin Avenue, Milwaukee, WI 53226, USA
E-mail address: mharmelink@mcw.edu

Crit Care Clin 38 (2022) 271–285
https://doi.org/10.1016/j.ccc.2021.11.004
0749-0704/22/© 2021 Elsevier Inc. All rights reserved.

the circulation. These toxic products being exposed to other organ tissues results in systemic symptoms, most notably renal injury or failure.[4]

The terminal pathway can be initiated either from energy failure or from direct myocyte damage; both result in calcium influx and further myocyte damage.[4] Although the biochemical hallmark of rhabdomyolysis—an elevation in the serum creatine kinase (CK) level—is an indicator of this terminal pathway, not all CK elevations indicate rhabdomyolysis. Diseases that involve myocyte sarcolemma damage that do not result in initiation of this terminal pathway are not rhabdomyolysis. In diseases with underlying structural membrane abnormalities, such as in the muscular dystrophies, or in instances of transient injury, such as with exercise, serum CK levels are elevated without a risk of the systemic pathology seen in rhabdomyolysis. A child with Duchenne muscular dystrophy, for example, can live with significantly elevated CK levels for their entire life without any risk of renal failure.

The important part to note is that CK itself is not often the injurious chemical but a surrogate marker. However, of those measured, only electrolytes and myoglobin are able to be clinically obtained. Rhabdomyolysis results in the activation of calcium-dependent neutral proteases and phospholipases.[4] Secondarily, there is destruction of the myofibrils, cytoskeleton, and sarcolemma. The myocyte fiber contents are auto-phagocytosed by lysosomes, and there is a release into the blood stream of multiple intracellular products.[4]

CLINICAL DIAGNOSTIC CRITERIA

Currently, there are several different criteria systems for the diagnosis of rhabdomyolysis. Most use CK levels varying from 1000 to 5000 IU/L in the appropriate clinical setting of preceding injury, exposure, or underlying medical condition.[5] Labeling all CK elevations as rhabdomyolysis can cause confusion in patients who might suffer from hyperCKemia, the elevation of serum creatine kinase in the absence of active rhabdomyolysis; repeat CK level determination several months after a patient has convalesced from supposed rhabdomyolysis can help determine if baseline CK levels are elevated or in the normal range. Finally, in patients with focal rhabdomyolysis, in which muscle breakdown is confined to a restricted site or in which total muscle bulk is low relative to total body volume, the serum CK will be normal despite the presence of an ongoing focal destructive process.

CK does not start to rise for about 24 hours after a monophasic injury. The half-life of CK under physiologic circumstances is 24 to 36 hours. This contrasts with myoglobin, which often will start to rise within a few hours of the injury, peak, and then mostly clear by 24 to 48 hours after the injury. These variances are important, as patients after longer delays can lack myoglobin and make timing of the inciting injury difficult.

PATTERNS

A summary of common causes of rhabdomyolysis is shown in **Box 1** for adults and **Box 2** for children. Although the most common causes of rhabdomyolysis are exercise, drugs, and alcohol, some characteristic patterns suggest other etiologies.

Exertional rhabdomyolysis may occur after a sudden increase in strenuous activity from the patient's baseline. A natural consequence of exercising is the breakdown of the myocyte sarcolemma, which often results in a mild CK elevation.[6] This elevation is often only up to a few hundred IU/L or maybe in the case of running a marathon, up to a few thousand; exertion-related elevations in CK will oftentimes quickly abate, although they sometimes can be sustained.[6,7] However, if the amount of exercise is beyond

---

Box 1
Common adult causes of nonrecurrent rhabdomyolysis

Alcohol and illicit substances

Muscle compression or trauma

Seizures

Excessive exercise

---

what the patient can tolerate, myocytes will start down an apoptotic pathway rather than recovering.

Exertional rhabdomyolysis differs from underlying genetic or metabolic muscle disease, as often the amount of exercise needed to cause rhabdomyolysis in patients with genetic or metabolic disease can be much milder, sometimes within the range of typical daily activities. In severe cases, just heat exposure alone has been enough to cause an episode. However, genetic etiologies should be suspected if a patient experiences multiple episodes of exertional rhabdomyolysis or has a family history of rhabdomyolysis. Muscle swelling after exercise and dark colored urine can be signs of an underlying disease and may represent episodes of rhabdomyolysis that did not rise to the level of requiring medical evaluation. When concerned for genetic causes, one of the best differentiating factors is obtaining a baseline CK. This baseline level determination needs to be done outside of the episode, often weeks to months after, when the patient has had no strenuous activity for the previous 48 to 72 hours, to avoid a false-positive elevation.

The typical clinical features for diffuse rhabdomyolysis are a proximal greater than distal weakness with pain and tenderness over the muscles, as well as possible muscle swelling. For those in whom exercise is involved, focal tenderness in the areas of activity can exist also. However, in the critical care unit, these symptoms are easily missed in a sedated patient, so serum testing is often warranted.

A patient's urine may be described as dark colored because of the visible presence of myoglobin (myoglobinuria), although in milder cases this may not be seen. Additionally, in patients who are receiving significant amounts of parenteral fluid, given that pigmentation is a feature of concentration, iatrogenically diluted urine may mask this feature. If the patient presents late after a monophasic event, given the short half-life of myoglobin, myoglobinuria may have cleared. For patients with renal injury, descriptions of oliguria or anuria may also be seen.

Given the potential toxicity of released intracellular substances, systemic features such as encephalopathy or cardiomyopathy may be seen; conversely, these features may be indicators of an underlying disease, of which rhabdomyolysis is one finding.

Box 2
Common pediatric causes of nonrecurrent rhabdomyolysis

Trauma

Nonketotic hyperosmolar coma

Viral

Excessive exercise

The approach to any patient with rhabdomyolysis should not only be to assess for rhabdomyolysis but also to ascertain the underlying etiology.

COMPLICATIONS

Although the injury to the muscle itself can be concerning, the muscle injury is often recoverable, whereas the systemic complications, if unrecognized and untreated, can result in permanent injury.

Local swelling of the muscle compartment can result in focal ischemia and injury to all structures within this compartment if the tissue pressure becomes greater than the perfusion/capillary pressure. In compartment syndrome, ischemia can start early with necrosis within 6 hours from onset.[8] For this reason, frequent distal neurovascular checks can be helpful in monitoring for this complication. Critically ill patients may be unable to relay the classic pain out of proportion on examination, as well as sensation abnormalities like burning or paresthesia or a feeling of tightness in the muscles. With any concerning features, emergent surgical consultation for compartment pressure determination and for possible fasciotomy is warranted.[9]

Renal failure can result from ferrihernate toxicity caused by dissociation from hemoglobin in an acidic environment and tubular obstruction caused by myoglobin cast precipitation.[10] For this reason, fluids are used aggressively to treat patients. Renal failure can also compound the hyperkalemia that can develop from muscle breakdown. Decreasing urine output, oliguria, or anuria in the setting of aggressive fluid administration is often a sign of progressive kidney damage.

TREATMENT

The treatment of rhabdomyolysis is supportive in nature unless it is warranted to treat the inciting etiology. Maintaining renal perfusion and output is important to avoid the complications. Often, use of normal saline infusions to maintain urine output is the standard of care, although there is little evidence to compare the specific criteria or methods. If patients have significant acidosis, including bicarbonate into the fluids is used by some centers as are diuretics if the urine output begins to drop despite good intake.[3,4]

The treatment of electrolyte abnormalities is warranted, but the use of glucose, carnitine and/or other drugs should be based on the etiology of the inciting disease.

SPECIFIC DISEASES

In the critical care setting, some of the underlying inciting events may not be feasibly diagnosed, whereas the lack of treatment of others could potentially be life-threatening. As such, uncommon causes of rhabdomyolysis will be discussed further. The list of all causes of rhabdomyolysis is extensive, and so, even the associated tables may not capture every possible cause. However, the underlying principles in each category should be helpful in identifying specific etiologies. General categories with examples are shown in **Table 1**.

Malignant Hyperthermia

Malignant hyperthermia (MH), a complication of certain anesthetics, often has an underlying genetic cause. There are 2 categories of diseases with high malignant hyperthermia risk: those with baseline abnormal clinical features and those without. Based on the nature of the underlying genetic abnormality, patients may have a myopathic phenotype where the associated myopathy is a clue to the risk of malignant

Table 1
Conditions predisposing to rhabdomyolysis

Etiology Category	Examples of Specific Diagnosis	History Features	Clinical Features	Laboratory Features
Malignant hyperthermia	Central core myopathy (RYR1)	May have a history of muscle pain or other symptoms	Some with muscle or other symptoms	Variable outside of the event
Glycogen metabolism	McArdle disease (myophosphorylase deficiency)	Rhabdomyolysis or myalgia within minutes of excising, second wind effect	May have pattern of weakness	Variable CK levels
Fatty acid, metabolic, and mitochondrial	Carnitine palmitoyltransferase II deficiency	Symptoms occur after prolonged fasting, infections, exercise, stress, or cold	Variable examination but may have baseline weakness or hypotonia	High lactate at rest or with mild exercise
Infection	Influenza B	Systemic infectious signs with muscle pain	Muscle pain, malaise, fever	Leukocytosis, positive viral testing
Toxin or illicit substance	Haff disease	Eating seafood	Gastrointestinal symptoms, sensory changes	None outside expected for rhabdomyolysis
Medications	Statin	Myalgia or muscle cramping	Myotonic discharges during rhabdomyolysis	Elevated creatine kinase at baseline

hyperthermia, or they may have no features except for malignant hyperthermia. Detailed elucidation of genotype-phenotype correlations is ongoing (**Table 2**). As such, it is nearly impossible to avoid every potential case of MH in an anesthetic-naïve patient.

General principles

In MH, potentially triggering anesthetics do not always precipitate a crisis; as such, previous anesthetic exposure history may be insufficient to assess risk.[11] Incidence is estimated at 1 in 100,000 hospitalized patients; while the overall incidence is therefore relatively common, the underlying genetic etiologies are less so.[12] Given that some of the underlying diseases affect the muscle contractile apparatus and not the muscle membrane itself, a normal baseline CK cannot be used to exclude MH risk. Although the most discussed causes are anesthetics such as inhalational agents and succinylcholine, some patients can develop mild MH from exercise in hot conditions, neuroleptic medications, infections, or even agents that are generally felt to be safe (e.g., ketamine, local anesthetics, or nitrous oxide).

Clinical features

The timing of onset of malignant hyperthermia ranges from immediately while under anesthesia to within 24 hours afterward. The onset is marked by a rise in end tidal CO_2 and/or core temperature as well as muscle contractures with rigidity, weakness, and possibly pain. Additional features include tachycardia, tachypnea, hyperhidrosis, and hemodynamic instability. Because of the continuous muscle contractions, fevers and cyanosis may develop. Eventually, these can lead to edema, cardiac arrest, and renal failure. Early diagnosis can help improve prognosis by addressing the hypermetabolism. The continued muscle contractions lead to increased oxygen consumption,

Table 2
Common causes of malignant hyperthermia

Name	Associated Gene or Genetic Locus
MH syndrome 1/central core disease/ King-Denborough Syndrome	RYR1
MH syndrome 2/periodic paralysis/ myotonia congenita	SCN4A
MH syndrome 3	Chromosome region 7q21-q22, likely CACNA2D1
MH syndrome 4	Chromosome region 3q13.1
MH syndrome 5	CACNA1S
MH syndrome 6	Chromosome 5p
STAC3 Myopathy	STAC3
Carnitine palmitoyltransferase II deficiency	CPTII
Dystrophinopathy (Duchenne or Becker)	Dystrophin
Myotonic dystrophy type 1	DMPK trinucleotide repeat
Schwartz-Jampel syndrome	Chromosome 1p36
Satoyoshi syndrome	Unknown, presumed autoimmune

Data from Rosenberg H, Sambuughin N, Riazi S, et al. Malignant hyperthermia susceptibility. 2003 Dec 19 [Updated 2020 Jan 16]. In: Adam MP, Ardinger HH, Pagon RA, et al, editors. GeneReviews [Internet]. Seattle (WA): University of Washington, Seattle; 1993-2021. Available from: https://www.ncbi.nlm.nih.gov/books/NBK1146/

rising CO_2, and lactic acidosis. Treatment with dantrolene is needed to bind to the ryanodine receptor 1, resulting in reduced excitation-contraction coupling and reduced intracellular calcium concentration.[13]

Diagnosis is via genetic sequencing though does not capture 100% of affected patients. In patients in whom clinical suspicion remains despite negative molecular genetic testing, functional testing by the halothane contracture test or caffeine contracture test can be done.[13] However, these assays need to be done on fresh muscle tissue and are not a standard procedure for most muscle laboratories; confirmation of the laboratory's ability to perform the test prior to obtaining the biopsy should be done, often in consultation with the patient's neuromuscular and/or genetic specialist.

Specific diseases
Specific diseases are associated with MH susceptibility. A brief description of the associated malignant hyperthermia syndromes follows.

Malignant hyperthermia syndrome type 1 (central core disease). In MH syndrome type 1 (MHS1), the ryanodine receptor 1 (*RYR1*) gene has a dominant pathogenic variant resulting in a high risk of MH. This gene controls intracellular movement of calcium and is large with various hot spots for pathogenic variants. Given the size of the gene and the variability in variants, in some phenotypes, patients will have myopathic features, whereas others carry only a risk for MH.[14,15] Additionally, the literature varies in the names of the disease so, although not all patients have central core disease caused by *RYR1* variants, all such patients without a genetic diagnosis and those with *RYR1* known pathogenic variants should be considered at risk for MH. Pathogenic variants in this gene underlie about half of the known MH syndrome cases.[13]

Malignant hyperthermia syndrome type 2. In MH syndrome type 2 (MHS2), a variant in the *SCN4A* gene results in a risk for MH.[16] Although this gene has been associated with myopathic features, it is also associated with all forms of periodic paralysis and congenital myasthenia gravis.[17] Given the former set of diseases can have a normal baseline examination outside of a spell, historic questioning for episodes of weakness, stiff gait, or limping should be performed in any patient with either MH or rhabdomyolysis.

Malignant hyperthermia syndrome type 3. In MH syndrome type 3 (MHS3), linkage studies identified that chromosomal locus 7q21-q22, which includes the *CACNA2D1* gene, is associated with a risk of MH. This genetic association has only been described in a few patients, however, and is not considered a common cause.[18]

Malignant hyperthermia syndrome 4. In MH syndrome type 4 (MHS4), a variant mapping to 3q13.1 in a single German pedigree was found to be associated with MH.[19]

Malignant hyperthermia syndrome type 5. In MH syndrome type 5 (MHS5), the *CACNA1S* gene has a dominant pathogenic variant that can result in hypokalemic periodic paralysis and is also associated with MH.[20] Accounting for about 1% of the MH syndromes, this gene also is involved in myocyte calcium regulation[13].

Malignant hyperthermia syndrome type 6. In MH syndrome type 6 (MHS6), a variant mapping to chromosome 6p has been described in a single Belgian pedigree as associated with malignant hyperthermia.[21]

STAC3 myopathy. Also known as Bailey-Bloch myopathy, STAC3 myopathy is an autosomal-recessive disease caused by variants in the *STAC3* gene. In this gene, patients present with myopathic features including abnormal facies, progressive scoliosis, and contractures, as well as short stature and palatal abnormalities.[13]

King-Denborough syndrome. This syndrome is caused by an *RYR1* variant. In this disease, patients present with proximal symmetric weakness, scapular winging, short stature, and early scoliosis (often in the first decade of life). Beyond the heat or anesthesia-triggered MH that can occur at any age, most patients present as children with the other associated features. Some of these children have dysmorphisms with malar hypoplasia, low-set ears, and micrognathia.[22,23]

Glycogen Metabolic Disorders

General principles
Glycogen metabolic disorders are a set of diseases that cause rhabdomyolysis because of a failure in energy production. All diseases in this category are characterized by a failure to either synthesize or degrade glycogen. Patients can present with many nonmuscle symptoms but often will have rhabdomyolysis triggered by some degree of either increased energy requirements (e.g., exercise, infection, certain medications, or illicit substances) or reduced substrate availability (e.g., fasting or vomiting), with the severity of the disease often associated with the severity of the trigger.

Clinical features
Overall, this is a large group of diseases with diverse symptoms. For those patients who have purely or predominantly myopathic features, muscle cramping, especially with or after exercise, is a common phenomenon. In some subtypes, if a patient starts to exercise, then takes a short break before restarting, he or she will have reduced or eliminated symptoms and increased endurance, the classic second wind phenomenon, wherein the rest allows muscle to start using fat as an energy source rather than glycogen for aerobic metabolism, thus alleviating the energy depletion.

Specific diseases
The most recognized of the myopathic glycogen storage diseases that cause rhabdomyolysis is McArdle disease (myophosphorylase deficiency). In this autosomal recessive condition, patients often present with episodes of cramping and/or rhabdomyolysis, with persistent proximal muscle weakness starting in their second decade. Because of an inability to initiate glycogenolysis in the skeletal muscle, patients will often have muscle pains after short intense exercise.[24] Baseline CK is elevated. The definitive diagnosis is now made via genetic sequencing, but patients can also undergo nonischemic forearm testing, during which following provocation, lactic acid does not rise as high as ammonia, demonstrating a defect in the metabolic pathway.[25] The treatment is to avoid high-intensity exercise and consider a high-protein diet to help with muscle recovery.

Other glycogen storage diseases to consider as causes of rhabdomyolysis are included in **Box 3**. Each of these diseases will have various nonrhabdomyolysis features but, in rhabdomyolysis, all revolve around the principle of energy failure.

Fatty Acid Oxidation, Lipid Metabolism, and Mitochondrial Disorders

General principles
Fatty acid oxidation disorders, lipid metabolism disease, and mitochondrial diseases all result in a failure of energy production. Although there are congenital forms that also present with systemic diseases, the purely myopathic forms can often present solely with rhabdomyolysis.

Box 3
Glycogen storage diseases associated with rhabdomyolysis

Phosphofructokinase

Aldolase A

Lactate dehydrogenase

Phosphoglycerate kinase

Phosphoglycerate mutase

Phosphorylase b kinase

Debrancher enzyme

Enolase-3

Myophosphorylase deficiency (McArdle disease)

In this category of diseases, patients often will have normal baseline CK levels that elevate when the patient is experiencing a metabolic stressor. Only in very severe cases, often resulting in myocyte injury outside of the episode of rhabdomyolysis, do these patients have baseline elevated CKs. However, unlike the glycogen storage diseases, these diseases have either elevated lactic acids at rest, or, in milder forms, significant elevations at times of stress. Additionally, given the pathways involved, some patients may have normal baseline examinations without signs of myopathy. The most common cause of rhabdomyolysis in a patient with a normal baseline CK in this category is the late-onset myopathic form of carnitine palmitoyltransferase II deficiency.

Specific diseases

Carnitine palmitoyltransferase II deficiency. The carnitine palmitoyltransferase II (CPTII) enzyme is a key component of the beta-oxidation pathway. CPTII deficiency is an autosomal-recessive disorder with 3 forms. In the infantile and childhood-onset forms, patients often have symptoms other than muscle disease, whereas the adult form often presents solely with rhabdomyolysis. Exercise and sometimes fasting or other stressors will result in energy depletion. Patients will describe muscle pains with activity but can also develop rhabdomyolysis that may only be noticed as darkening of the urine historically. However, between episodes, many adults have no muscle symptoms and normal CK values. The diagnosis can be made either by sequencing, although often, prior to that, screening with acylcarnitine profiles will demonstrate an abnormal pattern.[26] Importantly, in patients with presumed or confirmed CPTII deficiency, valproic acid should be avoided because of its depletion of carnitine.[27]

Myocyte Structural Genetic Diseases

General principles

Although many of the previously mentioned heritable diseases are associated with malignant hyperthermia, there are nonmalignant hyperthermia causes of rhabdomyolysis, some of which are heritable.

Many of the dystrophinopathies (any muscle disease that affects the myocyte sarcolemma) have the potential to result in rhabdomyolysis. Although in many of these cases the patients will either have an established diagnosis or have features of muscle disease on physical examination, a classic case of Becker muscular dystrophy demonstrates the exception to this rule.

Specific diseases

The dystrophinopathies are caused by pathogenic variants in the dystrophin gene and are clinically heterogenous. In the most severe case, an affected boy may lose the ability to ambulate in the early second decade and die of cardiopulmonary failure in his early third decade, a pattern classically seen in Duchenne muscular dystrophy. On the other end of the severity spectrum, patients with milder dystrophinopathies will ambulate with minimal skeletal muscle and cardiac features until late adulthood, a pattern typical of mild Becker muscular dystrophy. However, even patients with the mildest phenotypic manifestations can present with rhabdomyolysis because of structural stress, often from exercise, due to their intrinsic sarcolemma abnormalities. Also of note, that although this is an X-linked disease, female symptomatic carriers can have similar presenting features, although often milder, based upon their ratio of X-inactivation. CK is often elevated in patients with baseline clinical symptoms or in men with the disease but can be normal in symptomatic carrier women.

Dietary Exposures and Illicit Substances

General principles

Dietary exposures and illicit substances are common triggers for rhabdomyolysis (**Table 3**), as any substance that can decouple the energy production from energy demands can trigger muscle breakdown. In these cases, the duration of the initial insult, and thus the risk for ongoing muscle breakdown and release of toxins in the final common pathway, will be related to the half-life of the drug. Often, other symptoms related to the pharmacologic profile of the ingested substance will be present.

The list of associated medications is long. Given the existence published articles specifically on the drugs of abuse, an exhaustive list is not provided here.[5,28] However, a few less common causes will be described.

Specific diseases

Hemlock toxicity from quail eggs has been demonstrated to cause rhabdomyolysis. In these cases, the quails eat hemlock and accumulate the toxin in their eggs, which are then eaten by patients as a delicacy.[29] As another example of dietary causes of rhabdomyolysis, Haff disease, a toxin-induced rhabdomyolysis from freshwater or seafood

Table 3
Illicit substances associated with rhabdomyolysis

Substance	Putative Mechanism
Cocaine	Vasospasm-induced ischemia Direct toxic effect on muscle
Alcohol	Immobilization, calcium accumulation in sarcoplasmic reticulum, changes in myocyte carbohydrate metabolism
Carbon monoxide	Hypoxia
Amphetamine	Agitation and overactivity
Ecstasy	Agitation and overactivity
Heroin	Immobilization

Data from Keltz E, Khan FY, Mann G. Rhabdomyolysis. The role of diagnostic and prognostic factors. Muscles Ligaments Tendons J 2014;3(4):303-312. Published 2014 Feb 24; and John R Richards. Rhabdomyolysis and drugs of abuse, The Journal of Emergency Medicine 2000;19(1): 51-56

ingestion, also occurs. Often the disease onset is 6 to 24 hours after ingestion, similar to other food poisonings.[30] Patients will present with significant pain to light touch and myalgia throughout their bodies; some patients have also described numbness.[30–33] Additionally, there is diffuse weakness with some increased tone. Rhabdomyolysis is a common feature, as are other signs of gastrointestinal distress (e.g., nausea, vomiting, abdominal pain, and diarrhea). The care is supportive, as it often resolves within a few days of onset.[30–33] Another uncommon cause of rhabdomyolysis is mushroom intoxication. There are various mushroom-derived toxins.[34,35] The time to onset varies by the toxin, with some being immediately after eating, whereas others can be days to a week after multiple ingestions. This leaves a broad range when considering how to investigate based on dietary or illicit substance use history.

Other ingestions, including rocket fuels,[36] moonwort,[37] and thorn apples,[38] often have effects related to their toxidrome. Given this, in cases of ingestions of uncommonly seen toxidromes or where there might be unidentified contaminants, obtaining an appropriately timed CK can be diagnostic.

Medications

General principles
Iatrogenic rhabdomyolysis presents similarly to toxin and illicit substance-induced rhabdomyolysis, although identification and removal of the offending medication can be confounded in cases where there are multiple new medications introduced in a short period of time, as can occur in a critically ill patient, such as someone with refractory status epilepticus (SE). Additionally, underlying predisposing factors for rhabdomyolysis, such as metabolic disease, can lead to SE and result in difficulty differentiating between whether the medication or the underlying disease caused the rhabdomyolysis.

Specific diseases
Although neuroleptic malignant syndrome and serotonin syndrome are common enough that they are often not missed, statin-induced muscle breakdown is less commonly appreciated. Although statin use is relatively common, the incidence of statin-induced rhabdomyolysis is low.[39] These medications can cause various levels of muscle injury including chronic myalgia, a necrotizing myositis, and overt rhabdomyolysis itself. In most cases, these symptoms are not acute but start weeks to months after the initiation of the medication. In diagnosing statin-associated

---

Box 4
Systemic diseases associated with rhabdomyolysis

Hypokalemia

Hypophosphatemia

Hypocalcemia

Hyponatremia

Hypernatremia

Adrenal insufficiency

Thyroid disease

Hyperaldosteronism

Diabetic ketoacidosis

Table 4
Infections associated with rhabdomyolysis

Viral	Bacterial	Rickettsial	Tick-Borne
Influenza A & B	Streptococci	Scrub typhus	Ehrlichiosis
Coxsackie	*Salmonella*	Mediterranean tick typhus	Anaplasmosis
Herpes	Staphylococci		Babesiosis
Adenovirus	Typhoid		Lyme disease
HIV-1	*Legionella*		Rocky Mountain spotted fever
West Nile Virus	Clostridia		
	Escherichia coli		

Data from Torres PA, Helmstetter JA, Kaye AM, Kaye AD. Rhabdomyolysis: pathogenesis, diagnosis, and treatment. Ochsner J. 2015;15(1):58-69; and Singh U, Scheld WM. Infectious etiologies of rhabdomyolysis: three case reports and review. Clin Infect Dis 1996 Apr;22(4):642-9.

rhabdomyolysis, the threshold for CK is defined at more than 11 times the upper limit of normal, given that chronic muscle disease with hyperCKemia is associated with statins also.[40] The treatment is withdrawal of the statin.

Many other medications have been associated with rhabdomyolysis, and such a discussion is outside the scope of this article. However, given the ongoing expansion of this list of associations, it would be beneficial for the clinician to be aware of these causes.[4,41]

Systemic Disease, Infection, and Inflammatory Disease

General principles
Rhabdomyolysis can be secondary to systemic disease, as well as isolated endocrine and electrolyte abnormalities. Additionally, infections and inflammatory disease can also present with rhabdomyolysis (**Box 4**, **Table 4**). For inflammatory disease, although hyperCKemia is common, rhabdomyolysis is relatively rare.

Venom
Finally, venom has been associated with rhabdomyolysis because of myocyte membrane injury. Bee and wasp stings, as well as snake and spider bites, have all been associated with rhabdomyolysis in various regions of the world.[42–44] Even the common yellow jacket wasp sting has been associated with rhabdomyolysis.[43]

SUMMARY

Rhabdomyolysis is a relatively common phenomenon, although most cases do not require intensive care unit level of care. Although most common causes can be easily identified, in encephalopathic or critically ill patients, symptoms can be easily missed, as can uncommon etiologies. Given the potential morbidity, it is important that in any patient with concern for rhabdomyolysis, evaluation and management occur expeditiously. A general framework for recognizing the presence of and identifying the cause of rhabdomyolysis includes recognizing historic and physical features associated with rhabdomyolysis, such as myoglobinuria, muscle rigidity, a personal or family history of malignant hyperthermia, genetic or metabolic disease, signs of longstanding myopathy or dystrophinopathy, toxidromes, or exposure to certain medications. States of energy failure should be addressed by providing substate and cofactors as indicated, and induced rhabdomyolysis should be addressed by withdrawing the offending agent. Hydration and monitoring for complications are the mainstays of therapy, regardless of cause.

DISCLOSURE

M. Harmelink has received research funding for participating in clinical trials from Capricor Therapeutics, Sarepta Therapeutics, PTC Therapeutics, Mallinckrodt Pharmaceuticals, and Wave Life Sciences. He has received a nonrestricted educational grant from Sarepta Therapeutics and infrastructure clinical grants from MDA, PPMD and research grants from Cure SMA. He has received honorarium for advisory boards and consulting from Biogen, AveXis/Novartis Gene Therapies, Sarepta Therapeutics, and PTC Therapeutics. He actively consults for Emerging Therapy Solutions. He serves without compensation on DuchenneXchange and as a Board Member for Three Gaits, Inc and as an advisor for Hopeful Together, Inc.

CLINICS CARE POINTS

- Rhabdomyolysis is a diverse set of symptoms resulting from multiple pathologic processes. Close monitoring of non-muscle symptoms can identify rare causes and avoid other complications.

- Being careful to differentiate creatine kinase and myoglobin trends based upon the physiology and pathophysiology of the drugs can help differentiate the course of the disease and avoid being confused by the clinical course.

- In patients with clear causes of the rhabdomyolysis, further etiologic diagnosis is not always needed unless there are recurrent episodes of atypical (ex: prolonged course) features.

REFERENCES

1. Giannoglou GD, Chatzizisis YS, Misirli G. The syndrome of rhabdomyolysis: pathophysiology and diagnosis. Eur J Intern Med 2007;18(2):90–100.
2. Melli G, Chaudhry V, Cornblath DR. Rhabdomyolysis: an evaluation of 475 hospitalized patients. Medicine (Baltimore) 2005;84(6):377–85.
3. Watemberg N, Leshner RL, Armstrong BA, et al. Acute pediatric rhabdomyolysis. J Child Neurol 2000;15(4):222–7.
4. Torres PA, Helmstetter JA, Kaye AM, et al. Rhabdomyolysis: pathogenesis, diagnosis, and treatment. Ochsner J 2015;15(1):58–69.
5. Keltz E, Khan FY, Mann G. Rhabdomyolysis. The role of diagnostic and prognostic factors. Muscles Ligaments Tendons J 2014;3(4):303–12.
6. Kenney K, Landau ME, Gonzalez RS, et al. Serum creatine kinase after exercise: drawing the line between physiological response and exertional rhabdomyolysis. Muscle Nerve 2012;45(3):356–62.
7. Siegel AJ, Silverman LM, Lopez RE. Creatine kinase elevations in marathon runners: relationship to training and competition. Yale J Biol Med 1980;53(4):275–9.
8. Mubarak SJ, Hargens AR, Owen CA, et al. The wick catheter technique for measurement of intramuscular pressure. A new research and clinical tool. J Bone Joint Surg Am 1976;58(7):1016–20.
9. Via AG, Oliva F, Spoliti M, et al. Acute compartment syndrome. Muscles Ligaments Tendons J 2015;5(1):18–22.

10. Matthai TP, Zachariah UG, Matthai SM. Recurrent episodic acute kidney injury as presenting manifestation of mitochondrial myopathy. Indian J Nephrol 2014;24(6): 387–9.
11. Rosenberg H, Pollock N, Schiemann A, et al. Malignant hyperthermia: a review. Orphanet J Rare Dis 2015;10:93.
12. Brady JE, Sun LS, Rosenberg H, Li G. Prevalence of malignant hyperthermia due to anesthesia in New York State, 2001–2005. Anesth Analg 2009;109(4):1162–6.
13. Rosenberg H, Sambuughin N, Riazi S, et al. Malignant hyperthermia susceptibility. In: Adam MP, Ardinger HH, Pagon RA, et al, editors. GeneReviews. Seattle (WA): University of Washington, Seattle; 2003. p. 1993–2021. Available at: https://www.ncbi.nlm.nih.gov/books/NBK1146/.
14. Riazi S, Kraeva N, Hopkins PM. Malignant hyperthermia in the post-genomics era: new perspectives on an old concept. Anesthesiology 2018;128(1):168–80.
15. Todd JJ, Sagar V, Lawal TA, et al. Correlation of phenotype with genotype and protein structure in RYR1-related disorders. J Neurol 2018;265(11):2506–24.
16. Moslehi R, Langlois S, Yam I, et al. Linkage of malignant hyperthermia and hyperkalemic periodic paralysis to the adult skeletal muscle sodium channel (SCN4A) gene in a large pedigree. Am J Med Genet 1998;76(1):21–7.
17. Liu XL, Huang XJ, Luan XH, et al. Mutations of SCN4A gene cause different diseases: 2 case reports and literature review. Channels (Austin) 2015;9(2):82–7.
18. Sudbrak R, Golla A, Hogan K, et al. Exclusion of malignant hyperthermia susceptibility (MHS) from a putative MHS2 locus on chromosome 17q and of the alpha-1, beta-1, and gamma subunits of the dihydropyridine receptor calcium channel as candidates for the molecular defect. Hum Mol Genet 1993;2:857–62.
19. Sudbrak R, Procaccio V, Klausnitzer M, et al. Mapping of a further malignant hyperthermia susceptibility locus to chromosome 3q13.1. Am J Hum Genet 1995; 56:684–91.
20. Monnier N, Procaccio V, Stieglitz P, et al. Malignant-hyperthermia susceptibility is associated with a mutation of the alpha-1-subunit of the human dihydropyridine-sensitive L-type voltage-dependent calcium-channel receptor in skeletal muscle. Am J Hum Genet 1997;60:1316–25.
21. Robinson RL, Monnier N, Wolz W, et al. A genome wide search for susceptibility loci in three European malignant hyperthermia pedigrees. Hum Mol Genet 1997; 6:953–61.
22. King JO, Denborough MA, Zapf PW. Inheritance of malignant hyperpyrexia. Lancet 1972;299:365–70.
23. Isaacs H, Badenhorst ME. Dominantly inherited malignant hyperthermia (MH) in the King-Denborough syndrome. Muscle Nerve 1992;15:740–2.
24. Hicks J, Wartchow E, Mierau G. Glycogen storage diseases: a brief review and update on clinical features, genetic abnormalities, pathologic features, and treatment. Ultrastruct Pathol 2011;35(5):183–96.
25. Kazemi-Esfarjani P, Skomorowska E, Jensen TD, et al. A nonischemic forearm exercise test for McArdle disease. Ann Neurol 2002;52(2):153–9.
26. Sigauke E, Rakheja D, Kitson K, et al. Carnitine palmitoyltransferase II deficiency: a clinical, biochemical, and molecular review. Lab Invest 2003;83:1543–54.
27. Kottlors M, Jaksch M, Ketelsen UP, et al. Valproic acid triggers acute rhabdomyolysis in a patient with carnitine palmitoyltransferase type II deficiency. Neuromuscul Disord 2001;11(8):757–9.
28. Richards JR. Rhabdomyolysis and drugs of abuse. J Emerg Med 2000; 19(1):51–6.

29. Korkmaz I, Kukul Güven FM, Eren SH, et al. Quail consumption can be harmful. J Emerg Med 2011;41(5):499–502.
30. Bandeira AC, Campos GS, Ribeiro GS, et al. Clinical and laboratory evidence of Haff disease - case series from an outbreak in Salvador, Brazil, December 2016 to April 2017. Euro Surveill 2017;22(24):30552.
31. Krishna N, Wood J. It looked like a myocardial infarction after eating crawfish. Ever heard of Haff disease? Louisiana Morbidity Report 2001;12(3):1–2.
32. Zhang B, Yang G, Yu X, et al. Haff disease after eating crayfish in east China. Intern Med 2012;51(5):487–9.
33. Tolesani Júnior O, Roderjan CN, do Carmo Neto E, et al. Haff disease associated with the ingestion of the freshwater fish Mylossoma duriventre (pacu-manteiga). Rev Bras Ter Intensiva 2013;25(4):348–51.
34. Bedry R, Baudrimont I, Deffieux G, et al. Wild-mushroom intoxication as a cause of rhabdomyolysis. N Engl J Med 2001;345(11):798–802.
35. Laubner G, Mikulevičienė G. A series of cases of rhabdomyolysis after ingestion of Tricholoma equestre. Acta Med Litu 2016;23(3):193–7.
36. Nguyen HN, Chenoweth JA, Bebarta VS, et al. The toxicity, pathophysiology, and treatment of acute hydrazine propellant exposure: a systematic review. Mil Med 2021;186(3-4):e319–26.
37. Li F, Chen AB, Duan YC, et al. Multiple organ dysfunction and rhabdomyolysis associated with moonwort poisoning: report of four cases. World J Clin Cases 2020;8(2):479–86.
38. Trancă SD, Szabo R, Cociș M. Acute poisoning due to ingestion of Datura stramonium - a case report. Rom J Anaesth Intensive Care 2017;24(1):65–8.
39. Boccuzzi SJ, Bocanegra TS, Walker JF, et al. Long-term safety and efficacy profile of simvastatin. Am J Cardiol 1991;68(11):1127–31.
40. Pasternak RC, Smith SC, Bairey-Merz CN, et al. American College of Cardiology. American Heart Association. National Heart, Lung and Blood Institute. ACC/AHA/NHLBI clinical advisory on the use and safety of statins. Stroke 2002;33(9):2337–41.
41. Coco TJ, Klasner AE. Drug-induced rhabdomyolysis. Curr Opin Pediatr 2004;16(2):206–10.
42. Denis D, Lamireau T, Llanas B, et al. Rhabdomyolysis in European viper bite. Acta Paediatr 1998;87(9):1013–5.
43. Akdur O, Can S, Afacan G. Rhabdomyolysis secondary to bee sting. Case Rep Emerg Med 2013;2013:258421.
44. Hubbard JJ, James LP. Complications and outcomes of brown recluse spider bites in children. Clin Pediatr (Phila) 2011;50(3):252–8.

Common Presentations of Rare Drug Reactions and Atypical Presentations of Common Drug Reactions in the Intensive Care Unit

Justinn M. Tanem, MD[a,b], John P. Scott, MD[a,b],*

KEYWORDS

• Adverse drug reactions • Medication errors • Pediatric critical care

KEY POINTS

• Adverse drug reactions (ADRs) are extremely common.
• Outcomes range from mild symptoms to death.
• Every organ system may be involved.
• Children are at unique risk of ADRs because of age-dependent changes in pharmacokinetics and off-label prescribing.
• These risks are magnified in critical illness.

INTRODUCTION

Clinicians in the intensive care unit (ICU) must be facile in the diagnosis and management of rare disorders. The pace and complexity of patient care in this environment can create a burdensome cognitive load, which increases the risk of errors.[1] Diagnostic errors occur in approximately 5% to 20% of all patient encounters because of many systemic factors, and have been discovered in 28% of autopsies of patients who died in the intensive care unit.[2,3] The lethality of these errors directly correlates with the level of patient acuity.[4] Unintended secondary consequences of diagnostic

Conflicts: J.M Tanem and J.P. Scott reported no conflicts of interest.
[a] Department of Anesthesiology, Section of Pediatric Anesthesiology, Medical College of Wisconsin, 9000 W Wisconsin Avenue, Milwaukee, WI 53122, USA; [b] Department of Pediatrics, Section of Pediatric Critical Care, Medical College of Wisconsin, 9000 W Wisconsin Avenue, Milwaukee, WI 53122, USA
* Corresponding author. Anesthesiology and Pediatrics, Medical College of Wisconsin, 9000 W Wisconsin Avenue, Milwaukee, WI 53122.
E-mail address: scottjake@mcw.edu

Crit Care Clin 38 (2022) 287–299
https://doi.org/10.1016/j.ccc.2021.11.005   **criticalcare.theclinics.com**
0749-0704/22/© 2021 Elsevier Inc. All rights reserved.

errors and adverse patient outcomes include cognitive strain and burnout among intensivists, further increasing the risk of future medical errors and safety events.[5–8]

Adverse drug reactions (ADRs) represent a common form of iatrogenic injury. Left undetected, ADRs may significantly impact patient outcomes. As with diagnostic errors, there is a relationship between acuity of illness and the likelihood of ADR occurrence.[9] It is estimated that patients in the ICU experience 1.7 errors per day, and most experience a potentially life-threatening error during their ICU stay.[10,11]

Critically ill children are at unique risk for ADRs because of age-dependent changes in drug pharmacokinetics, especially volume of distribution and plasma clearance. These age-dependent differences in drug pharmacokinetics and pharmacodynamics are most pronounced in the first few years of life.[12] Many medications administered to children are prescribed off label because of inadequate testing in the pediatric age group.[13] These factors serve to increase ADR risk in children, even more so in critically ill children with coexistent organ dysfunction that impacts drug clearance. This article describes common ADRs in critically ill children according to the organ system involvement.

NEUROLOGIC

Acute neurologic dysfunction in critical illness encompasses a spectrum of conditions ranging from delirium to brain death. Features include acute alterations in mental status and consciousness that are not psychogenic in nature.[14] Although acute neurologic dysfunction is infrequently the chief complaint, over 80% of mechanically ventilated patients experience delirium during their ICU stay, increasing the risk of prolonged hospital length of stay, mortality, and cost.[15,16]

Delirium, defined as an acute disturbance of consciousness, attentiveness, cognition, or perception that fluctuates over time, can be categorized as hyperactive, hypoactive, or mixed.[17] Delirium is the most frequently observed form of acute neurologic dysfunction in the ICU and is frequently medication induced. The list of underlying etiologies is broad and includes systemic conditions as well as primary neurologic insults, injuries, and drug reactions. Medication exposure represents one of the few modifiable causes of delirium, as sedative-hypnotic medications, especially benzodiazepines, have been linked to the development of delirium.[15,18] Because of this association, the Society of Critical Care Medicine recently released the ICU Liberation Bundle, aimed at reducing medication-associated delirium, specifically focusing on benzodiazepines.[19] The results have been mixed, as a recent meta-analysis including 26,384 patients failed to demonstrate a decrease in incidence or duration of delirium in the ICU.[20] Treatment of medication-induced delirium includes discontinuation of the inciting medications and administration of antipsychotic medications. A Cochrane review demonstrated efficacy of antipsychotic medications in the postoperative period; however, more recent data question this conclusion.[21,22] The adverse effect profile of antipsychotic medications also poses problems for the intensivist, as high-dose haloperidol has been linked to extrapyramidal symptoms (EPS).[22] Additionally, hyperactive delirium may confound the picture, as the physical manifestations of EPS may mimic worsening delirium.[23]

Although seizures and status epilepticus (SE) occur frequently in critically ill patients, drug-induced seizures account for less than 5% of cases.[24] Various drug classes have been implicated in the development of seizures, including gamma-aminobutyric acid (GABA) antagonists (e.g., flumazenil). Antiepileptic drugs (AEDs) that occasionally exhibit paradoxic proconvulsant properties include phenytoin, carbamazepine, and lamotrigine, particularly in the setting of inappropriately treated idiopathic generalized epilepsies.[24] Antidepressant medications work through antagonism of GABA, hista-mine, or adenosine; stimulation of cholinergic or glutaminergic receptors; or the pre-vention of biogenic amine degradation resulting in increased concentration of excitatory neurotransmitters in the brain with resultant risk of seizures.[25] When consid-ering antidepressant-induced SE, the intensivist must take into account the half-life of the culprit medication, as certain medications may require treatment over several days.[26] Over 80% of patients admitted to the ICU are prescribed antibiotics, especially cephalosporins.[27] Cephalosporin-induced neurotoxicity has been well documented, with seizures occurring in over 10% of patients, and the mechanism likely resulting from a decrease in the release of GABA from presynaptic nerve terminals.[24,28] Other implicated medications include quinolones, macrolides, and multiple immunologic and chemotherapeutic agents.[24]

CARDIOVASCULAR

Cardiogenic shock represents the most severe form of circulatory failure, with a re-ported incidence of approximately 6%. Associated mortality rates have declined but remain over 40%.[29] The most common etiologies of cardiogenic shock include decompensated heart failure, cardiac arrest, and acute myocardial infarction (AMI). The intensivist must also consider other causes of myocardial dysfunction including cardiomyopathies, which can be drug induced. Drug-induced myocardial dysfunction may be secondary to deleterious effects on preload, afterload, or cardiac contrac-tility.[30] Many medications administered in the ICU, especially sedative-hypnotic agents, impact cardiac output and oxygen delivery through changes in vascular tone (e.g., preload or afterload) and myocardial contractility.

Patients with malignancies who have received anthracycline chemotherapeutic agents (e.g., doxorubicin and daunorubicin) may present to the ICU because of heart failure.[31] The pathogenesis of heart failure in this population is caused by oxygen radical formation, intracellular calcium overload, and interruption of aerobic metabolism, and has been described in detail elsewhere.[32] Despite the clinical benefits of chemothera-peutic regimens, there is no safe dose of anthracyclines, which cause irreversible car-diac toxicity in a dose-dependent fashion.[31,33] Although anthracyclines are the classic cardiotoxic chemotherapeutic agent, others have been linked to cardiac toxicity including cyclophosphamide, paclitaxel, mitoxantrone, 5-flurouracil, and cytarabine.[30]

Medications used to treat cardiovascular conditions are also associated with the development of cardiac dysfunction. Of these, antiarrhythmics must be treated with caution by the intensivist, with class I, II, and IV implicated because of their effects on intracellular calcium concentration.[34] Large randomized controlled trials demon-strate increased risk of heart failure in patients treated with antiarrhythmics. This poses therapeutic challenges, as many patients with heart failure require antiar-rhythmic therapy to control ventricular and supraventricular dysrhythmias.[35–37] Cal-cium channel blockers also intrinsically compromise cardiac function and result in the activation of the renin-angiotensin system.[38] Beta-blockers, now widely used in the treatment of congestive heart failure, can have a direct myocardial depressant ef-fect in the acute setting, and require deliberate titration by the clinician.[39,40] Conversely, beta-agonism may paradoxically augment myocardial dysfunction, with case reports of acute myocardial infarction and Takotsubo cardiomyopathy resulting from excessive albuterol administration.[41,42] Takotsubo cardiomyopathy is typified by systolic apical ballooning, which initially was thought to resemble a Japanese octopus fishing pot, or takotsubo. This cardiomyopathy is hypothesized to be stress induced, as two-thirds of patients experienced a physical or psychological stressor before developing cardiac dysfunction.[43] The exact causative physiologic mechanism is still unknown, but supraphysiologic levels of catecholamines have been observed in these patients, which raises plausible explanations such as catecholamine-induced vasospasm, sympathetically mediated microcirculatory dysfunction, or direct catecholamine-induced myocyte injury through cyclic-AMP-mediated calcium overload and the generation of reactive oxygen species.[44] Treatment is primarily supportive; however, exogenous catecholamines, including albuterol, should be used with caution given the postulated pathophysiology.

Procedural sedation for invasive procedures (e.g., tracheal intubation or central venous line placement) in children requires administration of sedative hypnotic and analgesic medications that may compromise cardiovascular function. Although the volatile anesthetics universally depress myocardial function, they are rarely used in the ICU.[45] The cyclohexamine ketamine has gained popularity and works primarily via noncompetitive antagonism of the NMDA receptor and is classified as a dissociative amnestic because of its ability to preserve airway reflexes and respiratory drive while providing adequate analgesia and sedation during painful procedures.[46] Ketamine prevents catecholamine reuptake, which may preserve hemodynamics following administration; however, the drug also possesses direct myocardial depressant properties.[46–48] Thus, ketamine should be used with caution in critically ill patients with depleted endogenous catecholamine stores.[49]

Brugada syndrome is a genetic cardiomyopathy linked to increased risk of ventricular arrhythmias and sudden cardiac death (SCD) in the absence of structural heart disease with an incidence of approximately 1/5 to 10,000.[50] Pathogenic variants in the *SCN5A* gene, which encodes the alpha-subunit of the cardiac sodium channel, result in inactivation of the channel, and a decrease in sodium trafficking during the initiation of an action potential (phase 0); they are implicated in approximately 30% of patients with Brugada syndrome. However, several other genes have also been implicated.[51] Precipitation of arrhythmias in patients with Brugada syndrome can occur with hyperthermia/fever (most common), hyperkalemia, hypokalemia, hypercalcemia, and alcohol. Medications utilized in the ICU setting can also precipitate arrhythmias, with cocaine, sodium channel blockers, tricyclic antidepressants, and certain local anesthetics (e.g., bupivacaine) implicated; such medications should be avoided in patients with Brugada syndrome.[51] Although propofol has been reported to precipitate arrhythmias when administered as an infusion in patients with Brugada syndrome, the use of a single induction dose of propofol likely does not increase the risk of ventricular arrhythmia.[51,52] Symptomatic patients should be treated with an implantable automatic defibrillator (ICD).

PULMONARY

The epidemiology, pathogenesis, and treatment of acute respiratory failure have taken on a new and special interest following the global pandemic caused by SARS-CoV-2. Acute respiratory failure historically is a common disease state with a prevalence of over 50% in adult ICUs.[53] The incidence of the most severe manifestation, acute respiratory distress syndrome (ARDS) in adults and pediatric acute respiratory distress syndrome (pARDS) in children, is 78.9 cases per 100,000 person years and 3.5 cases per 100,000 person years, respectively.[54,55] The underlying etiology of ARDS is predominantly caused by pneumonia (40%), with additional significant contributors being sepsis (32%) and aspiration pneumonia/pneumonitis (9%); however, several rare pathologies and medication adverse effects must be considered when a patient presents with ARDS to the ICU.[56]

Pulmonary alveolar proteinosis (PAP) is a rare disease characterized by accumulation of pulmonary surfactants within the alveoli.[57] In general, PAP can be categorized into 3 groups: congenital, secondary, and acquired, with the acquired form accounting for over 90% of cases.[58] Drugs that cause immunosuppression and impair alveolar macrophages are primarily implicated, including chemotherapeutic regimens.[57] Clinically, these patients may present with dyspnea that is insidious in onset along with nonproductive cough and tachypnea; however, approximately 15% of patients require intubation and mechanical ventilation at presentation.[59]

Amiodarone, a class III antiarrhythmic widely used in the treatment of ventricular and supraventricular tachycardias, has been associated with the development of significant pulmonary toxicity.[60] Lung toxicity occurs in up to 5% of patients who receive amiodarone, which has a prolonged half-life of 8 to 102 days.[60] Clinically, toxicity can occur as early as 2 days following administration and can cause a spectrum of disease ranging from bronchospasm, diffuse alveolar hemorrhage, lipoid pneumonia, and pulmonary fibrosis, to ARDS.[61] Risk factors for developing pulmonary toxicity include age, total dose, cardiothoracic surgery, and high fraction of inspired oxygen.[61] Careful patient selection, including precreening diffusion capacity, has been advocated, along with monitoring for pulmonary toxicity including chest roentgenograms following administration.[60] Treatment includes discontinuation of amiodarone and corticosteroids in severe cases.[62]

In August of 2019, the US Centers for Disease Control and Prevention (CDC), the US Food and Drug Administration, and state/local health departments began investigating an outbreak of e-cigarette vaping-associated lung injury (EVALI).[63] Clinically, this entity consists of dyspnea, chest pain, coughing, hemoptysis, nausea, vomiting, abdominal pain, fever, and malaise within 90 days of electronic cigarette use, with pulmonary infiltrates on chest imaging and absence of alternative etiologies.[64] As of Feb. 18, 2020, 2807 patients were hospitalized with EVALI, with approximately one-third of patients requiring intubation and mechanical ventilation at presentation; 68 died.[64–66] A pathophysiological correlation has been identified through bronchoalveolar lavage samples between vitamin E acetate, used as a thickening agent in tetrahydrocannabinol (THC)-containing products, and development of EVALI.[67] Vitamin E acetate interacts with phospholipids contained within surfactant, which may increase alveolar permeability and decrease surfactant function with subsequent generation of an inflammatory cascade.[63] Treatment of EVALI is largely supportive; however, systemic corticosteroids have been demonstrated to improve respiratory status in 65% of patients.[64] The diagnosis of EVALI has been significantly complicated with the concomitant coronavirus 2019 (COVID-19) pandemic, as both entities present similarly. Additionally, given the evolving demands of the pandemic, the CDC stopped issuing updates on the EVALI outbreak.[66] These 2 evolving public health crises may be related in certain populations and must be carefully considered, as demonstrated by the five-fold increase in COVID-19 disease in patients who report electronic cigarette use.[68]

HEPATIC

The liver functions as a major organ of drug metabolism and clearance. Critically ill patients may have hepatic dysfunction of an acute or chronic nature, with resultant alterations in drug metabolism and subsequent risk of ADR development. Furthermore, developmental changes in hepatic enzymatic activity and plasma-binding protein synthesis are responsible for age-dependent differences in drug clearance.[69] These processes are immature in infants and toddlers and increase the risk of ADRs in these age groups.

Medications administered in the ICU may be directly hepatoxic. Drug-induced liver injury (DILI) is particularly important to consider in the setting of acute liver injury in the absence of previous liver disease. The development of DILI depends on patient- and drug-related factors. The classic medication implicated in acute DILI is acetaminophen, with toxicity occurring in a dose-dependent fashion. Other hepatotoxic medications include antibiotics, nonsteroidal anti-inflammatory drugs (NSAIDs), and antiepileptic drugs. The spectrum of DILI ranges from mild elevation in transaminases to fulminant hepatic failure requiring liver transplant. Diagnosis relies on the biochemical assays, advanced imaging, and liver biopsy, as well as exclusion of other mechanisms of injury. Pathologic features of DILI include hepatocellular injury and cholestatic or mixed patterns of injury.[70] Left unrecognized and untreated, DILI may progress to fulminant hepatic failure with end-stage liver disease and necessitate liver transplantation.

METABOLIC

Metabolic derangements, frequent in critical illness, may be the manifestation of ADRs and include hypermetabolic syndromes (malignant hyperthermia, serotonin syndrome, and neuroleptic malignant syndrome) as well as drug-induced mitochondrial dysfunction.

Malignant Hyperthermia

Malignant hyperthermia (MH) is a hypermetabolic syndrome provoked by sustained release of calcium from the sarcoplasmic reticulum of skeletal muscle following exposure to a triggering agent including volatile anesthetic agents or the depolarizing neuromuscular blocking agent succinylcholine.[71] The most common responsible pathogenic variant is inherited in autosomal-dominant fashion and involves the gene encoding the ryanodine receptor of skeletal muscle. Males tend to be more susceptible than females; most cases occur in otherwise phenotypically normal patients.[72] Following exposure to a triggering agent, sustained contraction of skeletal muscle leads to cellular energy depletion and rhabdomyolysis. Left untreated, MH may progress to multiorgan dysfunction, ventricular arrhythmias, and death. Observed biochemical abnormalities include combined respiratory and metabolic acidosis, hyperkalemia, and increased creatine phosphokinase. A review of the North American Malignant Hyperthermia Registry revealed that the most common presenting signs and symptoms in children are tachycardia, hypercarbia, and hyperthermia, with some age-dependent variation in clinical characteristics.[72] Older children tend to have higher peak temperature and serum potassium levels, while the youngest children demonstrate more profound metabolic acidosis.[72]

The incidence of MH has declined over time with the reduced use of the depolarizing neuromuscular blocker succinylcholine, especially during the conduct of pediatric anesthesia care. More importantly, mortality rates have declined to less than 5% from over 70%, because of improved recognition and development of a definitive treatment with dantrolene.[73] Management of MH starts with prompt discontinuation of all triggering agents and administration of dantrolene (2.5 mg/kg intravenously every 5 minutes up to 10 mg/kg until abatement of symptoms). Other supportive interventions include hyperventilation with 100% oxygen, active cooling, and management of hyperkalemia with insulin, bicarbonate, and glucose.

Patients at risk for developing MH include those who have a muscle biopsy positive for a caffeine halothane contracture test, previous episode of MH, first-degree relative with history of MH, and children with myopathies or central core disease. Anesthetic management of patients at risk for MH should include strict avoidance of succinylcholine and volatile anesthetics, with intravenous induction agents including propofol, benzodiazepines, opiates, and depolarizing muscle relaxants considered safer. Pretreatment with dantrolene is not recommended in MH-susceptible individuals.

Serotonin Syndrome

Increased prescribing of selective serotonin reuptake inhibitors (SSRIs) and selective serotonin/norepinephrine reuptake inhibitors (SNRIs) for the management of psychiatric illness and nonpsychiatric conditions (e.g., migraines) has been associated with increased incidence of serotonin syndrome. Although SSRIs and SNRIs increase serum serotonin levels through prevention of reuptake at the synapse, other medications increase serotonin activity through amplified release of stored serotonin, production of serotonin, stimulation of serotonin receptors, or prevention of serotonin metabolism. Signs and symptoms of serotonin syndrome include altered mental status, autonomic changes (e.g., tachycardia, hypertension, or hyperthermia) and muscle rigidity.[74] Outcomes range from mild disease to death. Treatment includes discontinuation of all serotonergic agents and other supportive therapies.

Neuroleptic Malignant Syndrome

Similar to serotonin syndrome, neuroleptic malignant syndrome (NMS) is a rare consequence of treatment with psychiatric medications, most commonly observed in patients receiving atypical antipsychotic medications. Presenting signs and symptoms consist of hypermetabolic findings including tachycardia, muscle rigidity, and autonomic lability.[75] Treatment incudes prompt discontinuation of triggering medications and administration of bromocriptine, which has been shown to shorten duration of symptoms.[75] As with serotonin syndrome, outcomes may be fatal in severe cases; however, unlike serotonin syndrome, symptoms may persist following the discontinuation of triggering medications.[76]

Drug-Induced Mitochondrial Dysfunction

Mitochondrial dysfunction in critically ill patients is common even in the absence of diagnosed mitochondrial disorders.[77,78] Mitochondria are essential elements of cellular energy production generating adenosine triphosphate via the electron transport chain. Mitochondria contain their own DNA, which is released following cellular injury in critical illnesses such as sepsis and trauma. This mitochondrial cell-free DNA (mcfDNA) functions as a component and trigger of inflammation. Mitochondria also play a critical role in the manifestation of many ADRs,[79] as many commonly prescribed medications negatively impact mitochondrial function. Mechanisms of drug-induced mitochondrial dysfunction include direct inhibition of mitochondrial respiration with the electron transport chain and ATP generation, or indirectly through reactive oxygen species that alter mitochondrial DNA. Drugs that have been shown to have negative impact on mitochondrial function include NSAIDs, antibiotics, antipsychotics, antidepressants, and general and local anesthetic agents. Organ systems affected by drug-induced mitochondrial dysfunction include the heart, liver, and kidneys.[80]

Propofol is an short-acting intravenous anesthetic used in the ICU to produce hypnosis and sedation in a dose-dependent fashion.[81] Despite its utility, prolonged administration can result in propofol infusion syndrome (PRIS).[82] PRIS is characterized by acute metabolic acidosis, rhabdomyolysis, renal failure, and hypertriglyceridemia, culminating in cardiac dysfunction.[82] The pathophysiology stems from inhibition of mitochondrial oxidative phosphorylation and free fatty acid utilization, resulting in lactic acidosis and cellular injury.[83] Because of low baseline glycogen stores and reliance on fat metabolism, children are at increased risk for propofol infusion syndrome.[84] Risk factors for PRIS include infusions exceeding 4 mg/kg/h for greater than 48 hours, sepsis, elevated catecholamine states, elevated glucocorticoid levels, and low carbohydrate energy substrate levels.[85] The inhibition of oxidative phosphorylation requires consideration when providing sedation to patients with mitochondrial disorders, although propofol has been used with success in this vulnerable patient population.[86] Treatment is largely supportive, and the clinical focus should be on prevention with monitoring of blood lactate, creatinine kinase, and triglyceride levels; however, elevations may be a late finding in the development of this syndrome.[82,87]

CUTANEOUS

Cutaneous reactions are the most common ADRs in children, ranging from simple rashes to potentially life-threatening blistering skin reactions with systemic disease such Steven Johnson Syndrome (SJS) and toxic epidermal necrolysis (TEN). The diagnosis of cutaneous ADRs is complicated by the high frequency of viral infections in children, who may often present with exanthems.[88]

Stevens Johnson Syndrome and Toxic Epidermal Necrolysis

The spectrum of severe cutaneous ADRs that involve blistering of the skin and mucous membranes and systemic disease include SJS and TEN. These are delayed drug hypersensitivity reactions that present several days after constitutional symptoms that may be mistaken for a viral prodrome[89] and lead to a delay in diagnosis. The rash characteristically begins along the trunk and face before spreading to the extremities. The presence of pseudo-Nikolsky sign is pathognomonic for TEN and SJS, demonstrated when gentle pressure with a finger on skin denudes the upper layer of the epidermis because of underlying necrosis.[90] The pathophysiologic mechanism of SJS/TEN development involves activation of CD8+ T lymphocytes, triggering an immunologic response with cytokine activation against keratinocytes leading to cell death and the development of extensive bullae.

The percent of total body surface area (TBSA) involvement is used to differentiate SJS from TEN; less than 10% of TBSA is consistent with SJS, and greater than 30% is consistent with TEN, with SJS-TEN syndrome overlap for TBSA involvement ranging from 10% to 30%. Because of the greater TBSA involvement, the mortality rate associated with TEN approaches 25%. Drugs implicated include certain antibiotics (e.g., sulfonamides, penicillin, and isoniazid) and anticonvulsants (e.g., phenytoin, phenobarbital, carbamazepine, and valproic acid). Treatment of involves prompt discontinuation of the responsible medication and supportive treatment.

SUMMARY

The pathophysiology of ADRs in the critically ill patient is multifactorial and may affect every organ system, with a spectrum of severity ranging from mild symptoms to lethality. It is therefore incumbent on the ICU clinician to remain vigilant to maintain patient safety through the efficient and effective diagnosis and treatment of ADRs.

CLINICS CARE POINTS

- Adverse drug events (ADRs) represent one of the most common forms of iatrogenic injury.
- Critically ill children have increased risk for ADRs because of age-dependent changes in drug pharmacokinetics and off-label prescribing.

REFERENCE

1. Monsell S. Task switching. Trends Cogn Sci 2003;7(3):134–40.
2. Ball JR, Balogh E. Improving diagnosis in health care: highlights of a report from the national academies of sciences, engineering, and medicine. Ann Intern Med 2016;164(1):59–61.
3. Winters B, et al. Diagnostic errors in the intensive care unit: a systematic review of autopsy studies. BMJ Qual Saf 2012;21(11):894–902.
4. Saber Tehrani AS, et al. 25-Year summary of US malpractice claims for diagnostic errors 1986-2010: an analysis from the National Practitioner Data Bank. BMJ Qual Saf 2013;22(8):672–80.
5. Moss M, et al. An official critical care societies collaborative statement: burnout syndrome in critical care healthcare professionals: a call for action. Crit Care Med 2016;44(7):1414–21.
6. Shanafelt TD, et al. Burnout and medical errors among American surgeons. Ann Surg 2010;251(6):995–1000.
7. Bergl PA, Nanchal RS, Singh H. Diagnostic error in the critically iii: defining the problem and exploring next steps to advance intensive care unit safety. Ann Am Thorac Soc 2018;15(8):903–7.
8. Rothschild JM, et al. The Critical Care Safety Study: the incidence and nature of adverse events and serious medical errors in intensive care. Crit Care Med 2005; 33(8):1694–700.
9. Giraud T, et al. Iatrogenic complications in adult intensive care units: a prospective two-center study. Crit Care Med 1993;21(1):40–51.
10. Donchin Y, et al. A look into the nature and causes of human errors in the intensive care unit. Crit Care Med 1995;23(2):294–300.
11. Pronovost PJ, et al. Defining and measuring patient safety. Crit Care Clin 2005; 21(1):1–19, vii.
12. Lu H, Rosenbaum S. Developmental pharmacokinetics in pediatric populations. J Pediatr Pharmacol Ther 2014;19(4):262–76.
13. Napoleone E. Children and ADRs (adverse drug reactions). Ital J Pediatr 2010; 36:4.
14. Stevens RD, Pronovost PJ. The spectrum of encephalopathy in critical illness. Semin Neurol 2006;26(4):440–51.
15. Ely EW, et al. Delirium as a predictor of mortality in mechanically ventilated patients in the intensive care unit. JAMA 2004;291(14):1753–62.
16. Milbrandt EB, et al. Costs associated with delirium in mechanically ventilated patients. Crit Care Med 2004;32(4):955–62.
17. Miller RR 3rd, Ely EW. Delirium and cognitive dysfunction in the intensive care unit. Semin Respir Crit Care Med 2006;27(3):210–20.
18. Pandharipande P, et al. Lorazepam is an independent risk factor for transitioning to delirium in intensive care unit patients. Anesthesiology 2006;104(1):21–6.
19. Ely EW. The ABCDEF bundle: science and philosophy of how icu liberation serves patients and families. Crit Care Med 2017;45(2):321–30.
20. Zhang S, et al. Effectiveness of bundle interventions on ICU delirium: a meta-analysis. Crit Care Med 2021;49(2):335–46.
21. Girard TD, et al. Haloperidol and ziprasidone for treatment of delirium in critical illness. N Engl J Med 2018;379(26):2506–16.
22. Lonergan E, et al. Antipsychotics for delirium. Cochrane Database Syst Rev 2007;(2):CD005594.

23. Caroff SN, Campbell EC. Drug-induced extrapyramidal syndromes: implications for contemporary practice. Psychiatr Clin North Am 2016;39(3):391–411.
24. Cock HR. Drug-induced status epilepticus. Epilepsy Behav 2015;49:76–82.
25. Judge BS, Rentmeester LL. Antidepressant overdose-induced seizures. Psychiatr Clin North Am 2013;36(2):245–60.
26. Madi L, O'Brien AA, Fennell J. Status epilepticus secondary to fluoxetine. Postgrad Med J 1994;70(823):383–4.
27. Anand N, et al. Antimicrobial agents' utilization and cost pattern in an intensive care unit of a teaching hospital in South India. Indian J Crit Care Med 2016; 20(5):274–9.
28. Grill MF, Maganti R. Cephalosporin-induced neurotoxicity: clinical manifestations, potential pathogenic mechanisms, and the role of electroencephalographic monitoring. Ann Pharmacother 2008;42(12):1843–50.
29. Puymirat E, et al. Cardiogenic shock in intensive care units: evolution of prevalence, patient profile, management and outcomes, 1997-2012. Eur J Heart Fail 2017;19(2):192–200.
30. Feenstra J, et al. Drug-induced heart failure. J Am Coll Cardiol 1999;33(5): 1152–62.
31. Rhoden W, Hasleton P, Brooks N. Anthracyclines and the heart. Br Heart J 1993; 70(6):499–502.
32. Fu LX, Waagstein F, Hjalmarson A. A new insight into adriamycin-induced cardiotoxicity. Int J Cardiol 1990;29(1):15–20.
33. Saini J, Rich MW, Lyss AP. Reversibility of severe left ventricular dysfunction due to doxorubicin cardiotoxicity. Report of three cases. Ann Intern Med 1987;106(6): 814–6.
34. Schlepper M. Cardiodepressive effects of antiarrhythmic drugs. Eur Heart J 1989;10(Suppl E):73–80.
35. Hammermeister KE. Adverse hemodynamic effects of antiarrhythmic drugs in congestive heart failure. Circulation 1990;81(3):1151–3.
36. Pharand C, et al. Lidocaine prophylaxis for fatal ventricular arrhythmias after acute myocardial infarction. Clin Pharmacol Ther 1995;57(4):471–8.
37. Greene HL, et al. Congestive heart failure after acute myocardial infarction in patients receiving antiarrhythmic agents for ventricular premature complexes (Cardiac Arrhythmia Pilot Study). Am J Cardiol 1989;63(7):393–8.
38. Packer M. Pathophysiological mechanisms underlying the adverse effects of calcium channel-blocking drugs in patients with chronic heart failure. Circulation 1989;80(6 Suppl):IV59–67.
39. Packer M, et al. Double-blind, placebo-controlled study of the effects of carvedilol in patients with moderate to severe heart failure. The PRECISE Trial. Prospective Randomized Evaluation of Carvedilol on Symptoms and Exercise. Circulation 1996;94(11):2793–9.
40. Packer M, et al. The effect of carvedilol on morbidity and mortality in patients with chronic heart failure. U.S. Carvedilol Heart Failure Study Group. N Engl J Med 1996;334(21):1349–55.
41. Fisher AA, Davis MW, McGill DA. Acute myocardial infarction associated with albuterol. Ann Pharmacother 2004;38(12):2045–9.
42. Patel B, et al. Repeated use of albuterol inhaler as a potential cause of takotsubo cardiomyopathy. Am J Case Rep 2014;15:221–5.
43. Gianni M, et al. Apical ballooning syndrome or takotsubo cardiomyopathy: a systematic review. Eur Heart J 2006;27(13):1523–9.

44. Wittstein IS, et al. Neurohumoral features of myocardial stunning due to sudden emotional stress. N Engl J Med 2005;352(6):539–48.
45. McKinney MS, Fee JP, Clarke RS. Cardiovascular effects of isoflurane and halothane in young and elderly adult patients. Br J Anaesth 1993;71(5):696–701.
46. Hurth KP, et al. The reemergence of ketamine for treatment in critically ill adults. Crit Care Med 2020;48(6):899–911.
47. Sprung J, et al. Effects of ketamine on the contractility of failing and nonfailing human heart muscles in vitro. Anesthesiology 1998;88(5):1202–10.
48. Pagel PS, et al. Ketamine depresses myocardial contractility as evaluated by the preload recruitable stroke work relationship in chronically instrumented dogs with autonomic nervous system blockade. Anesthesiology 1992;76(4):564–72.
49. Dewhirst E, et al. Cardiac arrest following ketamine administration for rapid sequence intubation. J Intensive Care Med 2013;28(6):375–9.
50. Antzelevitch C, et al. Brugada syndrome: report of the second consensus conference. Heart Rhythm 2005;2(4):429–40.
51. Brugada J, et al. Present status of Brugada syndrome: JACC state-of-the-art review. J Am Coll Cardiol 2018;72(9):1046–59.
52. Flamee P, et al. Electrocardiographic effects of propofol versus etomidate in patients with Brugada syndrome. Anesthesiology 2020;132(3):440–51.
53. Franca SA, et al. The epidemiology of acute respiratory failure in hospitalized patients: a Brazilian prospective cohort study. J Crit Care 2011;26(3):330.e1-8.
54. Schouten LR, et al. Incidence and mortality of acute respiratory distress syndrome in children: a systematic review and meta-analysis. Crit Care Med 2016;44(4):819–29.
55. Rubenfeld GD, et al. Incidence and outcomes of acute lung injury. N Engl J Med 2005;353(16):1685–93.
56. Zilberberg MD, Epstein SK. Acute lung injury in the medical ICU: comorbid conditions, age, etiology, and hospital outcome. Am J Respir Crit Care Med 1998;157(4 Pt 1):1159–64.
57. Trapnell BC, Whitsett JA, Nakata K. Pulmonary alveolar proteinosis. N Engl J Med 2003;349(26):2527–39.
58. deMello DE, Lin Z. Pulmonary alveolar proteinosis: a review. Pediatr Pathol Mol Med 2001;20(5):413–32.
59. Hildebrandt J, et al. Characterization of CSF2RA mutation related juvenile pulmonary alveolar proteinosis. Orphanet J Rare Dis 2014;9:171.
60. Mason JW. Amiodarone. N Engl J Med 1987;316(8):455–66.
61. Papiris SA, et al. Amiodarone: review of pulmonary effects and toxicity. Drug Saf 2010;33(7):539–58.
62. Esinger W, et al. [Steroid-refractory amiodarone-induced pulmonary fibrosis. Clinical features and morphology after an amiodarone-free interval of 3 months]. Dtsch Med Wochenschr 1988;113(42):1638–41.
63. Winnicka L, Shenoy MA. EVALI and the pulmonary toxicity of electronic cigarettes: a review. J Gen Intern Med 2020;35(7):2130–5.
64. Layden JE, et al. Pulmonary illness related to E-cigarette use in Illinois and Wisconsin - final report. N Engl J Med 2020;382(10):903–16.
65. Werner AK, et al. Hospitalizations and deaths associated with EVALI. N Engl J Med 2020;382(17):1589–98.
66. The Lancet Respiratory, M., the EVALI outbreak and vaping in the COVID-19 era. Lancet Respir Med 2020;8(9):831.

67. Blount BC, et al. Evaluation of bronchoalveolar lavage fluid from patients in an outbreak of e-cigarette, or vaping, product use-associated lung injury - 10 states, August-October 2019. MMWR Morb Mortal Wkly Rep 2019;68(45): 1040–1.

68. Callahan SJ, et al. Diagnosing EVALI in the time of COVID-19. Chest 2020;158(5): 2034–7.

69. Krekels EHJ, et al. Chapter 8 - hepatic drug metabolism in pediatric patients. In: Xie W, editor. Drug metabolism in diseases. Boston: Academic Press; 2017. p. 181–206.

70. Licata A. Adverse drug reactions and organ damage: the liver. Eur J Intern Med 2016;28:9–16.

71. Ellinas H, Albrecht MA. Malignant hyperthermia update. Anesthesiol Clin 2020; 38(1):165–81.

72. Nelson P, Litman RS. Malignant hyperthermia in children: an analysis of the North American malignant hyperthermia registry. Anesth Analg 2014;118(2): 369–74.

73. Rosero EB, et al. Trends and outcomes of malignant hyperthermia in the United States, 2000 to 2005. Anesthesiology 2009;110(1):89–94.

74. Kant S, Liebelt E. Recognizing serotonin toxicity in the pediatric emergency department. Pediatr Emerg Care 2012;28(8):817–21 [quiz: 822–4].

75. Neuhut R, Lindenmayer JP, Silva R. Neuroleptic malignant syndrome in children and adolescents on atypical antipsychotic medication: a review. J Child Adolesc Psychopharmacol 2009;19(4):415–22.

76. Silva RR, et al. Neuroleptic malignant syndrome in children and adolescents. J Am Acad Child Adolesc Psychiatry 1999;38(2):187–94.

77. Supinski GS, Schroder EA, Callahan LA. Mitochondria and critical illness. Chest 2020;157(2):310–22.

78. Mantzarlis K, Tsolaki V, Zakynthinos E. Role of oxidative stress and mitochondrial dysfunction in sepsis and potential therapies. Oxid Med Cell Longev 2017;2017: 5985209.

79. Szewczyk A, Wojtczak L. Mitochondria as a pharmacological target. Pharmacol Rev 2002;54(1):101–27.

80. Varga ZV, et al. Drug-induced mitochondrial dysfunction and cardiotoxicity. Am J Physiol Heart Circ Physiol 2015;309(9):H1453–67.

81. Fulton B, Sorkin EM. Propofol. An overview of its pharmacology and a review of its clinical efficacy in intensive care sedation. Drugs 1995;50(4):636–57.

82. Fudickar A, Bein B. Propofol infusion syndrome: update of clinical manifestation and pathophysiology. Minerva Anestesiol 2009;75(5):339–44.

83. Schenkman KA, Yan S. Propofol impairment of mitochondrial respiration in isolated perfused Guinea pig hearts determined by reflectance spectroscopy. Crit Care Med 2000;28(1):172–7.

84. Short TG, Young Y. Toxicity of intravenous anaesthetics. Best Pract Res Clin Anaesthesiol 2003;17(1):77–89.

85. Bray RJ. Propofol infusion syndrome in children. Paediatr Anaesth 1998;8(6): 491–9.

86. Niezgoda J, Morgan PG. Anesthetic considerations in patients with mitochondrial defects. Paediatr Anaesth 2013;23(9):785–93.

87. Veldhoen ES, Hartman BJ, van Gestel JP. Monitoring biochemical parameters as an early sign of propofol infusion syndrome: false feeling of security. Pediatr Crit Care Med 2009;10(2):e19–21.

88. Ramien M, Goldman JL. Pediatric SJS-TEN: where are we now? F1000Res 2020; 9. https://doi.org/10.12688/f1000research.20419.1.
89. Lerch M, et al. Current perspectives on Stevens-Johnson syndrome and toxic epidermal necrolysis. Clin Rev Allergy Immunol 2018;54(1):147–76.
90. Maity S, et al. Nikolsky's sign: a pathognomic boon. J Fam Med Prim Care 2020; 9(2):526–30.

Pediatric Acute Liver Failure

Catherine Larson-Nath, MD[a], Bernadette Vitola, MD, MPH[b],*

KEYWORDS

- Acute liver failure • Pediatric • Transplant

KEY POINTS

- Pediatric acute liver failure is a life-threatening process with many different causes that differ based on the age of the patient.
- Early supportive care and identification of the underlying cause of acute liver failure is paramount in optimizing outcomes and survival.
- Identification and management of hepatic encephalopathy is critical for children with acute liver failure.

Abbreviations	
ALF	acute liver failure
PALF	pediatric acute liver failure

INTRODUCTION

Pediatric acute liver failure (PALF) is a complex, life-threatening process characterized by coagulopathy and impaired hepatic function. The exact pathophysiology depends on the underlying cause, which can include infectious, toxic, immune-mediated, metabolic, and genetic causes. In up to 50% of cases the cause of PALF is unknown.[1,2]

Approximately 12% of liver transplants in the United States are for cases of ALF.[3] Any suspicion for PALF should lead to prompt referral to a pediatric liver transplant center. Although there is no specific definition for PALF, the following criteria established by the Pediatric Acute Liver Failure Study can be used as a guideline[4]:

- No known chronic liver disease and
- Hepatic encephalopathy (HE) and an international normalized ratio (INR) greater than 1.5 that does not correct with vitamin K administration or

a Department of Pediatrics, Division of Pediatric Gastroenterology, Hepatology, and Nutrition, University of Minnesota, 2450 Riverside Avenue, Minneapolis, MN 55454, USA; b Transplant Institute, Medstar Georgetown University Hospital, 3800 Reservoir Road, NW 2 PHC, Washington, DC 20007, USA
* Corresponding author.
E-mail address: bernadette.vitola@medstar.net

Crit Care Clin 38 (2022) 301–315
https://doi.org/10.1016/j.ccc.2021.11.015

- No HE and an INR greater than 2 that does not correct with vitamin K administration

Once identified, supportive care is paramount. When applicable, therapy directed at the underlying cause of liver failure can also improve outcomes.

PRESENTATION

PALF often has an insidious onset over days to weeks. Clinically PALF may present with evidence of failure of hepatic metabolic functions including jaundice, hypoglycemia, and encephalopathy. At other times PALF is diagnosed during evaluation for other symptoms such as abdominal pain or fever. PALF may present at any age, with 37% of cases being in children younger than 3 years.[1,4]

The cause of PALF varies with age. Younger children are more likely to develop liver failure from underlying metabolic disease, whereas teenagers are more likely to present with acetaminophen toxicity.[4] PALF may also present in the setting of decompensated underlying chronic liver disease. Signs that suggest chronic liver disease include a small hard liver, ascites, telangiectasias, and signs of portal hypertension including splenomegaly, thrombocytopenia, and varices.

The presence of coagulopathy secondary to hepatic synthetic dysfunction is a requisite to diagnose PALF. Other biochemical tests such as transaminases, bilirubin, and ammonia may have different patterns in PALF depending on the underlying cause. Recognition of these patterns, combined with the history and examination, help point to specific causes of liver failure (**Table 1**). For instance, severe hepatitis is most often associated with ischemia, acetaminophen toxicity, and amanita mushroom poisoning, whereas minimal elevations in transaminases is most often associated with some metabolic diseases and Wilson disease.

Hepatic Encephalopathy

Approximately 50% of children with PALF will have HE at presentation and another 10% will develop HE during their disease course.[5] Symptoms of early HE may be subtle, especially in infants and young children, and can include irritability, inconsolable crying, changes in feeding or sleep patterns, and declines in school performance. These symptoms progress to somnolence and coma as encephalopathy worsens (**Table 2**).[6,7]

Many children with HE will have elevated ammonia. The level of ammonia alone does not correlate with the severity of HE; therefore, both ammonia level and clinical signs are considered when diagnosing encephalopathy.[8] The subtle and nonspecific nature of symptoms of HE in infants and young children may easily be missed. Providers must have a high suspicion for its presence and a low threshold for using electroencephalogram to help with diagnosis.

Encephalopathy is more common at presentation and over the course of illness in children with nonacetaminophen causes of PALF compared with those with encephalopathy secondary to acetaminophen toxicity.[4] Children who have HE at presentation are more likely to undergo liver transplantation or die.[5] The absence of HE does not negate the possibility of negative outcomes although, as in one large study, 11% of children with PALF without encephalopathy underwent liver transplantation or died.[5]

DIFFERENTIAL DIAGNOSIS

A wide variety of pathologies lead to PALF (see **Table 1**). A detailed history and physical examination and comprehensive laboratory evaluation are critical for accurate and

Table 1
Etiology of and findings in pediatric acute liver failure (PALF)

		Age	ALT/AST	Labs Bilirubin	INR	Other	Clinical Findings	Biopsy	Disease Specific Treatment	% of PALF cases
Drugs and Toxins	Acetaminophen	Any Peak in adolescents from intentional overdose	↑↑↑	↑ - ↑↑↑	↑↑↑	+Tylenol level (not always detectable depending on timing of ingestion)	+/- history of overdose or chronic acetaminophen use	Centrilobular hepatic necrosis	N-acetylcysteine	13.3[a]
	Antiepileptics	Any	↑↑ - ↑↑↑	↑ - ↑↑↑	↑ - ↑↑↑		History of ingestion	Variable depending on drug	Supportive care Stop offending medication	3.2[a]
	Antibiotics	Any	↑↑ - ↑↑↑	↑ - ↑↑↑	↑ - ↑↑↑		History of ingestion	Variable depending on drug	Supportive care Stop offending medication	
	Iron	Any	↑ - ↑↑↑	↑ - ↑↑↑	↑ - ↑↑↑	Elevated blood iron level	Gastrointestinal symptoms	Periportal zone-1 necrosis Iron deposition	Deferoxamine	<1[b]
	Amanita phalloides	Any	↑↑↑	↑ - ↑↑↑	↑↑ - ↑↑↑	Diarrhea, vomiting Renal failure	History of ingestion	Massive hepatic necrosis	Supportive care	1[b]
Metabolic and Genetic	Wilson's disease	Peak 6-20 years of age	Normal to ↑ AST>ALT	↑↑	↑↑ - ↑↑↑	↓ alkaline phosphatase Non-immune hemolytic anemia ↓ ceruloplasmin	Renal failure Kayser-Fleischer rings Neuropsychiatric changes	Non-specific findings Portal and peri-portal inflammation Steatosis Elevated hepatic copper	Chelation with trientine or D-penicillamine Low copper diet Most patients with fulminant liver disease need liver transplant	3.2[a]
	Ornithine transcarbamylase (OTC) deficiency	Males with severe phenotype in infancy Any age for people with less severe phenotype	↑ - ↑↑↑ AST>ALT	Normal	↑ - ↑↑↑	↑↑-↑↑↑ NH4 Elevated urine orotic acid	Altered mental status Seizures Often precipitated by illness or systemic stress	Non-specific changes in young patients Some fibrosis in older patients	Protein restriction Dialysis	1[b]

(continued on next page)

Table 1
(continued)

	Age	Labs				Clinical Findings	Biopsy	Disease Specific Treatment	% of PALF cases
		ALT/AST	Bilirubin	INR	Other				
Mitochondrial disease	Neonatal liver failure, Young child	+/-↑	+/-↑	↑	Lactate: pyruvate >20, ↑lactate	Often multisystemic disease	Microvesicular steatosis	Supportive care	1.5-3.5[a]
Tyrosinemia	<6 months	↑↑	↑	↑↑-↑↑↑	Urine succinylacetone	Renal dysfunction, Boiled cabbage odor, Neurologic crisis, Hepatocellular carcinoma	Macronodular cirrhosis, Steatosis, cholestasis	Low tyrosine diet, Nitisinone	1b
Galactosemia	<6 months	↑	↑↑	↑	+ Urine reducing substances	Association with *E. coli* sepsis	Fibrosis, cirrhosis, Steatosis, cholestasis, Bile ductular proliferation, bile plugs	Avoidance of galactose in the diet	1.3[a]
Febrile liver failure syndromes	Infant and young child (most <2 years) Episode frequency decreases with age	↑↑-↑↑↑	+/-↑	↑↑-↑↑↑		Fever	Microvesicular steatosis	Aggressive antipyresis, High protein provision for infant liver failure syndrome type 1	Data not available
Immune-Mediated — Autoimmune hepatitis	Any	↑↑	+/-↑	↑-↑↑↑	↑Immunoglobulin G, ↑auto-antibodies	Other autoimmune disease is sometimes present	Interface hepatitis, Centrilobular necrosis, Plasma cell infiltrate	Corticosteroids, Antimetabolites	6.6[a]
Gestational alloimmune liver disease	Newborn	Normal to ↑	↑	↑↑-↑↑↑	↑Ferritin, ↑transferrin and ↓transferrin saturation, ↑alpha-fetoprotein	Iron deposition (liver, salivary glands, brain, heart, pancreas), Mom with history of previous late miscarriages/still births	Marked hepatocyte loss, Siderosis in remaining hepatocytes, Fibrosis +/- regenerative nodules	Intravenous immunoglobulin, Double-volume exchange transfusion	3.2[a], 13.5 in infants 0-90 days[c]
Hemophagocytic lymphohistio-cytosis	Familial: infant; Secondary: any	↑↑-↑↑↑	↑-↑↑↑	↑-↑↑	Cytopenia in >2 lineages, Elevated triglyceride, Low fibrinogen, Elevated ferritin	Fever, Splenomegaly	Variable, Endotheliatis of central veins, Hemophagocytosis	Based on underlying etiology, usually chemotherapy and/or bone marrow transplant	3-6.3[a]

Category	Cause	Age				Diagnostic test	Clinical features	Histology	Treatment	Frequency
Infectious	Enterovirus	Any			↑ - ↑↑	Enterovirus PCR	May also have nausea, vomiting, diarrhea	Lymphohistiocytic inflammation; Hepatocellular necrosis	Supportive care	<1[b]; 2.7 in infants 0-90 days[c]
	Epstein-Barr virus (EBV)	Any	↑	+/-↑	↑ - ↑↑	EBV PCR	Immunocompromised	Sinusoidal lymphocytosis; Immunohistochemical stains +	Supportive care; Consider rituximab for immuno-compromised	2b
	Herpes simplex virus (HSV)	Most common cause of acute liver failure in infants. Can happen at any age	↑↑ - ↑↑↑	+/-↑	↑ - ↑↑	HSV PCR in blood; Viral culture or PCR of vesicle	Maternal fetal transmission; Immunocompromised	"Ground glass" nuclear inclusions; Coagulative necrosis; Immunohistochemical stains +	Acyclovir	2b; 12.8 in infants 0-90 days[c]
	Cytomegalovirus (CMV)	Any	↑↑ - ↑↑↑	+/-↑	↑ - ↑↑	CMV PCR	Immunocompromised	CMV viral inclusions; Immunohistochemical stains +	Can consider ganciclovir or valganciclovir	<1[b]; 0.7 in infants 0-90 days[c]
	Adenovirus	Any	↑↑ - ↑↑↑	+/-↑	↑ - ↑↑	Adenovirus PCR	Immunocompromised	Immunohistochemical stains +	Cidofovir	1b
	Hepatitis A	Any	↑↑ - ↑↑↑	+/-↑	↑ - ↑↑	Hepatitis A IgM	Diarrhea illness common	Portal and periportal inflammation	Supportive care	1b
Other	Ischemia	Any	↑↑ - ↑↑↑ Peaks after 48-72 hours	+/-↑	↑ - ↑↑		History of hypoxic insult	Centrilobular hepatic necrosis	Supportive care, assure return of hepatic blood flow	3.5-6.3[a]

[a] Narkewicz MR, Horslen S, Hardison RM, et al. A Learning Collaborative Approach Increases Specificity of Diagnosis of Acute Liver Failure in Pediatric Patients. Clin Gastroenterol Hepatol Off Clin Pract J Am Gastroenterol Assoc. 2018;16(11):1801-1810.e3.

[b] Squires RH, Shneider BL, Bucuvalas J, et al. Acute Liver Failure in Children: The First 348 Patients in The Pediatric Acute Liver Failure Study Group. J Pediatr. 2006;148(5):652-658.

[c] Sundaram SS, Alonso EM, Narkewicz MR, Zhang S, Squires RH. Characterization and Outcomes of Young Infants with Acute Liver Failure. J Pediatr. 2011;159(5):813-818.e1. Pathology descriptions mostly from Iacobuzio-Donahue CA, Montgomery E, Goldblum JR, eds. Gastrointestinal and Liver Pathology. A Volume in the Series Foundations in Diagnostic Pathology. Philadelphia, Elsevier, 2005, pp 503-563.

Table 2
Hepatic encephalopathy

Stage	Clinical	Reflexes	Neurologic Signs	EEG Changes
0	None	Normal	None	None
I: Infant/child	Inconsolable, crying, inattention to task, parents describe child as "not acting like self"	Normal or hyperreflexia	Difficult or impossible to assess	Normal or diffuse slowing to theta rhythm, triphasic waves
Adolescent/ young adult	Confused, mood changes, altered sleep habits, forgetful	Normal	Tremor, apraxia, impaired handwriting	
II: Infant/child	Inconsolable, crying, inattention to task, parents describe child as "not acting like self"	Normal or hyperreflexia	Difficult or impossible to assess	Abnormal, generalized slowing, triphasic waves
Adolescent/ young adult	Drowsy, inappropriate behavior, decreased inhibitions	Hyperreflexia	Dysarthria, ataxia	
III: Infant/child	Somnolence, stupor, combativeness	Hyperreflexia	Difficult or impossible to assess	Abnormal, generalized slowing, triphasic waves
Adolescent/ young adult	Stuporous, obeys simple commands	Hyperreflexia, (+) Babinski	Rigidity	
IV: Infant/child	Comatose, arouses with painful stimuli (IVa) or no response (IVb)	Absent	Decerebrate or decorticate	Abnormal, very slow, delta activity
Adolescent/ young adult	Comatose, arouses with painful stimuli (IVa) or no response (IVb)	Absent	Decerebrate or decorticate	

From Squires JE, McKiernan P, Squires RH. Acute Liver Failure. *Clin Liver Dis.* 2018;22(4):773-805; with permission. (Table 3 in original)

timely diagnosis.[1] A complete history must include the timing of symptoms, recent travel, infectious exposures, any current or recent medications, and any possible toxin exposures, including herbal supplements and over-the-counter medications. Key aspects of the family history include neuropsychiatric disorders (seen with Wilson disease), autoimmune diseases, consanguinity (seen with some metabolic and genetic disorders), and miscarriages and premature births associated with gestational alloimmune liver disease.

Drug- and Toxin-Induced Liver Injury

Toxic ingestions account for 19% of cases of PALF in the United States (14% from acetaminophen and 5% from other toxic ingestions).[4] Databases such as LiverTox through the National Institutes of Health (https://livertox.nlm.nih.gov) help with identification of medications associated with hepatic toxicity. The Poison Control system in the United States is also a valuable resource for providers to help with understanding the risk of hepatic toxicity for medications and other substances.

Acetaminophen

Acetaminophen is the most common cause of PALF accounting for 12% of all cases and 21% of cases in children older than 3 years.[4] PALF secondary to acetaminophen can occur with both acute overdose and chronic ingestion. Hepatic toxicity is rare with appropriately dosed acetaminophen (75 mg/kg/d for children or 4 g/d for adults).[9] Liver injury in the setting of acetaminophen ingestion occurs secondary to saturation of its metabolic pathways and subsequent depletion of glutathione and build-up of a toxic metabolite.[10] Children with liver failure secondary to acetaminophen may have significantly elevated transaminases (aspartate transaminase [AST] and alanine transaminase [ALT] >6000) and INR.

With early administration of N-acetylcysteine therapy, ideally within 8 to 12 hours of ingestion, transplant-free recovery from PALF secondary to acetaminophen ingestion is upward of 94% although outcomes are worse in those with chronic exposure.[4,11]

Other drugs and toxins

Non–acetaminophen-induced drug-induced liver injury accounts for 3.2% to 4.9% of cases of PALF.[1] Some of the more common drugs associated with PALF include minocycline, tetracycline, amoxicillin/clavulanic acid, sulfamethoxazole/trimethoprim, valproic acid, and iron, among others. Herbal supplements also may precipitate ALF, and therefore, a detailed history of accessible medications and supplements is paramount when a child presents with liver failure.

Metabolic and Genetic

Metabolic and genetic diseases account for up to 10% of PALF cases with a known cause.[1] Galactosemia, mitochondrial disease, tyrosinemia, and urea cycle disorders are the most common causes of PALF in infants and young children.[12,13] In older children, Wilson disease is the most common cause of metabolic liver disease. Other metabolic causes of PALF include febrile liver failure syndromes, fatty acid oxidation defects, hereditary fructose intolerance, and Niemann-Pick type C.[4]

Wilson disease

Wilson disease is caused by a pathogenic variant in the *ATP7B* gene that impairs the incorporation of copper into ceruloplasmin, limiting the excretion of copper in the biliary system and resulting in copper accumulation throughout the body over time. Wilson disease can present as a chronic process or with fulminant hepatic failure. Symptomatic Wilson disease is rarely diagnosed before 5 years of age but may be diagnosed with screening for causes of transaminase elevation before that time.[14] Laboratory findings common in fulminant Wilson disease include low ceruloplasmin, elevated urinary copper, low alkaline phosphatase, and Coombs-negative hemolytic anemia in the setting of a mild elevation of transaminases with AST greater than ALT and moderate elevation in bilirubin.[15,16] Renal failure is also common in fulminant Wilson disease.[16] Other common clinical findings that suggest Wilson disease include Kayser-Fleischer rings, mood or behavior changes, and declining school performance.[14] Confirmatory diagnosis of Wilson disease is made through genetic testing or through a positive Wilson disease diagnosis score greater than 4.[14,17]

Most children who present with fulminant Wilson disease will ultimately undergo liver transplant. Treatment specific to Wilson disease includes chelation therapy with trientine or D-penicillamine in the absence of renal failure. There are reports of successful plasma exchange therapy for fulminant Wilson diseases.[18] Successful chelation therapy and plasma exchange is the exception rather than the rule. Therefore, early evaluation for liver transplantation and careful monitoring of the King's College Criteria to predict prognosis without liver transplantation are paramount.[19]

Febrile liver failure syndromes

Febrile liver failure syndromes are a diverse group of disorders wherein fever results in episodes of fulminant liver failure. These disorders include neuroblastoma amplified sequence (NBAS) deficiency,[20] infant liver failure type 1,[21] and SCYL1 deficiency.[22] NBAS and SCYL1 deficiency result in abnormal function of the Golgi apparatus,[20,22] and infant liver failure type 1 results in abnormal leucine utilization.[22] Treatment of these disorders includes aggressive antipyresis and supportive care. In the case of infant liver failure type 1 the use of high protein provision (total parenteral nutrition with 2.5 g/kg/d) during acute episodes may help recovery.[21] For all of these syndromes, the frequency and severity of liver failure episodes decrease with age.[20–22] Successful liver transplant without reoccurrence of disease has been reported for NBAS and SCYL1 deficiency.

Mitochondrial disease

Mitochondrial diseases are a set of disorders with variable but often severe systemic effects.[23] PALF is most often associated with mitochondrial depletion syndromes related to pathogenic variants in DGOUK, POLG, MPV17, and PEO1.[24] Mitochondrial disease accounts for 1.5% to 3.5% of PALF cases.[1] Definitive diagnosis is based on genetic testing and/or demonstration of abnormal tissue respiratory chain function or mitochondrial DNA loss.[24] Children who present with PALF secondary to mitochondrial disease often present with an elevated lactate level and multisystem dysfunction.[25] Treatment of this group of disorders most often is supportive care.

Urea cycle disorders/ornithine transcarbamylase deficiency

Urea cycle disorders are a group of inborn errors of metabolism that result in abnormal clearance of the products of protein digestion, most commonly ammonia. OTC deficiency is the most common urea cycle disorder associated with PALF. There are case reports of citrullinemia type 1 presenting with liver failure.[26]

OTC deficiency may present at any age; up to 52% of patients will meet the criteria for PALF at the time of diagnosis or at some point in their illness course.[27,28] Because OTC deficiency is an X-linked disorder, male children with a severe phenotype present in early infancy with hyperammonemia; female and male children with some residual enzyme function may present at any age, often during times of metabolic stress such as with illness or surgery. When in a metabolic crisis, children with OTC deficiency and liver failure have significant hyperammonemia and coagulopathy.

Transaminase elevation during episodes of PALF ranges from mild (around 100) to significant (around 1000).[27] Diagnosis of OTC deficiency is made through a combination of genetic testing, classic patterns on plasma/serum amino acids, and/or elevated urine orotic acid.[29] Acute treatment is with protein restriction and dialysis to remove ammonia. Liver transplant is a curative option for many urea cycle disorders.

Tyrosinemia
Tyrosinemia type 1 results from the lack of fumarylacetoacetate hydrolase required for tyrosine metabolism due to a pathogenic variant in the *FAH* gene.[30] Tyrosinemia most often presents in the first weeks to months of life and is associated with liver failure and kidney disease.[30] It accounts for 3% to 4% of cases of ALF in infants.[4,12] Diagnosis is based on newborn screening results or genetic testing. Children with tyrosinemia will have an elevated urine succinylacetone.[30] Treatment is through protein restriction and nitisinone supplementation, which prevents formation of 4-maleylacetoacetic acid and fumarylacetoacetic acid, precursors to succinylacetone.[30]

Galactosemia
Galactosemia accounts for 1% of all cases of PALF and up to 8% of cases in infants.[31] Galactosemia results from absent activity of galactose-1-phosphate uridyltransferase (GALT), galactokinase, or uridine diphosphate galactose epimerase enzymes.[32] There is universal newborn screening for galactosemia in the United States through measurement of red blood cell GALT activity. These results are unreliable if the baby has been transfused before assessment.[32] Urine-reducing substances are also positive for children with galactosemia who are receiving galactose in their diet. Confirmatory diagnosis is through genetic testing, and treatment is avoidance of galactose in the diet.[32]

Immune-Mediated Liver Disease

Immune-mediated liver disease accounts for approximately 12% of cases of PALF.[1] Causes of immune-mediated liver failure include autoimmune hepatitis, gestational alloimmune liver disease, and hemophagocytic lymphohistiocytosis.

Autoimmune hepatitis
Autoimmune hepatitis may present at any age. It accounts for 7% of cases of PALF.[1,4] As the name suggests, autoimmune hepatitis results from immune dysregulation most likely involving the stimulation of Th1 and Th2 cells.[33] Biochemical tests consistent with autoimmune hepatitis include elevation in autoantibodies, the most common being antismooth muscle antibody, antiliver kidney microsomal antibody, soluble liver antigen, anticytosol type 1 antibody, and antinuclear antibody, with elevation in total immunoglobulin G (IgG) and transaminases.[33,34] Autoantibodies may also be elevated in other causes of PALF; therefore, other causes of PALF must also be considered. In addition, children may present with seronegative autoimmune hepatitis, so the absence of autoantibodies does not rule out autoimmune hepatitis.[35] Classic biopsy findings in autoimmune hepatitis include an interface hepatitis with plasma cell infiltrate and centrilobular necrosis.[33] Diagnosis of autoimmune hepatitis is made through a combination of clinical, pathologic, and laboratory findings. Steroids are the mainstay of the acute management of autoimmune hepatitis, and therefore, practitioners should have a low threshold for starting steroid therapy in the setting of PALF of unknown cause.

Gestational alloimmune liver disease
Gestational alloimmune liver disease results from fetal antigen that causes production of maternal antibodies that cross the placenta and cause hepatic injury. The most common cause is neonatal hemochromatosis (NH).[36] In NH this immune process

leads to iron deposition in the liver, pancreas, heart, brain, and salivary glands. Children present most often in the first days of life with a very elevated INR, mild elevation in bilirubin, and normal to mildly elevated transaminases.[36] In addition, alpha-fetoprotein and ferritin are often elevated. NH accounts for up to 14% of cases of neonatal liver failure with an identified cause.[12,31] NH can have a rapidly progressive course, so early diagnosis and treatment is critical. Diagnosis is through clinical suspicion, laboratory abnormalities, and evidence of extrahepatic siderosis on MRI or salivary gland biopsy.[36] Treatment is with intravenous (IV) immunoglobulin (IG) and exchange transfusion. Recurrence with subsequent pregnancies is high, and antenatal IVIG helps prevent recurrence.[36]

Hemophagocytic lymphohistiocytosis

Hemophagocytic lymphohistiocytosis (HLH) accounts for 3% to 6% of PALF cases.[1,31] Familial HLH often presents in the first days to weeks of life, whereas secondary HLH is most often the result of an infectious trigger and may present at any age.[37] Fever and splenomegaly are almost universal. Diagnosis is made through fulfilling HLH-2004 diagnostic criteria (**Box 1**).[38] Treatment is based on the underlying cause and often includes chemotherapy and/or bone marrow transplant.[38] Liver transplant is typically not necessary once a diagnosis is made and treatment is initiated.

Infectious

Infectious hepatitis accounts for 6% to 13% of cases of PALF across all ages and 16% of cases of ALF in the newborn,[1,4,31] although this figure is likely an underestimation of the true prevalence, given the high percentage of cases of PALF without a cause.[1] The most common infectious cause of ALF in infants and newborns is herpes simplex virus (HSV) followed by enteroviral infections.[31] In older children Epstein-Barr virus and hepatitis A also account for a significant proportion of PALF from infectious causes.[6] Other possible causes include cytomegalovirus, adenovirus, human herpesvirus 6, parvovirus, hepatitis E, and, rarely, hepatitis B, among others. Infants with viral-induced liver failure often have transaminases greater than 1000.[39] Broad serologic testing for infectious causes of PALF is important, especially for infants and those with any suspicious lesions. Acyclovir therapy should be started for potential HSV-associated disease due to the high mortality rate of HSV liver failure.

Other

Ischemia

Hepatic ischemia accounts for 6% of cases of ALF across all ages and up to 30% of cases in infants younger than 30 days.[1,12,31,39] Risk factors include cardiogenic shock, hypovolemia, and right-sided heart failure. Laboratory testing often shows dramatically elevated transaminases (>6000) with the AST greater than ALT and mild elevation in bilirubin.[40] Transaminases tend to peak 48 to 72 hours after the ischemic event.[40] Transplant is rarely needed, as hepatic recovery occurs with restoration of hepatic blood flow.

MANAGEMENT

The backbone of management for PALF is supportive care. Disease-targeted treatment should be initiated as applicable on determination of a cause of PALF.

Fluids/Electrolytes

Fluid and electrolyte derangements are common in PALF. Both hypernatremia and hyponatremia may occur, and extremes should be avoided. Hypophosphatemia is common in PALF and may be a sign of hepatic recovery.[41]

Box 1
Revised diagnostic guidelines for hemophagocytic lymphohistiocytosis (HLH)

The diagnosis of HLH can be established if one of either 1 or 2 of the following is fulfilled:
1. A molecular diagnosis consistent with HLH
2. Diagnostic criteria for HLH fulfilled (5 out of the 8 criteria)
   a. Initial diagnostic criteria (to be evaluated in all patients with HLH)
      - Fever
      - Splenomegaly
      - Cytopenias (affecting >2 of 3 lineages in the peripheral blood):
        ○ Hemoglobin less than 90 g/L (in infants <4 weeks: hemoglobin <100 g/L)
        ○ Platelets less than 100 x 109/L
        ○ Neutrophils less than 1.0 x 109/L
      - Hypertriglyceridemia and/or hypofibrinogenemia:
        ○ Fasting triglycerides greater than 3.0 mmol/L (ie, >265 mg/dL)
        ○ Fibrinogen less than 1.5 g/L
      - Hemophagocytosis in bone marrow or spleen or lymph nodes
      - No evidence of malignancy
   b. New diagnostic criteria
      - Low or absent NK cell activity (according to local laboratory reference)
      - Ferritin greater than 500 μg/L
      - Soluble CD25 (ie, soluble IL-2 receptor) > 2400 U/mL

Comments: (1) if hemophagocytic activity is not proved at the time of presentation, further search for hemophagocytic activity is encouraged. If the bone marrow specimen is not conclusive, material may be obtained from other organs. Serial marrow aspirates over time may also be helpful. (2) The following findings may provide strong supportive evidence for the diagnosis: (a) spinal fluid pleocytosis (mononuclear cells) and/or elevated spinal fluid protein, (b) histologic picture in the liver resembling chronic persistent hepatitis (biopsy). (3) Other abnormal clinical and laboratory findings consistent with the diagnosis are cerebromeningeal symptoms, lymph node enlargement, jaundice, edema, and skin rash. Hepatic enzyme abnormalities, hypoproteinemia, hyponatremia, and VLDL increased and HDL decreased.

Abbreviations: HDL, high-density lipoprotein; IL-2, interleukin-2; NK, natural killer; VLDL, very-low-density lipoprotein.

- Avoid extreme hyper/hyponatremia. Some hypernatremia is tolerable to decrease cerebral edema.
- Maintain total fluids at 80% to 90% of maintenance.
- Carefully monitor phosphorus due to a risk of hypophosphatemia.

Glucose Homeostasis

Impaired gluconeogenesis and depletion of glycogen stores lead to hypoglycemia in acute liver failure.

- Maintain normoglycemia of 90 to 120 mg/dL; may require a glucose infusion rate of 10 to 15 mg/kg/min.
- Monitor serum glucose frequently.

Nutrition

Children with ALF are at risk of catabolism. Adequate protein and energy provision are important. Unless hyperammonemia is present, protein restriction is not needed.

- Initiate oral or enteral nutrition as soon as possible. If unable to safely provide enteral nutrition, parenteral nutrition should be provided.
- Provide 2 to 3 g/kg per day of protein, reduce to 1 g/kg per day if hyperammonemia is present.

Neurologic

HE and cerebral edema are life-threatening complications of PALF. HE occurs in up to 60% of cases of PALF at some point in the disease course.[5] The primary objective in managing HE is to prevent brain edema and increased intracranial pressure. Factors that worsen HE include shock, sepsis, gastrointestinal bleeding, and electrolyte imbalances.[7]

- Carefully monitor for signs of HE.
- Conduct serial assessment of ammonia levels.
- Initiate early use of lactulose (via NG tube or enema) and consider rifaximin to reduce ammonia production by intestinal flora.
- Minimize stimulation.
- Avoid sedating or paralytic medications when possible.
- Consider intracranial pressure monitoring for stage III or IV HE and electroencephalogram showing slowing, the need for intubation, or signs of edema on head imaging.

Coagulopathy

Coagulopathy that is not correctable with vitamin K is a hallmark of PALF. This coagulopathy results from hepatic synthetic dysfunction. Bleeding in PALF is rare, and an elevated INR does not represent the bleeding risk in PALF due to decreased production of both procoagulants and anticoagulants.[42]

In addition to an elevated INR, other findings may include low factor V and VII levels with normal or increased factor VIII due to compensatory endothelial production.

- Administer vitamin K, as this is part of the assessment of liver failure.
- Administer blood products only for procedures or active bleeding.
- Start acid suppression to decrease risk of gastrointestinal bleeding.
- Consider the use of thromboelastography to assess bleeding risk.

Infectious Disease

Children with PALF are at increased risk for infection due to immune dysfunction. In addition, infectious complications account for 11% to 20% of the morbidity associated with PALF.[43]

- Obtain blood culture on admission and with any clinical deterioration.
- Initiate empirical acyclovir for possible HSV disease for any infant with ALF and any child with a suspicion of HSV disease.
- Have a low threshold for starting empirical broad-spectrum antibiotics and antifungals at presentation or for any clinical deterioration.

OUTCOMES

Approximately 10% to 15% of pediatric liver transplantations in the United States are for PALF.[4] Survival and need for liver transplant vary based on the underlying diagnosis. With appropriate supportive care and treatment (when applicable and directed at a specific underlying diagnosis) most children will recover from an episode of PALF. The rate of spontaneous recovery without transplant depends on the cause and presenting clinical factors.[4,31] In infants younger than 30 days with liver failure, 33% were alive at 1 year of age.[39] Overall transplant-free survival for children with acetaminophen-induced ALF is approximately 94%.[4] In non–acetaminophen-related liver failure, 21 days after diagnosis 55% of patients had spontaneous recovery,

34% of patients underwent liver transplant, and 11% of patients died.[5] Worsening HE and grade III to IV HE are associated with higher likelihood of needing liver transplant and death, with only 25% of patients demonstrating spontaneous recovery.[5] The absence of HE does not eliminate the possibility of a negative outcome, with 4% of patients dying having never developed HE.[5] The most common causes of death in PALF include multisystem organ failure, brain herniation, cardiac failure, and sepsis.[5]

PALF is a life-threatening diagnosis with many causes. With appropriate diagnosis, support, and treatment, recovery is possible for many children. However, rapid referral to a pediatric liver transplant center is recommended for management and evaluation for liver transplantation if required for survival.

CLINICS CARE POINTS

- PALF from acetaminophen toxicity has the highest rate of spontaneous recovery.
- Infectious complications cause up to 20% of the morbidity associated with PALF.
- HE has a significant effect on outcomes. Only 25% of patients with persistent high-grade (III–IV) encephalopathy demonstrate spontaneous recovery.
- Bleeding is an uncommon complication despite significant coagulopathy.
- Hypoglycemia is common and can be profound. Patients may require glucose infusion rates of 5 to 6 mg/kg/min or higher.

DISCLOSURE

The authors have nothing to disclose.

REFERENCES

1. Narkewicz MR, Horslen S, Hardison RM, et al. A learning collaborative approach increases specificity of diagnosis of acute liver failure in pediatric patients. Clin Gastroenterol Hepatol 2018;16(11):1801–10.e3.
2. Narkewicz MR, Olio DD, Karpen SJ, et al. Pattern of diagnostic evaluation for the causes of pediatric acute liver failure: an opportunity for quality improvement. J Pediatr 2009;155(6):801–6.e1.
3. Elisofon SA, Magee JC, Ng VL, et al. Society of pediatric liver transplantation: current registry status 2011-2018. Pediatr Transplant 2020;24(1):e13605.
4. Squires RH, Shneider BL, Bucuvalas J, et al. Acute liver failure in children: the first 348 patients in the pediatric acute liver failure study group. J Pediatr 2006;148(5): 652–8.
5. Ng VL, Li R, Loomes KM, et al. Outcomes of children with and without hepatic encephalopathy from the pediatric acute liver failure (PALF) study group. J Pediatr Gastroenterol Nutr 2016;63(3):357–64.
6. Squires RH. Acute liver failure in children. Semin Liver Dis 2008;28(02):153–66.
7. Squires JE, McKiernan P, Squires RH. Acute liver failure. Clin Liver Dis 2018; 22(4):773–805.
8. Toney NA, Bell MJ, Belle SH, et al. Hepatic encephalopathy in children with acute liver failure – utility of serum neuromarkers. J Pediatr Gastroenterol Nutr 2019; 69(1):108–15.
9. James LP, Wilson JT, Simar R, et al. Evaluation of occult acetaminophen hepatotoxicity in hospitalized children receiving acetaminophen. Pediatric pharmacology research unit network. Clin Pediatr (Phila) 2001;40(5):243–8.

10. Suchy FJ, Sokol RJ, Balistreri WF, editors. Liver disease in children. 5th edition. Cambridge University Press; 2021.
11. Leonis MA, Alonso EM, Im K, et al. Chronic acetaminophen exposure in pediatric acute liver failure. Pediatrics 2013;131(3):e740–6.
12. Bitar R, Thwaites R, Davison S, et al. Liver failure in early infancy. J Pediatr Gastroenterol Nutr 2017;64(1):70–5.
13. Durand P, Debray D, Mandel R, et al. Acute liver failure in infancy: a 14-year experience of a pediatric liver transplantation center. J Pediatr 2001;139(6):871–6.
14. Socha P, Janczyk W, Dhawan A, et al. Wilson's disease in children: a position paper by the hepatology Committee of the European Society for Paediatric Gastroenterology, Hepatology and Nutrition. J Pediatr Gastroenterol Nutr 2018;66(2):334–44.
15. Tissières P, Chevret L, Debray D, et al. Fulminant Wilson's disease in children: appraisal of a critical diagnosis. Pediatr Crit Care Med J Soc Crit Care Med 2003;4(3):338–43.
16. Roberts EA, Schilsky ML. Diagnosis and treatment of Wilson disease: an update. Hepatology 2008;47(6):2089–111.
17. Ferenci P, Caca K, Loudianos G, et al. Diagnosis and phenotypic classification of Wilson disease1. Liver Int 2003;23(3):139–42.
18. Proost R, Cassiman D, Levtchenko E, et al. Fulminant wilson disease in children: recovery after plasma exchange without transplantation. J Pediatr Gastroenterol Nutr 2020;71(6):720–5.
19. Dhawan A, Taylor RM, Cheeseman P, et al. Wilson's disease in children: 37-Year experience and revised King's score for liver transplantation. Liver Transpl 2005;11(4):441–8.
20. Staufner C, Peters B, Wagner M, et al. Defining clinical subgroups and genotype–phenotype correlations in NBAS-associated disease across 110 patients. Genet Med 2020;22(3):610–21.
21. Casey JP, Slattery S, Cotter M, et al. Clinical and genetic characterisation of infantile liver failure syndrome type 1, due to recessive mutations in LARS. J Inherit Metab Dis 2015;38(6):1085–92.
22. Schmidt WM, Rutledge SL, Schüle R, et al. Disruptive SCYL1 mutations underlie a syndrome characterized by recurrent episodes of liver failure, peripheral neuropathy, cerebellar atrophy, and ataxia. Am J Hum Genet 2015;97(6):855–61.
23. Alston CL, Rocha MC, Lax NZ, et al. The genetics and pathology of mitochondrial disease. J Pathol 2017;241(2):236–50.
24. McKiernan P, Ball S, Santra S, et al. Incidence of primary mitochondrial disease in children younger than 2 years presenting with acute liver failure. J Pediatr Gastroenterol Nutr 2016;63(6):592–7.
25. Molleston JP, Sokol RJ, Karnsakul W, et al. Evaluation of the child with suspected mitochondrial liver disease. J Pediatr Gastroenterol Nutr 2013;57(3):269–76.
26. Faghfoury H, Baruteau J, de Baulny HO, et al. Transient fulminant liver failure as an initial presentation in citrullinemia type I. Mol Genet Metab 2011;102(4):413–7.
27. Gallagher RC, Lam C, Wong D, et al. Significant hepatic involvement in patients with ornithine transcarbamylase deficiency. J Pediatr 2014;164(4):720–5.e6.
28. Laemmle A, Gallagher RC, Keogh A, et al. Frequency and pathophysiology of acute liver failure in ornithine transcarbamylase deficiency (OTCD). PLoS ONE 2016;11(4):e0153358.
29. Summar M. Urea cycle disorders. In: Sarafoglou K, Hoffmann GF, Roth KS, editors. Pediatric endocrinology and inborn errors of metabolism. 2nd edition. 1st edition. McGraw-Hill Companies; 2009. p. 141–52.

30. Chinsky JM, Singh R, Ficicioglu C, et al. Diagnosis and treatment of tyrosinemia type I: a US and Canadian consensus group review and recommendations. Genet Med 2017;19(12):1–16.
31. Sundaram SS, Alonso EM, Narkewicz MR, et al. Characterization and outcomes of young infants with acute liver failure. J Pediatr 2011;159(5):813–8.e1.
32. Demirbas D, Coelho AI, Rubio-Gozalbo ME, et al. Hereditary galactosemia. Metabolism 2018;83:188–96.
33. Mack CL, Adams D, Assis DN, et al. Diagnosis and management of autoimmune hepatitis in adults and children: 2019 practice guidance and guidelines from the american association for the study of liver diseases. Hepatology 2020;72(2): 671–722.
34. Mieli-Vergani G, Vergani D, Baumann U, et al. Diagnosis and management of pediatric autoimmune liver disease: ESPGHAN Hepatology Committee position Statement. J Pediatr Gastroenterol Nutr 2018;66(2):345–60.
35. Maggiore G, Socie G, Sciveres M, et al. Seronegative autoimmune hepatitis in children: spectrum of disorders. Dig Liver Dis 2016;48(7):785–91.
36. Whitington PF. Gestational alloimmune liver disease and neonatal hemochromatosis. Semin Liver Dis 2012;32(04):325–32.
37. Al-Samkari H, Berliner N. Hemophagocytic lymphohistiocytosis. Annu Rev Pathol Mech Dis 2018;13(1):27–49.
38. Henter J-I, Horne A, Aricó M, et al. HLH-2004: diagnostic and therapeutic guidelines for hemophagocytic lymphohistiocytosis. Pediatr Blood Cancer 2007;48(2): 124–31.
39. Borovsky K, Banc-Husu AM, Saul SA, et al. Applying an age-specific definition to better characterize etiologies and outcomes in neonatal acute liver failure. J Pediatr Gastroenterol Nutr 2021;73(1):80–5.
40. Garland JS, Werlin SL, Rice TB. Ischemic hepatitis in children: diagnosis and clinical course. Crit Care Med 1988;16(12):1209–12.
41. Quirós-Tejeira RE, Molina RA, Katzir L, et al. Resolution of hypophosphatemia is associated with recovery of hepatic function in children with fulminant hepatic failure. Transpl Int 2005;18(9):1061–6.
42. Kawada PS, Bruce A, Massicotte P, et al. Coagulopathy in children with liver disease. J Pediatr Gastroenterol Nutr 2017;65(6):603–7.
43. Cochran JB, Losek JD. Acute liver failure in children. Pediatr Emerg Care 2007; 23(2):129–35.

Uncommon Causes of Acute Kidney Injury

Cassandra L. Formeck, MD, MS[a,b], Carlos L. Manrique-Caballero, MD[b,c], Hernando Gómez, MD[b,d], John A. Kellum, MD, MCCM[b,e,f],*

KEYWORDS

- AKI • Critically ill • Immune mediated • Microangiopathy • Obstruction

KEY POINTS

- Uncommon causes of acute kidney injury (AKI) can include structural, immune-mediated, and microvascular disease, many of which are associated with high morbidity and mortality when diagnosis and initiation of disease-specific therapy are delayed.
- The presence of oliguria and abdominal or flank pain should alert practitioners to potential structural causes of AKI, including urinary tract obstruction, renal infarction, or abdominal compartment syndrome, and should be evaluated with renal imaging and intravesical pressure measurement.
- In hospitalized patients biopsied for AKI of uncertain cause, acute tubulointerstitial nephritis (TIN) accounts for up to one-third of cases, with drug-associated TIN being the most common cause of TIN in critically ill patients.
- Glomerulonephritis is an immune-mediated disease characterized by glomerular inflammation that results in hematuria with or without the presence of proteinuria and is frequently associated with dark colored urine, hypertension, and edema.
- Thrombotic microangiopathy is characterized by the clinical triad of thrombocytopenia, microangiopathic hemolytic anemia, and acute organ dysfunction and encompasses a variety of diseases including thrombocytopenic purpura, hemolytic uremic syndrome, and the hemolysis, elevated liver enzymes, and low platelets syndrome.

[a] Division of Nephrology, Department of Pediatrics, UPMC Children's Hospital of Pittsburgh, 4401 Penn Avenue, Faculty Pavilion, 4th Floor, Pittsburgh, PA 15224, USA; [b] Center for Critical Care Nephrology, University of Pittsburgh, Pittsburgh, PA 15261, USA; [c] Renal-Electrolyte Division, Department of Medicine, University of Pittsburgh, A919 Scaife Hall, 3550 Terrace Street, Pittsburgh, PA 15261, USA; [d] Department of Critical Care Medicine, University of Pittsburgh School of Medicine, 3550 Terrace Street, Scaife Hall, Suite 612c, Pittsburgh, PA 15261, USA; [e] Department of Critical Care Medicine, University of Pittsburgh School of Medicine, Pittsburgh, PA, USA; [f] Center for Critical Care Nephrology, 3347 Forbes Avenue, Suite 220, Pittsburgh, PA 15213, USA
* Corresponding author. Center for Critical Care Nephrology, Department of Critical Care Medicine, University of Pittsburgh School of Medicine, 3550 Terrace Street, 600 Scaife Hall, Pittsburgh, PA 15261, USA
E-mail address: kellum@pitt.edu

Crit Care Clin 38 (2022) 317–347
https://doi.org/10.1016/j.ccc.2021.11.010
0749-0704/22/© 2021 Elsevier Inc. All rights reserved.
criticalcare.theclinics.com

INTRODUCTION

Acute kidney injury (AKI) is one of the most important complications of critical illness. It is defined as an increase in serum creatinine (sCr), decreased urine output, or both.[1] AKI occurs in approximately 55% to 60% of critically ill patients. This number may seem high until one realizes that the rates of respiratory and cardiovascular failure among the critically ill are similar—being critically ill usually means multiorgan dysfunction. Some estimates of AKI incidence and rates among hospitalized patients have used only sCr changes, but this approach fails to recognize more than one-third of cases.[2,3] Among the critically ill stage 2 or 3 AKI occurred in 18% without any changes in sCr sufficient to make the diagnosis, and these patients had an 8.6% hospital mortality. Conversely only 3% had stage 2 or 3 AKI by sCr without any urine output criteria, and hospital mortality was only slightly higher at 11.4% (17).[2]

Given how frequent AKI occurs in the critical care setting, it is easy for it to seem to be part of the background clinical picture. Furthermore, general supportive care efforts and treatment of underlying disease conditions that result in AKI are often the only available interventions. AKI is commonly associated with 3 potentially overlapping conditions: sepsis, cardiac dysfunction, and exposure to nephrotoxic medications, with sepsis being the most common condition associated with AKI in the critically ill. Cardiac dysfunction in the context of either myocardial infarction[4] or cardiac surgery is the next most prevalent association. Importantly, nephrotoxic medications complicate both sepsis and cardiac disease, and this form of AKI is a particularly prevalent condition in these populations.

When one adds major surgery, trauma and burns, and advanced liver disease to the list, virtually every patient admitted to the intensive care unit (ICU) will have experienced one or more of these exposures. As such, it is tempting to think of AKI as part of the baggage of critical illness. Because therapy for AKI arising from these conditions is nonspecific (except for removing nephrotoxins), identification of the precise cause infrequently alters management. However, certain less common causes of AKI have specific treatments, and missing these diagnoses can be devastating to patient outcomes. These conditions fall into 3 large categories: structural (ie, urinary tract obstruction, renal infarction, and abdominal compartment syndrome), immune mediated (ie, glomerulonephritis and interstitial nephritis), and microvascular (ie, thrombotic microangiopathies). Because the last category can represent the most significant diagnostic challenges, the authors focus mainly on it. However, this article begins by briefly discussing the first two.

STRUCTURAL DISEASES

Anatomic abnormalities are important contributors to AKI in the ICU. Obstructive nephropathy accounts for 5% to 10% of cases of AKI in the ICU[5] but accounts for up to a quarter of cases in critically ill patients older than 80 years.[6] Unilateral obstruction can be easily missed, as urine volume may be preserved. Hence, a high index of suspicion should be maintained particularly in patients with a history of nephrolithiasis.

AKI is often the first clinical manifestation of intraabdominal hypertension (IAH) and abdominal compartment syndrome (ACS), with the prevalence of ACS ranging from 5% to 56% among patients admitted to the medical or surgical ICU worldwide.[7,8] Renal infarction, although relatively uncommon, is associated with AKI in more than one-third of cases.[9] Together, structural abnormalities are important to consider in the critically ill patient with AKI.

Clinical Manifestations and Risk Factors

Patients with urinary outflow obstruction may present with pelvic pain, flank pain, dysuria, urinary frequency, urinary hesitancy, and/or enuresis.[10] In addition to AKI, metabolic acidosis and hyperkalemia are frequently observed as a result of distal tubular dysfunction. Common causes of obstructive nephropathy include cancer, benign prostatic hyperplasia, prostate adenomas, lithiasis, retroperitoneal or ureteral fibrosis, and bladder dysfunction.[5,10] Prostate cancer accounts for half of cancer-related obstructive AKI in adults, with uterine and bladder cancer also being frequent contributors.[5] Radiation is a known risk factor for urethritis, bladder dysfunction, and pelvic or retroperitoneal fibrosis leading to urinary obstruction.[5] In patients exhibiting urinary retention without a clear anatomic abnormality, medication-associated urinary retention should be considered and potential offending agents discontinued when medically able.

Oliguria and AKI are often presenting symptoms in the critically ill patients with IAH or ACS.[11,12] Other symptoms may include abdominal bloating/distention, abdominal pain, malaise, lightheadedness, and dyspnea. Physical examination is universally notable for a tensely distended abdomen but may also include jugular venous distension, peripheral edema, poor peripheral perfusion, and acute respiratory decompensation. Primary causes of ACS include, but are not limited to, trauma, pancreatitis, ileus, bowel obstruction, hemo- or pneumoperitoneum, intrabdominal infection, and space occupying lesion. Secondary causes can include large volume fluid resuscitation, sepsis, prone positioning, hypothermia, elevation of the head of the bed, and capillary leak.[7,13]

In comparison, acute renal infarction usually presents with acute onset of flank or abdominal pain, accompanied by gastrointestinal symptoms including nausea and vomiting. In some patients, fever is also a presenting symptom.[14,15] In addition to AKI, common laboratory features may include hematuria, proteinuria, increased lactate dehydrogenase (LDH), leukocytosis, and elevated C-reactive protein levels. Hematuria is observed in approximately one-third of patients, whereas proteinuria is less common, occurring in less than a quarter of patients.[16] Risk factors for renal infarction include renal artery injury, cardiovascular disease including hypertension, older age, smoking history, atrial fibrillation, and valvular disease, along with diabetes mellitus and hypercoagulable states.[16] Renal artery injury may occur from a trauma or intervention or may be secondary to underlying disease states including Marfan syndrome, vasculitis, fibromuscular dysplasia, or Ehlers-Danlos syndrome.[9]

Pathophysiology

The primary mechanism of kidney injury from urinary obstruction occurs as a result of increased intraluminal pressure. This pressure transfers to the renal tubules and then Bowman space, causing decreased filtration pressure in the glomerular capillary wall. These changes ultimately lead to increased production of angiotensin II and thromboxane A2, resulting in afferent and efferent arteriolar vasoconstriction and decreased glomerular filtration.[17] Comparatively, the pathophysiology of ACS starts with increasing intraabdominal pressure that compresses arterial and venous vasculature. Compression of the intraabdominal vasculature leads to decreased arterial pressure and venous congestion, resulting in compromised arterial perfusion pressure, organ edema, and end organ injury.[7] In addition to decreased renal artery blood flow and venous congestion, ACS may also lead to direct compression of the renal parenchyma, resulting in decreased glomerular filtration pressure, impaired microvascular flow, and decreased oxygen delivery, causing AKI.[7] In patients with renal infarction, direct damage or occlusion of a main, segmental, or subsegmental renal artery leads to hypoperfusion and ischemia of either the entire kidney or a segment of the kidney parenchyma.

Diagnosis

When structural AKI is suspected, renal ultrasonography (US) or computed tomography (CT) should be performed. Renal US should include Doppler evaluation of the renal vasculature when renal arterial or venous thrombosis or renal vascular injury is suspected. In patients with urinary tract obstruction, the diagnosis is usually established by the presence of hydronephrosis.[10] Urinary bladder postvoid residual volumes greater than 150 mL suggest bladder outlet obstruction.[10] Dopplers can also be used to assess for the presence or absence of ureteral jets, with absence or decreased frequency suggesting ureteral obstruction. CT of the abdomen is useful in the identification of lithiasis, pelvic masses, renal vascular injury, and renal infarction. For renal infarction, classic findings on CT include a wedge-shaped perfusion defect. In patients with concerns for renal infarction, MRI is an alternative imagine modality and avoids exposure to CT contrast.

IAH is defined as an intraabdominal pressure greater than 12 mm Hg, and ACS is characterized by sustained IAH, leading to new organ dysfunction.[18] The current gold standard for IAH is measurement of intravesical (ie, bladder) pressure.[7] Although commercially available kits are available, bladder pressure can be measured with routine ICU supplies using a Foley catheter and a pressure transducer.

Prognosis and Management

The mainstay of treatment of obstructive AKI is to relieve the urinary obstruction, which may include Foley catheterization, suprapubic catheterization, nephrostomy tube placement, or urinary diversion in some instances. Medical providers should observe closely for postobstruction diuresis, which can place patients at risk for dehydration, electrolyte derangements, and worsening AKI.[5] Importantly, obstructive AKI can be a significant contributor to morbidity and mortality in critically ill patients. In a cohort study by Hamdi and colleagues, out of 62 adults with obstructive AKI, 40% of individuals required renal replacement therapy (RRT), 21% had persistent kidney dysfunction, and 6% developed end-stage kidney disease (ESKD) at 3-month follow-up.[5] In this cohort, volume of diuresis after the relief of the urinary obstruction was fairly predictive of renal recovery, with a greater than 7000 mL diuresis in the first 24 hours correlating with a 79% chance of recovering renal function within 3 months. As such, high clinical suspicion and early identification are critical for optimizing outcomes in this population.

In patients with ACS, nonsurgical or surgical treatment options can be considered. Medical treatment options to reduce intraabdominal pressure can include sedation, analgesia, and neuromuscular blockade to improve abdominal wall compliance; paracentesis or percutaneous drainage to remove ascites; nasogastric or rectal decompression to remove intraluminal contents; correction of fluid balance with diuretics, fluid restriction, and/or use of RRT; optimizing blood pressure with vasopressor support; and improving alveolar recruitment and ventilation.[13] If conservative management is unsuccessful, then surgical decompression with laparotomy may be considered.[19] If left untreated, ASC is fatal, and delays in treatment are associated with high mortality, with rates of mortality reaching as high as 70%.[19,20]

For patients with renal infarction, evidence regarding management is limited by lack of comparative studies. Although most patients are managed conservatively, for those with thromboembolic disease, thrombosis, or renal artery dissection, current approaches for treatment include systemic anticoagulation, percutaneous endovascular treatment including thrombolysis, thrombectomy, or stent placement, and open surgery. Benefits from revascularization surgery are time limited and high suspicion is required.[21] Surgical intervention can be considered in patients with infarction from traumatic renal artery occlusion or in patients with arterial dissection; however, evidence for his approach is mixed.[21–23] Importantly, patients should be monitored for the development of acute hypertension, which is observed in more than half of the patients.[24]

IMMUNE-MEDIATED ACUTE KIDNEY INJURY
Tubulointerstitial Nephritis

Tubulointerstitial nephritis (TIN) is an immune-mediated disease commonly associated with AKI, characterized by infiltration of the renal interstitium by inflammatory cells. In hospitalized patients biopsied for AKI of uncertain cause, acute TIN accounts for up to one-third of cases.[25] Although common and well described, the diagnosis of TIN is often delayed due to its nonspecific findings.

Most cases of TIN are secondary to medication exposure. A wide variety of medications have been identified as causing TIN, with antibiotics, nonsteroidal antiinflammatory drugs, and proton pump inhibitors being the most common culprits (**Table 1**).[17,26,27] Notably, in drug-induced TIN, no dose dependance is observed, and TIN will often reoccur if the patient is reexposed to the offending agent. Although numerous antibiotics have been identified to cause TIN, beta-lactams have been cited as the most common cause.[26]

TIN has also been associated with a variety of pathogens including cytomegalovirus (CMV), polyomavirus, adenovirus, Epstein-Barr virus (EBV), and *Mycoplasma pneumoniae* and most recently SARS-CoV-2.[28] Some systemic diseases have also been linked with TIN such as systemic lupus erythematous (SLE), inflammatory bowel disease, sarcoidosis, Sjögren disease, autoimmune pancreatitis, and tubulointerstitial nephritis and uveitis syndrome to name a few.[27,29–32] Several genetic factors have also been associated with occurrence of TIN but these are generally associated with more chronic forms of interstitial nephritis.[33,34]

Table 1
Medications commonly associated with tubulointerstitial nephritis

Antibiotics	Antivirals	Diuretics	Neuropsychiatric	Others
Beta-lactams	Abacavir	Amiloride	Carbamazepine	Allopurinol
Cephalosporins	Acyclovir	Furosemide	Lamotrigine	Alendronate
Ciprofloxacin	Atazanavir	Thiazides	Levetiracetam	Azathioprine
Doxycycline	Indinavir	Tienilic acid	Lithium	Antiangiogenesis drugs
Ethambutol		Triamterene	Phenobarbital	Captopril
Fluoroquinolones			Phenytoin	Interferon
Gentamicin				Sulfasalazine
Isoniazid				
Macrolides				
Nitrofurantoin				
Rifampin				
Sulfonamides				
Vancomycin				

Clinical Manifestations and Risk Factors

In addition to AKI, the clinical manifestations can include flank pain, rash, and fever.[27] Although helpful in establishing a diagnosis when present, these symptoms are relatively infrequent and occur in less than a quarter of patients.[27] Flank pain is secondary to kidney edema and swelling, which is occasionally observed on renal US.[17] Symptoms generally occur within a few days of drug initiation; however, onset of TIN may occur weeks or months following the start of a medication. As such, kidney injury may be acute or present as gradual loss of kidney function over time. Eosinophilia may be present but is observed in less than one-third of patients.[27] Proximal tubular dysfunction may result in tubular wasting of bicarbonate and other electrolytes leading to metabolic acidosis and low serum electrolyte levels, whereas distal nephron injury may result in abnormal renal acidification and defects in potassium secretion, resulting in acidosis and hyperkalemia.[26] Urine studies may also be notable for sterile pyuria, glucosuria, hematuria, and mild proteinuria.[27]

Pathophysiology

The exact pathophysiology of TIN is influenced by the underlying cause, but ultimately results from inflammation in the tubulointerstitial space. Infiltration of lymphocytes and plasma cells into the interstitium is associated with the development of interstitial edema, leading to compromised blood flow to the region,[35] and this results in tubular dysfunction and reduced glomerular filtration rate. Prolonged inflammation subsequently leads to accumulation of extracellular matrix causing irreversible interstitial fibrosis and tubular atrophy. Some growth factors, including transforming growth factor-beta may mediate profibrotic changes in the interstitium.[35,36]

Diagnosis

Urinalysis and urine microscopy can provide helpful evidence in establishing and diagnosing TIN. Sterile pyuria is observed in roughly half of the patients, along with mild proteinuria and occasionally microscopic hematuria.[27] Although eosinophiluria is classically associated with TIN, studies show a 67% sensitivity and 83% specificity in patients with AKI.[17] However, to establish a definitive diagnosis of TIN, renal biopsy is required.[27]

Prognosis and Management

The first line of treatment of drug-induced TIN is discontinuation of the offending agent. The likelihood of renal recovery following medication discontinuation depends on the duration and severity of kidney injury, with approximately one-third of patients progressing to chronic kidney disease (CKD).[27] If an infectious cause is identified, then treatment of underlying infection should be undertaken when able. In patients with solid organ or bone marrow transplant with TIN secondary to viral infection (CMV, polyomavirus, adenovirus, EBV), reduction in immunosuppressive medications may be beneficial.[37] For idiopathic or other causes of TIN, there remains a paucity of evidence-based studies to guide treatment recommendations. Although corticosteroids have traditionally been used in the management of TIN, no prospective randomized controlled trials have evaluated efficacy in reducing AKI severity or progression to CKD. Retrospective studies that have examined the effectiveness of corticosteroids for the management of drug-associated AKI have shown mixed results, with many showing no difference in renal outcomes.[38] Despite lack of prospective data, many investigators support a trial of corticosteroids in patients with persistent or worsening AKI, in particular when the duration of AKI is less than 3 weeks, and renal biopsy shows minimal interstitial fibrosis or tubular atrophy.[27,39] In some populations, other steroid sparing agents have been used, including methotrexate, cyclosporine, mycophenolate mofetil, and azathioprine; however, the efficacy of these agent also remains unclear. Overall, older age and duration of kidney failure for more than 3 weeks have been associated with worse long-term outcomes.[27,38]

Glomerulonephritis

Glomerulonephritis (GN) is an inflammatory glomerular disease that results in hematuria with or without proteinuria. Inflammation can be limited to the kidney or can involve other organs. GN typically occurs as a result of 1 of 3 common mechanisms: linear antibody deposition (antiglomerular basement membrane [GBM] disease), pauci-immune disorders (small vessel vasculitis), and granular immune complex disorders.[40] GN can occur acutely or can take a slow or chronic course. Acute nephritis can also range from self-limited disease, as frequently observed with postinfectious GN, to rapidly progressive deterioration of kidney function, as often seen with pauci-immune disorders such as antineutrophil cytoplasmic antibody (ANCA)-associated vasculitis or anti-GBM disease.[41]

Clinical Manifestations and Risk Factors

Acute GN is characterized by the sudden onset of painless, dark (cola- or tea-colored) urine. AKI, edema, and hypertension are common clinical findings and together with hematuria constitute the nephritic syndrome.[40,42] In addition to peripheral edema, other signs of volume overload may be present, including pulmonary crackles, dyspnea, and jugular venous distension. In patients with pulmonary-renal syndrome such as anti-GBM disease or granulomatosis with polyangiitis (GPA—formerly called Wegener granulomatosis), clinical manifestations may include cough, stridor, wheezing, hemoptysis, dyspnea, or respiratory failure.[43–45] Skin and musculoskeletal findings may indicate a systemic disease such as immunoglobulin A (IgA) vasculitis or SLE.[46–48] Risk factors for nephritis commonly include an infectious trigger. In patients with postinfectious GN (including poststreptococcal GN), upper respiratory symptoms, sore throat, or soft tissue infection are frequently reported in 2 to 3 weeks before the onset of gross hematuria.[49–51] In patients with IgA nephritis, concurrent respiratory or gastrointestinal infection is often observed. Various drugs (eg, hydralazine, minocycline, procainamide, and anti-tumor necrosis factor alpha, among others.)[52] have also been associated with GN and should be screened for and discontinued when clinically able. Familial or genetic risk factors may also contribute to some forms of GN, including SLE, ANCA-associated GN, anti-GBM disease, and C3 glomerulopathy, among others.[53–56]

Pathophysiology

Although incompletely understood, inflammation in GN is thought to be mediated by both the cellular and humoral immune systems.[42] In the case of GN, inflammatory infiltrates and cytokine release results in glomerular capillary damage, disruption of the GBM, and decreased glomerular filtration[40]; this leads to hematuria, proteinuria, oliguria, salt retention, and azotemia. Salt and water retention subsequently leads to intravascular volume expansion causing edema and hypertension. Damage to the GBM can occur by various mechanisms, depending on the underlying cause of nephritis. For example, in poststreptococcal GN, antibodies are produced against the nephrito-genic antigens of group A streptococcus,[57] and this leads to immune complex deposition in and around the GBM, resulting in activation of the complement cascade and recruitment of various immune cells.[57] Comparatively, in anti-GBM disease, an auto-antibody against a peptide within the alpha 3 chain of type IV collagen is produced, leading to direct damage to the GBM.[58] Direct damage to the endothelial cell layer or the podocyte cell layer can also occur in other forms of GN.[40]

Diagnosis
In all patients with AKI, a urinalysis should be obtained to assess for the presence of hematuria, proteinuria, and/or pyuria. The presence of hematuria or proteinuria may be a sign of glomerular or tubular disease and should prompt urine microscopy. The presence of dysmorphic red blood cells, along with red blood cell or mixed cellular casts on urine microscopy, indicates the presence of GN.

In patients with evidence of glomerulonephritis on urine microscopy, laboratory studies and clinical history are often sufficient to identify the underlying diagnosis. Complement levels, including C3 and C4, can often help differentiate between causes of nephritis.[40] Postinfectious, SLE, membranoproliferative, and infective endocarditis-associated GN often present with hypocomplementemia, whereas the most common causes of GN with normal complement include IgA nephropathy, IgA vasculitis, GPA, and anti-GBM disease. Additional serologic testing should include antistreptolysin O titers (ASO), ANAs, anti-dsDNA and anti-GBM antibody levels, ANCA, human immunodeficiency virus (HIV), hepatitis B surface antigen, and hepatitis C antibodies, along with rheumatoid factor, serum protein electrophoresis, and serum immunofixation in select cases.[40] In the setting of a recent sore throat or cellulitis, high ASO titers indicate recent streptococcal infection and a likely diagnosis of poststreptococcal GN, particularly in conjunction with low C3 levels.[50,59] Low C4 levels, along with a positive ANA and anti-dsDNA antibodies suggest SLE. Positive anti-GBM antibodies or positive ANCA are seen in anti-GBM disease and GPA, respectively. Rheumatoid factor can be obtained to screen for cryoglobulinemia in suspected patients, and serum electrophoresis and serum immunofixation can be used to help identify plasma cell disorders associated with some forms of GN.[40] If a new murmur or signs of systemic infection are present, infective endocarditis should be considered. Although the underlying cause of GN can often be determined with the previously mentioned serologic studies and a thorough patient history, in patients with AKI, nephrotic range proteinuria (>3 g/24h or a urine protein-to-creatinine ratio >2 mg/mg), or hypertension, a renal biopsy should be obtained to confirm diagnosis and guide therapy.

A rapid and progressive loss of kidney function in the setting of nephritis should raise concern for rapidly progressive glomerulonephritis (RPGN), also commonly referred to as crescentic GN.[41] This syndrome is clinically defined by loss of kidney function over a short period of time (days to weeks) and is morphologically characterized by extensive glomerular crescent formation. RPGN can be associated with any form of GN and is broadly classified based on histopathology and immune complex deposition into 3 categories: linear antibody deposition (anti-GBM disease), pauci-immune disorders (small vessel vasculitis), and granular immune complex disorders.[41,42] Serologic studies, as elaborated earlier, and a renal biopsy should be obtained in order to identify the underlying cause.

Prognosis and Management
The management of GN is primarily supportive, with specific attention to volume status and blood pressure. Because GN is associated with volume overload and hypertension, diuretics should be considered as first-line treatment.[40] In patients who are hemodynamically stable, intravenous fluids should be limited and given judiciously, as volume overload could result in respiratory distress or hypertensive emergency. In cases where blood pressure cannot be controlled solely with diuretics, or the patient is experiencing hypertensive urgency/emergency, other antihypertensive agents may be required. Disease-specific therapy should be informed by the results of serologic testing and renal pathology findings when available. In patients with autoimmune disease (SLE, anti-GBM disease, GPA), immunosuppressant treatment should be

initiated as soon as possible after a diagnosis is made.[41,60–62] Early recognition and initiation of disease-specific therapy following renal biopsy—or even after strong clinical suspicion—are essential to minimize irreversible kidney injury in the setting of RPGN.[41] This is particularly true in the setting of suspected pulmonary renal syndrome, where pulmonary involvement may be life threatening. Empirical therapy includes pulse intravenous glucocorticoids and consideration of therapeutic plasma exchange (TPE) in select patients, particularly patients with hemoptysis.[63,64]

Glomerulonephritis accounts for 10% to 15% of ESKD in the United States.[42] If left untreated, 90% of patients with RPGN will progress to ESKD within 6 months, but progression to ESKD can occur within days to weeks. Poor prognostic factors include high sCr level on initial evaluation, greater than 75% circumferential crescents or greater than 50% globally sclerosed glomeruli on renal biopsy, oliguria, and age greater than 60 years.[65] In patients with greater than 50% globally sclerosed glomeruli, renal recovery has been reported at less than 25% at 5-year follow-up.[65]

THROMBOTIC MICROANGIOPATHY

Thrombotic microangiopathy (TMA) is defined by the clinical triad of thrombocytopenia, microangiopathic hemolytic anemia (MAHA), and acute organ dysfunction.[66] TMA is a histopathologic term used to describe a variety of thrombotic vascular lesions that characterize a group of diseases that includes thrombotic thrombocytopenic purpura (TTP), hemolytic uremic syndrome (HUS), and the HELLP (hemolysis, elevated liver enzymes, and low platelets) syndrome.[67] Despite having different causes, TMA share similar pathologic and mechanistic features.

Traditionally TTP and HUS have been considered overlapping syndromes or even the same disease. However, experimental, genetic, and clinical studies have contributed to the understanding of the discrete pathophysiologic mechanisms of these disorders. Now, it is clear that TTP and HUS are distinct entities and that HUS encompasses several subtypes. By contrast, HELLP has always been considered a separate entity given its unique epidemiology. Although HELLP is exclusively a rare complication of pregnancy, TTP and HUS can be triggered by drugs, rheumatic disease (principally in children), and certain types of infection (viral being most common). In the context of infection, distinguishing TMA from sepsis may pose a difficult challenge to the medical provider.[68] Moreover, sepsis may lead to disseminated intervascular coagulation (DIC), which courses with both thrombocytopenia and microangiopathic hemolytic anemia.[69,70]

These advances in the understanding of TMA have led to the discovery and implementation of novel, targeted therapies that have had a significant effect on morbidity and mortality.[71] Here, the authors review the classification, epidemiology, pathophysiologic mechanisms, clinical presentation, and the current approach to management of TMA.

DISSEMINATED INTRAVASCULAR COAGULATION

Although not a TMA, DIC is the most frequent disorder confused with TMA. DIC is characterized by macro- and microvascular thrombosis, unlike TMA that is limited to capillary and small vessels.[72] Symptoms may include acute bleeding, bruising, shortness of breath, confusion, and hemodynamic instability. Risk factors include infection, malignancy, liver disease, surgery, anesthesia, severe tissue injury, blood products, pregnancy, and inflammation in solid organs such as pancreatitis, among others.[73] Notably, many of these risk factors have also been identified as triggers for HUS and other forms of TMA.

Diagnosis

DIC is a consumptive coagulopathy, leading to thrombocytopenia, organ dysfunction, and elevated prothrombin time- international normalized ratio (INR). In 2001 the International Society on Thrombosis and Haemostasis (ISTH) proposed diagnostic criteria centered on 4 laboratory variables, namely platelet count, PT/INR, fibrinogen, and fibrin degradation products or D-dimer (**Table 2**).[74,75] A score higher than 5 on the ISTH-DIC criteria is considered diagnostic of DIC. Notably, prothrombin time and/or INR are elevated in DIC, but not in TMA,[76] which often constitutes the first step in differentiating sepsis-associated DIC and TMA.

HEMOLYTIC UREMIC SYNDROME
Classification

HUS is a rare disorder characterized by MAHA, thrombocytopenia, and renal dysfunction. Traditionally, HUS was divided into 2 categories: diarrhea-positive and diarrhea-negative. However, current classification is based on the underlying pathophysiologic mechanisms (**Fig. 1**). Shiga-toxin (STX) HUS, formerly known as diarrhea-positive or "typical" HUS, is the most common cause of HUS worldwide. It can be caused by infection with either STX producing *Escherichia coli* (STEC) serotype 0157:H7 or *Shigella dysenteriae* type 1.[77–79] Other causes include infection with *Streptococcus pneumoniae* (SpHUS),[80–83] influenza,[84] H1N1,[85,86] HIV,[87] and inborn errors of metabolism including cobalamin C deficiency[88,89] and diacylglycerol kinase epsilon (DGKE) deficiency.[90,91] Secondary forms of HUS also occur in various disease states and conditions including bone marrow or solid organ transplant, malignancy, autoimmune disorders, malignant hypertension, and drug-associated HUS.[92–96] Comparatively, atypical HUS (aHUS) encompasses a group of disorders resulting from an inherited or acquired dysregulation of the alternative complement pathway.[97] A stepwise approach to diagnose and classify HUS is essential to differentiate HUS from other forms of TMA and other similar conditions such as sepsis and DIC.

Pathophysiology

The primary mechanism of HUS is endothelial injury in small arterioles and capillaries. This endothelial injury may result in thrombosis, platelet and fibrin aggregation, and nonthrombotic vascular lesions.[98] Buildup of thrombi on the endothelium consumes platelets and exerts shearing forces on erythrocytes, leading to hemolytic anemia.

Table 2
The International Society on Thrombosis and Haemostasis Scoring System for Overt Disseminated Intravascular Coagulation

Measure	Points	Criteria
Platelet count (x10⁹/L)	2	<50
	1	$\geq$50, <100
Prothrombin time elevation	2	$\geq$6 s
	1	$\geq$3, <6 s
Fibrinogen (g/mL)	1	<100
Fibrin degradation products or D-dimer	3	Strong increase
	2	Moderate increase
	1	—

Abbreviations: DIC, disseminated intravascular coagulation; INR, international normalized ratio; ISTH, International Society on Thrombosis and Haemostasis.

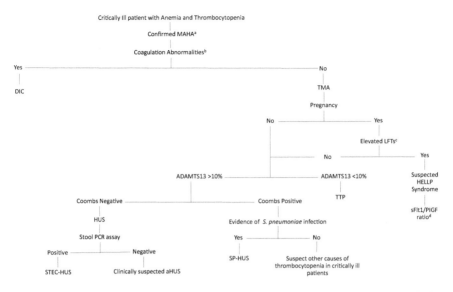

Fig. 1. Other causes of thrombocytopenia in critically ill patients. Pulmonary embolism, heparin-induced thrombocytopenia, idiopathic thrombocytopenic purpura, posttransfusion purpura, hemodilution, splenic sequestration, decreased production of platelets (chemotherapy, radiotherapy, bone marrow disorder, hematinic deficiency), laboratory artifacts. [a]Presence of hemoglobin level less than 10 g/dL, LDH level greater than 1.5 times the upper limit of normal, undetectable serum haptoglobin level, negative direct Coombs test, and evidence of either red blood cell hemolysis on peripheral blood smear or features of TMA on solid organ biopsy. [b]Elevated PT/INR, low fibrinogen, elevation in fibrin degradation products, or D-dimer. [c]Aspartate aminotransferase (AST) or alanine aminotransferase (ALT) greater than or equal to 2 times the upper limit of normal. [d]sFlt1/PlGF ratio greater than 85 before 34 weeks of gestations and greater than 110 after 34 weeks gestation strongly suggest HELLP syndrome in the setting of TMA and elevated liver function testing, whereas ratios less than 38 suggest another cause of TMA. ADAMTS13, a disintegrin and metalloproteinase with a thrombospondin type 1 motif, member 13; DIC, disseminated intravascular coagulation; HUS, hemolytic uremic syndrome; INR, international normalized ratio; LDH, lactate dehydrogenase; LFTs, liver function tests; MAHA, microangiopathic hemolytic anemia; PlGF, placental growth factor; PT, prothrombin time; sFlt-1, soluble FMS-like tyrosine kinase-1; TTP, thrombotic thrombocytopenic purpura.

In addition, endothelial swelling and mesangiolysis (necrosis of mesangial cells and dissolution of the mesangial matrix) are observed in the kidney.[99] Interestingly, overt thrombosis is not always present in renal biopsies of patients with aHUS, which has led some investigators to question if aHUS should be classified as a TMA.

SHIGA TOXIN–ASSOCIATED HEMOLYTIC UREMIC SYNDROME
Epidemiology

STX–associated HUS (ST-HUS) is the most common cause of HUS worldwide, accounting for up to 95% of HUS cases in the United States and Europe, with an annual incidence estimated at 1.9 to 2.9 cases per 100,000 children young than 5 years and 0.6 to 0.8 cases per 100,000 children younger than 15 to 18 years.[100] In North America and Europe, ST-HUS is most commonly caused by STEC.[77,78] Comparatively, *S. dysenteriae* type 1 remains the predominant cause of ST-HUS globally. Other enterohemorrhagic *E. Coli* (EHEC) serotypes that have been reported to cause HUS include O26, O45, O103, O111, O113, O121, and O145.[78,79,101–103] Among children and adults who develop EHEC enterocolitis, around 20% of children younger than 5 years and 5% of adults older than 60 years will develop HUS following STEC infection.[78,104,105]

Clinical Manifestations and Risk Factors

Following STEC exposure, symptoms of enterocolitis usually present within 2 to 12 days. Initial symptoms include watery diarrhea, after which nausea, vomiting, abdominal pain, and bloody stools develop over the following 72 hours.[77,102] Symptoms of HUS usually begin 2 to 14 days after the onset of diarrhea and may include fatigue, pallor, jaundice, and oliguria.[77] Signs of volume overload, including peripheral edema and shortness of breath, may accompany oliguria. Known risk factors for developing HUS include history of bloody diarrhea, young age, leukocytosis on presentation, and treatment with antibiotics or antimotility agents.[102,104] Extrarenal manifestations are relatively common, occurring in up to one-third of patients and affecting multiple organ systems. Neurologic symptoms have been documented in up to 50% of patients, ranging from headache to focal neurologic defects, seizures, and coma.[100,106] Cardiovascular symptoms may include myocarditis, myocardial infarction, and hypertension.[100,105] Further gastrointestinal complications can include pancreatitis, cholecystitis, and perforating colitis.[100,105] Rhabdomyolysis and ulcerative-necrotic skin lesions have also been reported.[107]

Pathophysiology

Following ingestion, STEC travels to the intestines where it binds receptors located on the surface of intestinal epithelial cells.[108] Once inside the cell, STX is released into the cytoplasm initiating an inflammatory response causing effacement of the luminal brush border, leading to secondary malabsorption and diarrhea.[109] STX is also secreted into the blood stream, where it binds to receptors on the surface of neutrophils, monocytes, erythrocytes, and platelets. When it reaches the renal vasculature, STX binds globotriaosylceramide (Gb3) receptors expressed on the endothelial cell surface where it initiates a proinflammatory and prothrombotic cascade mediated by cell-adhesion molecules such as P-selectin and von Willebrand factor.[108] Furthermore, STX upregulates expression of chemokine receptors on the cell surface and exerts a proapoptotic effect by hindering ribosomal activity, thereby inhibiting protein synthesis and ultimately resulting in cellular dysfunction and death.[67,102,110–113]

Although not primarily a result of complement dysregulation, complement activation play a role in the pathophysiology of ST-HUS. The upregulation of cell surface adhesion molecules leads to the formation of C3 convertase, a key regulator in both the classic and alternative complement pathways. In turn, formation of C3 convertase results in increased cleavage of C3. STX may also activate complement by binding complement factor H, an inhibitory factor in the alternative complement pathway.[110] Other studies have identified elevated levels of C3 and complement factor B in some cases of ST-HUS.[114] However, further research is needed to understand the contribution of complement activation in the development of ST-HUS.

Diagnosis

The clinical diagnosis of HUS is based on the triad of anemia (hemoglobin <8 g/dL or packed-cell volume <30%), thrombocytopenia (platelet count <150 × 10^9/L), and evidence of renal dysfunction, including hematuria, proteinuria, or an elevated sCr level.[115] ST-HUS is characterized by nonimmune MAHA, and as such direct Coombs testing and a peripheral blood smear should be obtained. In patients with ST-HUS, results of direct Coombs testing should be negative, and peripheral blood smear should show evidence of MAHA with findings of schistocytes, burr cells, or helmet cells.[78,116] A peripheral blood smear without evidence of MAHA would indicate other forms of Coombs-negative hemolytic anemia such as paroxysmal nocturnal hemoglobin-uria.[117] Other laboratory indicators of hemolysis are likely to be observed and may include elevated serum LDH and bilirubin levels, along with an undetectable serum haptoglobin.[115] Although the identification of STEC or STX in the stool is not required to make the diagnosis of ST-HUS, stool samples should be collected and sent for STEC and STX testing. Stool culture should be plated specifically using sorbitol-MacConkey medium to improve detection of STEC; alternately, molecular genetic assays can be used. Importantly, other signs of coagulopathy should not be present. In patients with ST-HUS, fibrinogen concentrations are normal or high, and prothrombin time/INR time is normal or only slightly elevated.[115] To differentiate HUS from TTP, ADAMTS13 activity level should be sent before administration of blood products and is low (<10%) in patients with TTP.[93] Additional information regarding the diagnosis of TTP are discussed later.

Prognosis and Management

Treatment of ST-HUS remains primarily supportive. Notably, early volume expansion has been associated with a lower incidence of oliguric AKI and need for RRT.[118] Close monitoring of urine output and fluid balance during fluid resuscitation is critical to maintain adequate intravascular volume while avoiding fluid overload. In patients who develop evidence of volume overload including cardiomegaly, pulmonary edema, or hypertension, fluid restriction should be used. Diuretics may be used judiciously to help correct volume overload, with close attention to avoid intravascular volume depletion, and thereby perpetuate microvascular thrombi formation.

The use of antibiotics for treatment of STEC infection remains a topic of debate. Early data suggested that treatment of EHEC-associated enteritis with bactericidal antibiotics was associated with an increased risk for developing HUS[119,120]; however, more recent data suggest that this may not be true. A meta-analysis by Safdar and colleagues in 2002 and a prospective observational study by Geerdes-Fenge and colleagues in 2013 showed no significant increase in the risk for developing HUS in patients who received antibiotics for EHEC infection,[121] whereas some studies suggest that the risk of developing HUS in patients with EHEC enterocolitis may be related to the specific antibiotic or the specific pathogen involved. Other data have shown that antimicrobial therapy in patients with ST-HUS may reduce the severity of HUS and shorten the duration of pathogen excretion.[122] Ultimately, at present, data regarding the efficacy and/or potential morbidity of antimicrobial therapy in patients with ST-HUS are inconclusive.

Platelet transfusions in patients with ST-HUS also remain controversial. Although some studies suggest harm, other studies have demonstrated no significant difference in the rates of thrombotic events, seizures, need for RRT, or mortality in patients with ST-HUS who did or did not receive platelets.[123,124] Notably, in a study looking at the consequences of platelet transfusions in patients with STEC-HUS during the 2011 *E. coli* outbreak in Germany, the investigators found that death occurred in 6 of 711 patients with STEC-HUS as a direct result of procedural-related bleeding.[123] Therefore, the potential risk versus benefit of platelet administration in patients with HUS undergoing invasive procedures should be considered on a case-by-case basis.

Although complement activation likely plays some role in the pathophysiology of ST-HUS, complement blockage with eculizumab, a monoclonal antibody against C5, has not been shown to improve outcomes.[125] However, evidence-based data and randomized control trials to evaluate the efficacy of eculizumab in patients with ST-HUS remain limited. The efficacy of other treatment modalities for management of ST-HUS, including TPE, also remains unclear. Limited evidence suggests that TPE may reduce mortality in patients with ST-HUS older than 60 years or in some pediatrics patients with severe disease; however, no definitive recommendations can be made at this time based on current literature.[126]

ATYPICAL HEMOLYTIC UREMIC SYNDROME
Epidemiology

Because of similarities in the clinical presentation of aHUS and more prevalent diseases including sepsis and DIC, the incidence and prevalence of aHUS has been challenging to define. In the United States, the incidence of aHUS is estimated at 1 in 500,000 per year.[116] The overall prevalence of aHUS has been shown to be highest among children younger than 4 years, at approximately 3 per 1 million children. Prevalence subsequently declines in higher age groups, with an estimated prevalence of 0.3 to 1 per million children aged 5 to 15 years. In adults, best estimates place the prevalence of aHUS around 2.4 to 5.8 per million people.[127]

Clinical Manifestations and Risk Factors

Atypical HUS is a complex disease with a wide range of clinical manifestations. Acute cases of aHUS will usually present with signs of MAHA and/or kidney injury including fatigue, pallor, jaundice, oliguria, and edema. Notably, abdominal pain, nausea, vomiting, and diarrhea are common presenting symptoms, with diarrhea occurring in approximately half of the patients with aHUS.[128–130] Therefore, the presence or absence of diarrhea cannot be used to differentiate between patients with ST-HUS and aHUS. Neurologic symptoms are also seen frequently, with central nervous system symptoms ranging from headaches to seizures, focal neurologic deficits, and even encephalopathy and coma.[97,129,131–134] The occurrence of ocular symptoms, cardiac injury including myocardial infarction, peripheral vascular symptoms, and skin lesions is also well described.[135]

PATHOPHYSIOLOGY

Atypical HUS is a group of disorders that results from dysregulation of the alternative complement pathway. Up to 60% of patients with aHUS have an identifiable pathogenic gain-of-function variant in an effector gene or loss-of-function variant in a regulatory gene in the complement pathway.[136] The list of genes involved in aHUS include complement factor H (CFH), membrane cofactor protein (MCP or CD46), C3, complement factor I (CFI), complement factor B (CFB), THBD (encoding thrombomodulin), and DGKE.[131,137]

Atypical HUS is known to have incomplete genetic penetrance, with only 40% to 50% of carriers with known pathogenic variants going on to develop TMA.[131] It is therefore proposed that aHUS occurs following a trigger event, such as infection, malignancy, systemic illness, solid organ or bone marrow transplantation, medication exposure, pregnancy, or other event that initiates the release of inflammatory mediators. These mediators cause an inflammatory response, leading to endothelial cell damage and further propagation of complement activity. Unregulated complement activation ultimately results in the formation of the C5b-C9 membrane attack complex (MAC), leading to more endothelial injury and the formation of vascular thrombi.[136]

Diagnosis

In patients with a Coombs-negative MAHA, thrombocytopenia, and renal dysfunction, further history and testing should be undertaken to rule out TTP and other causes of HUS. In pediatric patients, the primary differential diagnosis of aHUS is STEC-HUS, whereas in adults TTP and secondary forms of HUS are more common. Low C3 levels are found in approximately 40% of patients but are not diagnostic for aHUS.[138,139] Genetic testing should be obtained, although turnaround times may preclude the use of clinically actionable results during the index hospitalization. Evaluation of secondary forms of HUS should be undertaken including a thorough history and targeted laboratory evaluation. Causes of secondary HUS can include solid organ or bone marrow transplant, malignancy, viral (eg, HIV, CMV, EBV, influenza) or certain bacterial infections (eg, S. pneumoniae), and drug-associated HUS.[140,141] Transplant-associated HUS normally occurs within the first few weeks following transplantation and may be related to rejection or high-dose immunosuppressive therapy. Many medications have been reported to cause HUS including chemotherapeutic agents (eg, bleomycin, cisplatin, gemcitabine, mitomycin), immunotherapeutic agents (eg, cyclosporine, interferon, muromonab-CD3, quinine, tacrolimus), and antiplatelet agents (eg, clopidogrel, ticlopidine).[142,143] When likely causes of secondary HUS have been excluded, then a diagnosis and treatment of aHUS should be highly considered. Although not required to establish the diagnosis of aHUS, tissue biopsy (skin, kidney or heart) with extensive microvascular deposition of C5b-9 MAC supports the diagnosis of aHUS.[144] However, in the setting of thrombocytopenia and increased risk for bleeding, tissue biopsy should be considered judiciously.

Prognosis and Management

Many of the trigger events associated with aHUS are known risk factors for infection and sepsis, which as we have described, can closely mimic the presentation of TMA. In addition, sepsis and DIC share many of the proinflammatory, endothelial dysfunction and complement activation features of TMA, resulting in thrombocytopenia and thrombus formation. It is therefore imperative that health care providers have a high degree of clinical suspicion for TMA in critically ill patients presenting with kidney injury, thrombocytopenia, anemia, or multiorgan failure. The presence of thrombocytopenia and MAHA should alert health care providers to consider the diagnosis of TMA and perform the appropriate diagnostic tests to evaluate for these conditions. Given the exceptionally high morbidity and mortality associated with TMA, early identification and initiation of disease specific therapy is critical for patient survival.

Historically, plasma therapy, dialysis, and kidney transplantation were the mainstay of therapy for aHUS. In 2007, management of aHUS changed significantly with the release of eculizumab, a monoclonal humanized antibody directed against C5. Adoption of eculizumab as the first-line treatment of aHUS has been associated with a significant reduction in patient morbidity and mortality[145–148]; however, further studies are needed to assess the long-term outcomes with complement blockade therapies. Treatment with eculizumab or other terminal complement inhibitors has been associated with invasive infection with encapsulated bacteria, including meningococcal infection. Patients receiving eculizumab therapy should receive both the meningococcal conjugate and serogroup B meningococcal vaccines. Antibiotic prophylaxis against meningococcal infection is mandated during the first 2 weeks of eculizumab therapy and should be continued for a minimum of 2 weeks following meningococcal vaccination.[140] If complement blockage therapy is not available, then treatment with TPE can be used.[141,149] Duration of treatment with eculizumab remains controversial, and recommendations are largely based on expert option. In general, complement blockade should be continued for a minimum of 12 months after initiation of therapy and a minimum of 3 months following renal recovery,[140] after which discontinuation of therapy can be considered on case-by-case basis.

Clinical outcomes in aHUS are generally unfavorable, with mortality rates around 25% and progression to ESKD occurring in approximately half of the patients.[66] Although overall outcomes are generally poor, patient prognosis can vary significantly depending on the underlying pathogenic genetic variant. MCP variants generally carry the best prognosis, with a risk of ESKD of less than 25%. Comparatively, CFH, CFI, or C3 variants have been associated with mortality rates as high as 30% during the first episode of aHUS, with rates of ESKD or mortality reaching 75% at 5 years.[131,139] For patients who develop ESKD, the decision to pursue kidney transplantation should be considered in the context of the patient's underlying genetic abnormalities, response to therapy, and risk of relapse following transplantation.

THROMBOCYTOPENIC PURPURA
Classification and Epidemiology

TTP is an acquired or hereditary disorder that, as HUS, is characterized by the presence of MAHA and thrombocytopenia caused by reduced activity of the enzyme ADAMTS13. Classically, TTP was also defined by the presence of renal dysfunction, fever, and neurologic findings; however, the diagnosis of TTP may be made in the absence of these symptoms, with less than 5% of patients presenting with the full clinical pentad.[150,151] Occurrence of TTP is rare, with an incidence of acquired TTP around 3 in 1 million adults and 1 in 10 million children per year.[152]

Clinical Manifestations and Risk Factors

Symptoms of TTP most often include fatigue, petechial rash, and other bleeding. Other presenting symptoms may include easy bruising, dyspnea, weakness, fever, dizziness, arrhythmias, abdominal pain, nausea and/or vomiting, and neurologic findings including headache, confusion, altered mental status, transient focal abnormalities, seizures, stroke, or coma.[150,151] Neurologic symptoms are present in roughly 30% of patients, whereas gastrointestinal symptoms can occur in up to 70% of patients with TTP.[151] In a modern cohort, fever occurred in only 10% of patients.[151] Risk factors include female sex, with approximately 75% of cases occurring in women.[152,153]

Pathophysiology

TTP is caused by reduced activity of the von Willebrand factor (vWF) cleaving protease ADAMTS13. vWF is a procoagulant responsible for platelet adhesion. As such, reduced activity of ADAMTS13 leads to increased platelet adhesion and thrombi formation, particularly at the arteriole-capillary junction and at locations of vascular injury. Although hereditary TTP is secondary to an inherited pathogenic variant in ADAMTS13, acquired TTP is defined by the development of IgG autoantibodies against ADAMTS13.[154]

Diagnosis

TTP should be suspected in patients presenting with MAHA (hemoglobin <10 g/dL) and severe thrombocytopenia (platelet count <30 × 10^9/L). As in HUS, the presence of MAHA should be confirmed with a negative direct Coombs test and the presence of schistocytes, burr cells, or helmet cells on peripheral smear. Other laboratory studies consistent with hemolysis may include elevated serum LDH, free hemoglobin levels, and low serum haptoglobin level. ADAMTS13 activity and ADAMTS13 autoantibody testing ideally should be collected before administration of TPE or blood products. In patients with clinically significant TTP, ADAMTS13 activity is typically less than 10%.[151,155] Although ADAMTS13 activity of 10% to 20% has been reported in some patients with TTP (primarily those who have received therapy before ADAMTS13 testing), activity levels greater than 10% should prompt consideration of other forms of TMA. Importantly, evidence of DIC or other forms of coagulopathy should not be present.

The PLASMIC score (**Table 3**), developed in a cohort of adults with suspected TMA, can be used to estimate the probability that a patient presenting with MAHA and thrombocytopenia has TTP.[156] One point is given for the presence of each feature. A total score of 0 to 4 predicts a low probability, 5 an intermediate probability, and 6 to 7 a high probability of TTP. A 2020 systematic review and meta-analysis of the diagnostic accuracy of the PLASMIC score in patients with suspected TTP reported that a PLASMIC score greater than or equal to 5 provided 99% sensitivity and 57% specificity for the diagnosis of TTP.[157] The investigators therefore suggested that given the severity of the disease, all patients with clinical suspicion for TTP and a PLASMIC a score of greater than or equal to 5 should receive empirical treatment pending the results of ADAMTS13 testing. Overall, the ADAMTS13 level and the PLASMIC score should be interpreted in clinical context, and decisions regarding therapy should not solely rely on either measurement.

Prognosis and Management

The mainstay of treatment of all patients with presumed or confirmed TTP is TPE. TPE should be initiated urgently and continued daily until the platelet count normalizes or an alternative diagnosis is established. In addition, patients should receive glucocorticoids and rituximab, with the dose of glucocorticoids based on the severity of features at presentation. Treatment with caplacizumab, an anti-vWF antibody, should be considered for patients presenting with severe neurologic features or high serum troponin levels.[158] Platelet transfusions should be given in patients who develop clinically significant bleeding or for those who require a surgical or interventional procedure that may predispose to significant blood loss. Importantly, there is no evidence to

Table 3 Plasmic score	
Variable	Points
Platelet count <30 × 10⁹/L	1
Hemolysis variables • Reticulocyte count >2.5% • Undetectable haptoglobin • Bilirubin—indirect >2.0 mg/dL	1
No active cancer	1
No history of solid-organ or stem-cell transplant	1
Mean corpuscular volume (MCV) < 90 fL	1
INR <1.5	1
Creatinine <2.0 mg/dL	1
0–4 Low probability, 5 intermediate probability, and 6–7 high probability.	

suggest that administration of platelets in patients with TTP is associated with harm.[159]

Recovery of platelet counts normally occurs within 7 to 10 days of initiation of TPE. Approximately 15% to 20% of patients will have exacerbation of disease following discontinuation of TPE, most often characterized by a decrease in platelet count without new neurologic symptoms. Literature suggests that rates of relapse following remission are most dependent on treatment with rituximab, with relapse rates around 13% and 40% with and without rituximab treatment, respectively.[151,160] Relapse most often occurs within 2 years of the initial presentation but can occur as late as 20 years after the initial diagnosis. The potential benefit of long-term treatment with rituximab must be weighed against the potential risks in individual cases. Despite current therapies, mortality rates among patients with TTP remains as high as 10% to 20%. If left untreated, mortality is as high as 90%.[151,155]

PREGNANCY-ASSOCIATED THROMBOTIC MICROANGIOPATHY
Classification and Epidemiology

HELLP syndrome is a life-threating medical condition that is characterized by hemolysis, elevated liver enzyme tests, and low platelet count. HELLP is the most common subtype of TMA occurring in pregnancy and is most often observed in women with preeclampsia (PE)/eclampsia; however, HELLP can rarely occur in the absence of these conditions.[161] HELLP, as PE and eclampsia, is thought to be secondary to an imbalance of angiogenic and antiangiogenic factors although its pathogenesis is not well understood.[162] Although HELLP is a disease exclusive to pregnancy, pregnancy has also been identified as a risk factor for other forms of TMA including HUS and TTP. HELLP affects 0.2% to 0.6% of all pregnancies, occurring in 4% to 12% of woman with PE/eclampsia.[161] Comparatively, TTP and aHUS occur in less than 1 in 17,000 and 1 in 25,000 pregnancies, respectively.[163,164] Pregnancy-associated TTP accounts for 10% to 30% of adult TTP cases, whereas pregnancy-associated aHUS represents approximately 16% of aHUS cases in women aged 18 to 45 years.[164]

Clinical Manifestations and Risk Factors

Initial symptoms of HELLP are usually relatively nonspecific and may include fatigue, malaise, nausea, vomiting, epigastric or right upper quadrant (RUQ) pain, and headache.[161] Patients may also experience bleeding and visual disturbance.[165] On examination, affected patients may have edema, elevated blood pressure, jaundice, and RUQ tenderness.[161,165] HELLP is most often observed during the third trimester of pregnancy, but onset in the late second trimester or at term/postpartum is also common.[166] Onset before 20 weeks is rare, occurring in less than 3% of cases, whereas onset following delivery is observed in approximately 30% of cases with most patients being diagnosed within 48 hours of delivery.[166] Risk factors for HELLP include maternal age greater than 25 years, multiparity, PE/eclampsia, and a history of HELLP in a prior pregnancy. Various genetic variants/polymorphisms, both maternal and fetal, have also been associated with an increased risk for the development of HELLP. These include, but are not limited to, pathogenic variants in factor V Leiden coagulation factor, the Fas receptor, and vascular endothelial growth factor (VEGF).[167]

Pathophysiology

High circulating levels of antiangiogenic mediators are thought to underlie the endothelial dysfunction present in PE/eclampsia and HELLP. Increased levels of soluble FMS-like tyrosine kinase-1 (sFlt-1), a naturally occurring antagonist to VEGF and placental growth factor (PIGF), has been identified in patients with PE.[168] This in turn is accompanied by decreased levels of free VEGF and PIGF.[169] When administered in animal models, sFlt-1 can induce symptoms of PE, including hypertension and proteinuria. Other findings of generalized endothelial dysfunction in patients with PE include elevated concentrations of thrombomodulin and factor VIII antigen and decreased production of endothelial-derived vasodilators including nitric oxide and prostacyclin, along with enhanced vascular reactivity to angiotensin II and impaired flow-mediated vasodilation.[170] Some of these findings, including vascular oxidative stress and vascular sensitivity to angiotensin II, have been replicated in animal models following exposure to sFlt-1.[168,170] However, the trigger for increased production of sFlt-1 by the placenta remains unclear.

Preliminary evidence suggests that complement dysregulation may also play an important role in the pathogenesis of HELLP. In one study, plasma levels of soluble C5b-9 MAC were significantly higher in HELLP patients at the time of diagnosis when compared with healthy gestational age-matched controls.[171] Similarly, C5a plasma levels were also higher in cases compared with controls. Genetically, 22 genetic variants involved in complement-related diseases were identified, 17 among the 19 patients with HELLP and 5 among matched controls.[172] Other studies have similarly identified evidence of complement activation in patients with HELLP compared with unaffected pregnancy and nonpregnant controls.[173] Although these findings suggest that complement dysregulation may play a role in the pathogenesis of HELLP, its overall contribution remains unknown.

Diagnosis

Mild thrombocytopenia is commonly observed in pregnancy, with approximately 10% of patients with uncomplicated pregnancies having a platelet count less than 150 x10^9/L.[174,175] As such, the definition of TMA is modified in the setting of pregnancy and defined as a platelet count less than 100 x10^9/L, evidence of MAHA (hemoglobin <10 g/dL, LDH >1.5x the upper limit of normal, undetectable serum haptoglobin level, negative direct Coombs test, and evidence of either red blood cell hemolysis on peripheral blood smear or features of TMA on organ solid biopsy), and organ injury.[164] Diagnostic criteria or HELLP also require the presence of elevated liver enzymes, defined as an aspartate aminotransferase (AST) or alanine aminotransferase (ALT) greater than or equal to 2x the upper limit of normal. Evaluation for HELLP should also include measurement of sFlt1 and PIGF levels; sFlt1/PIGF ratio greater than 85 before 34 weeks of gestations and greater than 110 after 34 weeks gestation strongly suggest HELLP in the setting of TMA and elevated liver function testing, whereas ratios less than 38 suggest another cause of TMA.[169,176,177]

Prognosis and Management

Management of TMA during pregnancy should take into account the cause, timing of the TMA, patient symptoms, and laboratory findings. Maternal complications from HELLP can include placental abruption, ruptured liver hematoma, pulmonary edema, acute respiratory distress syndrome, AKI, and DIC.[166] For patients with HELLP, the primary treatment is delivery.[178,179] Patients requiring urgent assessment and intervention include those with severe hypertension, severe RUQ or epigastric pain, abnormal fetal heart rate tracing, low fetal biophysical profile scores, or any complication. Hypertension should be treated promptly to reduce the risk of stroke and seizure. Patients with severe RUQ or epigastric pain should undergo expedited imaging to evaluate for hepatic hematoma or rupture.[180–185] When available, management of a hematoma or an active bleed should be performed in consultation with a surgical team experienced in liver trauma surgery. Patients with pulmonary edema, AKI, or DIC should be stabilized and delivered.[178,179] Prompt delivery is indicated among those with pregnancies greater than or equal to 34 weeks of gestation or in those with placental abruption, fetal demise, or pregnancies less than the age of viability. In the absence of these scenarios and an estimated gestational age between the lower limits of viability and 34 weeks, delivery may be delayed following a course of betamethasone to promote fetal lung development.[178,179] Magnesium sulfate should be administrated for seizure prophylaxis at the time of admission and continued through delivery and the postpartum period. After delivery, laboratory studies may continue to worsen over the following 48 hours. If the patient has worsening thrombocytopenia and a continued increase in LDH at 4 days post partum, then an alternative diagnosis to HELLP should be considered. Maternal mortality rate in HELLP is around 1.1%, with an infant mortality rate as high as 60%.[161]

OVERVIEW OF THE DIAGNOSTIC APPROACH TO THE CRITICALLY ILL PATIENT WITH SUSPECTED TMA

DIC, HUS, TTP, and HELLP share common clinical features but can often be differentiated by their laboratory features (**Table 4**). The presence of coagulopathy is key to differentiate DIC from TMA. Although DIC is a systemic disorder of the coagulation system resulting in a consumptive coagulopathy, TMA is associated with normal coagulation profiles (see **Fig. 1**). After the presence of MAHA and thrombocytopenia have been confirmed, early differentiation between TTP, HUS, and HELLP is critical. In pregnant patients, the presence of elevated liver function testing should alert clinicians to the possibility of HELLP. Measurement of sFlt-1 and PIGF levels can help to differentiate HELLP from other forms of pregnancy-associated TMA. In pregnant patients with normal liver function testing and those who are not pregnant, evaluation for TTP or HUS should be undertaken.

Table 4
Laboratory profile in patient with suspected thrombotic microangiopathy

Disease/Condition[e]	Platelet Count	MAHA[a]	PT (INR)	PTT	Fibrinogen	Fibrin Marker[b]	ADAMTS13 Activity
HUS	↓	+	↔	↔	↔	↔ [c]	↔
DIC	↓	+	↓	↓	↓	↓	↔
TTP	↓	+	↔	↔	↔	↔	↓ [d]

↓ = decreased level; ↔ = normal level; + = present.

Abbreviations: ADAMTS13, A disintegrin and metalloproteinase with a thrombospondin type 1 motif, member 13; DIC, disseminated intravascular coagulation; HUS, hemolytic uremic syndrome; INR, international normalized ratio; LDH, lactate dehydrogenase; MAHA, microangiopathic hemolytic anemia; PIGF, placental growth factor; PT, prothrombin time; sFlt-1, soluble FMS-like tyrosine kinase-1; TTP, thrombotic thrombocytopenic purpura.

[a] Presence of any of the following: elevated indirect bilirubin and LDH, decreased hemoglobin and haptoglobin, presence of schistocytes in peripheral blood smear.
[b] Include D-dimer and fibrin degradation products.
[c] There can be activation of the fibrinolytic pathway with increased circulating levels of fibrin degradation products.
[d] Less than 10% activity of ADAMTS13 is consistent with TTP.
[e] sFlt1/PIGF ratio greater than 85 before 34 wk of gestations and greater than 110 after 34 wk gestation strongly suggest HELLP syndrome in the setting of TMA and elevated liver function testing, whereas ratios less than 38 suggest another cause of TMA.

ADAMTS13 activity level is the definitive test to distinguish between TTP and other forms of TMA, with an ADAMTS13 activity level less than 10% consistent with a diagnosis of TTP. However, the results of ADAMTS13 testing may take days or weeks to result, leading to potential delays in disease-specific treatment. As such, use of scoring systems such the PLASMIC score should be used to guide early disease-specific therapy. When risk for TTP is high, presumptive treatment (eg, therapeutic plasma exchange) should be initiated while awaiting test results.

When TTP has been ruled out or deemed unlikely, steps to differentiate between the various forms of HUS should be performed. In patients with a history of diarrhea, stool culture and stool PCR for STX should be obtained. Additional laboratory testing should include a direct Coombs test and body fluid cultures if localized infection is suspected. Coombs testing can help differentiate HUS from other forms hemolytic anemia. Although a positive Coombs test indicates an autoimmune hemolytic anemia and thereby excludes most forms of TMA, a positive direct Coombs test can be present in a select group of patients with *S pneumoniae*–associated HUS (SP-HUS). Although not discussed in depth in this review, SP-HUS should be suspected in young children presenting with features of HUS and evidence of invasive *S pneumoniae* infection. SP-HUS accounts for less than 5% of HUS cases in children, and as with sepsis, the mainstay of therapy is treatment of the underlying bacterial infection. In those in which stools studies are negative for STEC or STX, aHUS should be highly considered. Ultimately, the diagnosis of aHUS is made by exclusion of DIC and other forms of TMA. Screening for secondary causes of HUS including underlying malignancy, autoimmune disease, viral infection (hepatitis B and C, EBV, CMV, HIV, influenza), medication use commonly associated with TMA, or family history of TMA should be performed. Screening for pathogenic genetic variants associated with aHUS can assist in prognosis and long-term management but often is impractical in the acute setting when rapid diagnosis of aHUS is required; further improvements in molecular genetic technologies may result in decreased sequencing time and increased and more rapid availability of clinically actionable genetic results. In patients in whom a diagnosis is unclear, tissues biopsy (skin, kidney, heart) with extensive microvascular staining for terminal MAC can help support the diagnosis of aHUS.

SUMMARY

The uncommon causes of AKI discussed in this review have a significant contribution to patient morbidity and mortality in the ICU. High suspicion for TMA, immune-mediated, and structural causes of AKI is required to make a prompt diagnosis and thereby initiate disease-directed therapy, particularly in the critically ill patient. Kidney imaging, urine studies (urinalysis and urine microscopy), and serum hemolytic studies (LDH, unconjugated bilirubin, and haptoglobin levels) should be a routine part of the evaluation of AKI among critically ill patients. The presence of acute oliguria, hematuria, sterile pyuria, or thrombocytopenia should alert medical providers to the possibility of these disease entities and prompt further diagnostic evaluation.

DISCLOSURE

J.A. Kellum discloses grant support and consulting fees from Astute Medical/BioMerieuxand Baxter and is currently a full-time employee of Spectral Medical. H. Gómez discloses grant support and consulting fees from BioMerieux. All other authors declare no conflicts of interest.

CLINICS CARE POINTS

- The presence of acute oliguria, hematuria, sterile pyuria, or thrombocytopenia should alert clinicians to the possibility of an unusual cause of AKI and prompt further diagnostic evaluation.
- Microangiopathic hemolytic anemia is characterized by one or more of the following: elevated indirect bilirubin and LDH, decreased hemoglobin and haptoglobin, presence of schistocytes in peripheral blood smear.
- Immune-mediated tubulointerstitial nephritis is the most common finding on kidney biopsy when patients with AKI undergo this procedure.

REFERENCES

1. Ronco C, Bellomo R, Kellum JA. Acute kidney injury. Lancet 2019;394(10212): 1949–64.
2. Hoste EA, Bagshaw SM, Bellomo R, et al. Epidemiology of acute kidney injury in critically ill patients: the multinational AKI-EPI study. Intensive Care Med 2015; 41(8):1411–23.
3. Kellum JA, Sileanu FE, Murugan R, et al. Classifying AKI by urine output versus serum creatinine level. J Am Soc Nephrol 2015;26(9):2231–8.
4. Murugan R, Kellum JA. Acute kidney injury: what's the prognosis? Nat Rev Nephrol 2011;7(4):209–17.
5. Amin AP, Salisbury AC, McCullough PA, et al. Trends in the incidence of acute kidney injury in patients hospitalized with acute myocardial infarction. Arch Intern Med 2012;172(3):246–53.
6. Goldstein SL, Kirkendall E, Nguyen H, et al. Electronic health record identification of nephrotoxin exposure and associated acute kidney injury. Pediatrics 2013;132(3):e756–67.
7. Hamdi A, Hajage D, Van Glabeke E, et al. Severe post-renal acute kidney injury, post-obstructive diuresis and renal recovery. BJU Int 2012;110(11 Pt C): E1027–34.
8. Akposso K, Hertig A, Couprie R, et al. Acute renal failure in patients over 80 years old: 25-years' experience. Intensive Care Med 2000;26(4):400–6.
9. Patel DM, Connor MJ Jr. Intra-abdominal hypertension and abdominal compartment syndrome: an underappreciated cause of acute kidney injury. Adv Chronic Kidney Dis 2016;23(3):160–6.
10. Vidal MG, Ruiz Weisser J, Gonzalez F, et al. Incidence and clinical effects of intra-abdominal hypertension in critically ill patients. Crit Care Med 2008; 36(6):1823–31.
11. Yang J, Lee JY, Na YJ, et al. Risk factors and outcomes of acute renal infarction. Kidney Res Clin Pract 2016;35(2):90–5.
12. Chavez-Iniguez JS, Navarro-Gallardo GJ, Medina-Gonzalez R, et al. Acute kidney injury caused by obstructive nephropathy. Int J Nephrol 2020;2020: 8846622.
13. Malbrain ML, De Laet IE. Intra-abdominal hypertension: evolving concepts. Crit Care Nurs Clin North Am 2012;24(2):275–309.
14. Sugrue M, Buist MD, Hourihan F, et al. Prospective study of intra-abdominal hypertension and renal function after laparotomy. Br J Surg 1995;82(2):235–8.

15. Mohmand H, Goldfarb S. Renal dysfunction associated with intra-abdominal hypertension and the abdominal compartment syndrome. J Am Soc Nephrol 2011; 22(4):615–21.

16. Chu PL, Wei YF, Huang JW, et al. Clinical characteristics of patients with segmental renal infarction. Nephrology (Carlton) 2006;11(4):336–40.

17. Domanovits H, Paulis M, Nikfardjam M, et al. Acute renal infarction. Clinical characteristics of 17 patients. Medicine (Baltimore) 1999;78(6):386–94.

18. Oh YK, Yang CW, Kim YL, et al. Clinical characteristics and outcomes of renal infarction. Am J Kidney Dis 2016;67(2):243–50.

19. Perazella MA, Markowitz GS. Drug-induced acute interstitial nephritis. Nat Rev Nephrol 2010;6(8):461–70.

20. Matthew D, Oxman D, Djekidel K, et al. Abdominal compartment syndrome and acute kidney injury due to excessive auto-positive end-expiratory pressure. Am J Kidney Dis 2013;61(2):285–8.

21. Muresan M, Muresan S, Brinzaniuc K, et al. How much does decompressive laparotomy reduce the mortality rate in primary abdominal compartment syndrome?: a single-center prospective study on 66 patients. Medicine (Baltimore) 2017;96(5):e6006.

22. Eddy V, Nunn C, Morris JA Jr. Abdominal compartment syndrome. The Nashville experience. Surg Clin North Am 1997;77(4):801–12.

23. Ouriel K, Andrus CH, Ricotta JJ, et al. Acute renal artery occlusion: when is revascularization justified? J Vasc Surg 1987;5(2):348–55.

24. Haas CA, Spirnak JP. Traumatic renal artery occlusion: a review of the literature. Tech Urol 1998;4(1):1–11.

25. Haas CA, Dinchman KH, Nasrallah PF, et al. Traumatic renal artery occlusion: a 15-year review. J Trauma 1998;45(3):557–61.

26. Paris B, Bobrie G, Rossignol P, et al. Blood pressure and renal outcomes in patients with kidney infarction and hypertension. J Hypertens 2006;24(8):1649–54.

27. Farrington K, Levison DA, Greenwood RN, et al. Renal biopsy in patients with unexplained renal impairment and normal kidney size. Q J Med 1989;70(263): 221–33.

28. Baker RJ, Pusey CD. The changing profile of acute tubulointerstitial nephritis. Nephrol Dial Transplant 2004;19(1):8–11.

29. Joyce E, Glasner P, Ranganathan S, et al. Tubulointerstitial nephritis: diagnosis, treatment, and monitoring. Pediatr Nephrol 2017;32(4):577–87.

30. Ng JH, Zaidan M, Jhaveri KD, et al. Acute tubulointerstitial nephritis and COVID-19. Clin Kidney J 2021;14(10):2151–7.

31. Klaus R, Jansson AF, Griese M, et al. Case report: pediatric renal sarcoidosis and prognostic factors in reviewed cases. Front Pediatr 2021;9:724728.

32. Medhat BM, Behiry ME, Fateen M, et al. Sarcoidosis beyond pulmonary involvement: a case series of unusual presentations. Respir Med Case Rep 2021;34: 101495.

33. Ambruzs JM, Walker PD, Larsen CP. The histopathologic spectrum of kidney biopsies in patients with inflammatory bowel disease. Clin J Am Soc Nephrol 2014;9(2):265–70.

34. Mackensen F, Smith JR, Rosenbaum JT. Enhanced recognition, treatment, and prognosis of tubulointerstitial nephritis and uveitis syndrome. Ophthalmology 2007;114(5):995–9.

35. Ayasreh-Fierro N, Ars-Criach E, Lopes-Martin V, et al. Familial chronic interstitial nephropathy with hyperuricaemia caused by the UMOD gene. Nefrologia 2013; 33(4):587–92.

36. Devuyst O, Olinger E, Weber S, et al. Autosomal dominant tubulointerstitial kidney disease. Nat Rev Dis Primers 2019;5(1):60.
37. Hodgkins KS, Schnaper HW. Tubulointerstitial injury and the progression of chronic kidney disease. Pediatr Nephrol 2012;27(6):901–9.
38. Garcia-Sanchez O, Lopez-Hernandez FJ, Lopez-Novoa JM. An integrative view on the role of TGF-beta in the progressive tubular deletion associated with chronic kidney disease. Kidney Int 2010;77(11):950–5.
39. Storsley L, Gibson IW. Adenovirus interstitial nephritis and rejection in an allograft. J Am Soc Nephrol 2011;22(8):1423–7.
40. Rossert J. Drug-induced acute interstitial nephritis. Kidney Int 2001;60(2):804–17.
41. Moledina DG, Perazella MA. Drug-induced acute interstitial nephritis. Clin J Am Soc Nephrol 2017;12(12):2046–9.
42. Hashmi MS, Pandey J. Nephritic syndrome. Treasure Island (FL): StatPearls; 2021.
43. Naik RH, Shawar SH. Rapidly progressive glomerulonephritis. Treasure Island (FL): StatPearls; 2021.
44. Vinen CS, Oliveira DB. Acute glomerulonephritis. Postgrad Med J 2003;79(930):206–13, quiz: 212-203].
45. Gomez-Puerta JA, Hernandez-Rodriguez J, Lopez-Soto A, et al. Antineutrophil cytoplasmic antibody-associated vasculitides and respiratory disease. Chest 2009;136(4):1101–11.
46. Solans-Laque R, Bosch-Gil J, Canela M, et al. Clinical features and therapeutic management of subglottic stenosis in patients with Wegener's granulomatosis. Lupus 2008;17(9):832–6.
47. Lazor R, Bigay-Game L, Cottin V, et al. Alveolar hemorrhage in anti-basement membrane antibody disease: a series of 28 cases. Medicine (Baltimore) 2007;86(3):181–93.
48. Trapani S, Micheli A, Grisolia F, et al. Henoch Schonlein purpura in childhood: epidemiological and clinical analysis of 150 cases over a 5-year period and review of literature. Semin Arthritis Rheum 2005;35(3):143–53.
49. Greco CM, Rudy TE, Manzi S. Adaptation to chronic pain in systemic lupus erythematosus: applicability of the multidimensional pain inventory. Pain Med 2003;4(1):39–50.
50. Lee HJ, Sinha AA. Cutaneous lupus erythematosus: understanding of clinical features, genetic basis, and pathobiology of disease guides therapeutic strategies. Autoimmunity 2006;39(6):433–44.
51. Gilliam JN, Sontheimer RD. Distinctive cutaneous subsets in the spectrum of lupus erythematosus. J Am Acad Dermatol 1981;4(4):471–5.
52. Sanjad S, Tolaymat A, Whitworth J, et al. Acute glomerulonephritis in children: a review of 153 cases. South Med J 1977;70(10):1202–6.
53. Blyth CC, Robertson PW, Rosenberg AR. Post-streptococcal glomerulonephritis in Sydney: a 16-year retrospective review. J Paediatr Child Health 2007;43(6):446–50.
54. Nissenson AR, Baraff LJ, Fine RN, et al. Poststreptococcal acute glomerulonephritis: fact and controversy. Ann Intern Med 1979;91(1):76–86.
55. Hess EV. Drug-related lupus. Curr Opin Rheumatol 1991;3(5):809–14.
56. Martin B, Smith RJH. C3 glomerulopathy. In: Adam MP, Ardinger HH, Pagon RA, et al, editors. Gene Reviews®. Seattle (WA): University of Washington, Seattle; 1993-2022. p. 56–147.

57. Costa-Reis P, Sullivan KE. Genetics and epigenetics of systemic lupus erythe-matosus. Curr Rheumatol Rep 2013;15(9):369.

58. Alberici F, Martorana D, Bonatti F, et al. Genetics of ANCA-associated vasculit-ides: HLA and beyond. Clin Exp Rheumatol 2014;32(3 Suppl 82):S90–7.

59. Zhou XJ, Lv JC, Zhao MH, et al. Advances in the genetics of anti-glomerular basement membrane disease. Am J Nephrol 2010;32(5):482–90.

60. Rodriguez-Iturbe B, Haas M. Post-streptococcal glomerulonephritis. In: Ferretti JJ, Stevens DL, Fischetti VA, editors. Streptococcus pyogenes: basic biology to clinical manifestations. Oklahoma City (OK): University of Oklahoma Health Sci-ences Center; 2016.

61. Kalluri R, Wilson CB, Weber M, et al. Identification of the alpha 3 chain of type IV collagen as the common autoantigen in antibasement membrane disease and Goodpasture syndrome. J Am Soc Nephrol 1995;6(4):1178–85.

62. Eison TM, Ault BH, Jones DP, et al. Post-streptococcal acute glomerulonephritis in children: clinical features and pathogenesis. Pediatr Nephrol 2011;26(2):165–80.

63. Jones RB, Furuta S, Tervaert JW, et al. Rituximab versus cyclophosphamide in ANCA-associated renal vasculitis: 2-year results of a randomised trial. Ann Rheum Dis 2015;74(6):1178–82.

64. Appel GB, Contreras G, Dooley MA, et al. Mycophenolate mofetil versus cyclo-phosphamide for induction treatment of lupus nephritis. J Am Soc Nephrol 2009;20(5):1103–12.

65. Rovin BH, Furie R, Latinis K, et al. Efficacy and safety of rituximab in patients with active proliferative lupus nephritis: the lupus nephritis assessment with rit-uximab study. Arthritis Rheum 2012;64(4):1215–26.

66. Walsh M, Merkel PA, Peh CA, et al. Plasma exchange and glucocorticoids in se-vere ANCA-associated vasculitis. N Engl J Med 2020;382(7):622–31.

67. Levy JB, Turner AN, Rees AJ, et al. Long-term outcome of anti-glomerular base-ment membrane antibody disease treated with plasma exchange and immuno-suppression. Ann Intern Med 2001;134(11):1033–42.

68. Salmela A, Tornroth T, Poussa T, et al. Prognostic factors for survival and relapse in anca-associated vasculitis with renal involvement: a clinical long-term follow-up study. Int J Nephrol 2018;2018:6369814.

69. Noris M, Remuzzi G. Atypical hemolytic-uremic syndrome. N Engl J Med 2009;361(17):1676–87.

70. George JN, Nester CM. Syndromes of thrombotic microangiopathy. N Engl J Med 2014;371(7):654–66.

71. Gasser C, Gautier E, Steck A, et al. [Hemolytic-uremic syndrome: bilateral ne-crosis of the renal cortex in acute acquired hemolytic anemia]. Schweiz Med Wochenschr 1955;85(38–39):905–9.

72. Singer M, Deutschman CS, Seymour CW, et al. The third international consensus definitions for sepsis and septic shock (Sepsis-3). JAMA 2016;315(8):801–10.

73. Gotts JE, Matthay MA. Sepsis: pathophysiology and clinical management. BMJ 2016;353:i1585.

74. Iba T, Levi M, Levy JH. Sepsis-induced coagulopathy and disseminated intra-vascular coagulation. Semin Thromb Hemost 2020;46(1):89–95.

75. Kavanagh D, Goodship TH. Atypical hemolytic uremic syndrome. Curr Opin Hematol 2010;17(5):432–8.

76. Chang JC. Disseminated intravascular coagulation: new identity as endotheliopathy-associated vascular microthrombotic disease based on

in vivo hemostasis and endothelial molecular pathogenesis. Thromb J 2020; 18:25.

77. Levi M, Toh CH, Thachil J, et al. Guidelines for the diagnosis and management of disseminated intravascular coagulation. British Committee for Standards in Haematology. Br J Haematol 2009;145(1):24–33.

78. Toh CH, Hoots WK. The scoring system of the scientific and standardisation committee on disseminated intravascular coagulation of the international society on thrombosis and haemostasis: a 5-year overview. J Thromb Haemost 2007; 5(3):604–6.

79. Taylor FB Jr, Toh CH, Hoots WK, et al. Towards definition, clinical and laboratory criteria, and a scoring system for disseminated intravascular coagulation. Thromb Haemost 2001;86(5):1327–30.

80. Wada H, Matsumoto T, Suzuki K, et al. Differences and similarities between disseminated intravascular coagulation and thrombotic microangiopathy. Thromb J 2018;16(1):14.

81. Fakhouri F, Zuber J, Fremeaux-Bacchi V, et al. Haemolytic uraemic syndrome. Lancet 2017;390(10095):681–96.

82. Cody EM, Dixon BP. Hemolytic uremic syndrome. Pediatr Clin North Am 2019; 66(1):235–46.

83. Noris M, Remuzzi G. Hemolytic uremic syndrome. J Am Soc Nephrol 2005; 16(4):1035–50.

84. Castro VS, Figueiredo EES, Stanford K, et al. Shiga-Toxin producing escherichia coli in Brazil: a systematic review. Microorganisms 2019;7(5).

85. Loirat C, Fremeaux-Bacchi V. Atypical hemolytic uremic syndrome. Orphanet J Rare Dis 2011;6:60.

86. Constantinescu AR, Bitzan M, Weiss LS, et al. Non-enteropathic hemolytic ure-mic syndrome: causes and short-term course. Am J Kidney Dis 2004;43(6): 976–82.

87. Szilagyi A, Kiss N, Bereczki C, et al. The role of complement in streptococcus pneumoniae-associated haemolytic uraemic syndrome. Nephrol Dial Transpl 2013;28(9):2237–45.

88. Huang YH, Lin TY, Wong KS, et al. Hemolytic uremic syndrome associated with pneumococcal pneumonia in Taiwan. Eur J Pediatr 2006;165(5):332–5.

89. Krysan DJ, Flynn JT. Renal transplantation after streptococcus pneumoniae-associated hemolytic uremic syndrome. Am J Kidney Dis 2001;37(2):E15.

90. Kobbe R, Schild R, Christner M, et al. Case report - atypical hemolytic uremic syndrome triggered by influenza B. BMC Nephrol 2017;18(1):96.

91. Trachtman H, Sethna C, Epstein R, et al. Atypical hemolytic uremic syndrome associated with H1N1 influenza A virus infection. Pediatr Nephrol 2011;26(1): 145–6.

92. Rhee H, Song SH, Lee YJ, et al. Pandemic H1N1 influenza A viral infection complicated by atypical hemolytic uremic syndrome and diffuse alveolar hem-orrhage. Clin Exp Nephrol 2011;15(6):948–52.

93. Cervero Marti A, Martin J, Perez-Paya A, et al. Hemolytic-uremic syndrome associated with pancreatitis in an HIV-positive patient. Ann Hematol 1992; 65(5):236–7.

94. Cornec-Le Gall E, Delmas Y, De Parscau L, et al. Adult-onset eculizumab-resistant hemolytic uremic syndrome associated with cobalamin C deficiency. Am J Kidney Dis 2014;63(1):119–23.

95. Adrovic A, Canpolat N, Caliskan S, et al. Cobalamin C defect-hemolytic uremic syndrome caused by new mutation in MMACHC. Pediatr Int 2016;58(8):763–5.

96. Quaggin SE. DGKE and atypical HUS. Nat Genet 2013;45(5):475–6.
97. Mele C, Lemaire M, Iatropoulos P, et al. Characterization of a New DGKE intronic mutation in genetically unsolved cases of familial atypical hemolytic uremic syndrome. Clin J Am Soc Nephrol 2015;10(6):1011–9.
98. Favre GA, Touzot M, Fremeaux-Bacchi V, et al. Malignancy and thrombotic microangiopathy or atypical haemolytic and uraemic syndrome? Br J Haematol 2014;166(5):802–5.
99. Shibagaki Y, Fujita T. Thrombotic microangiopathy in malignant hypertension and hemolytic uremic syndrome (HUS)/thrombotic thrombocytopenic purpura (TTP): can we differentiate one from the other? Hypertens Res 2005;28(1):89–95.
100. Govind Babu K, Bhat GR. Cancer-associated thrombotic microangiopathy. Ecancermedicalscience 2016;10:649.
101. Martis N, Jamme M, Bagnis-Isnard C, et al. Systemic autoimmune disorders associated with thrombotic microangiopathy: a cross-sectional analysis from the French National TMA registry: systemic autoimmune disease-associated TMA. Eur J Intern Med 2021;93:78–86.
102. Medina PJ, Sipols JM, George JN. Drug-associated thrombotic thrombocytopenic purpura-hemolytic uremic syndrome. Curr Opin Hematol 2001;8(5):286–93.
103. Siegler R, Oakes R. Hemolytic uremic syndrome; pathogenesis, treatment, and outcome. Curr Opin Pediatr 2005;17(2):200–4.
104. Brocklebank V, Wood KM, Kavanagh D. Thrombotic microangiopathy and the kidney. Clin J Am Soc Nephrol 2018;13(2):300–17.
105. Ohanian M, Cable C, Halka K. Eculizumab safely reverses neurologic impairment and eliminates need for dialysis in severe atypical hemolytic uremic syndrome. Clin Pharmacol 2011;3:5–12.
106. Salvadori M, Bertoni E. Update on hemolytic uremic syndrome: diagnostic and therapeutic recommendations. World J Nephrol 2013;2(3):56–76.
107. Council of State and Territorial Epidemiologists. Public health reporting and national notification for Shiga toxin-producing Escherichia coli (STEC). Atlanta (GA): Council of State and Territorial Epidemiologists; 2017.
108. Gould LH, Demma L, Jones TF, et al. Hemolytic uremic syndrome and death in persons with Escherichia coli O157:H7 infection, foodborne diseases active surveillance network sites, 2000-2006. Clin Infect Dis 2009;49(10):1480–5.
109. Scheiring J, Andreoli SP, Zimmerhackl LB. Treatment and outcome of Shiga-toxin-associated hemolytic uremic syndrome (HUS). Pediatr Nephrol 2008;23(10):1749–60.
110. Tarr PI, Gordon CA, Chandler WL. Shiga-toxin-producing Escherichia coli and haemolytic uraemic syndrome. Lancet 2005;365(9464):1073–86.
111. Nathanson S, Kwon T, Elmaleh M, et al. Acute neurological involvement in diarrhea-associated hemolytic uremic syndrome. Clin J Am Soc Nephrol 2010;5(7):1218–28.
112. Khalid M, Andreoli S. Extrarenal manifestations of the hemolytic uremic syndrome associated with Shiga toxin-producing Escherichia coli (STEC HUS). Pediatr Nephrol 2019;34(12):2495–507.
113. Mayer CL, Leibowitz CS, Kurosawa S, et al. Shiga toxins and the pathophysiology of hemolytic uremic syndrome in humans and animals. Toxins (Basel) 2012;4(11):1261–87.

114. Griffin PM, Olmstead LC, Petras RE. Escherichia coli O157:H7-associated colitis. A clinical and histological study of 11 cases. Gastroenterology 1990;99(1): 142–9.

115. Orth D, Khan AB, Naim A, et al. Shiga toxin activates complement and binds factor H: evidence for an active role of complement in hemolytic uremic syndrome. J Immunol 2009;182(10):6394–400.

116. Liu F, Huang J, Sadler JE. Shiga toxin (Stx)1B and Stx2B induce von Willebrand factor secretion from human umbilical vein endothelial cells through different signaling pathways. Blood 2011;118(12):3392–8.

117. Petruzziello-Pellegrini TN, Marsden PA. Shiga toxin-associated hemolytic uremic syndrome: advances in pathogenesis and therapeutics. Curr Opin Nephrol Hypertens 2012;21(4):433–40.

118. Morigi M, Galbusera M, Gastoldi S, et al. Alternative pathway activation of complement by Shiga toxin promotes exuberant C3a formation that triggers microvascular thrombosis. J Immunol 2011;187(1):172–80.

119. Monnens L, Molenaar J, Lambert PH, et al. The complement system in hemolytic-uremic syndrome in childhood. Clin Nephrol 1980;13(4):168–71.

120. Talarico V, Aloe M, Monzani A, et al. Hemolytic uremic syndrome in children. Minerva Pediatr 2016;68(6):441–55.

121. Borowitz MJ, Craig FE, Digiuseppe JA, et al. Guidelines for the diagnosis and monitoring of paroxysmal nocturnal hemoglobinuria and related disorders by flow cytometry. Cytometry B Clin Cytom 2010;78(4):211–30.

122. Hickey CA, Beattie TJ, Cowieson J, et al. Early volume expansion during diarrhea and relative nephroprotection during subsequent hemolytic uremic syndrome. Arch Pediatr Adolesc Med 2011;165(10):884–9.

123. Smith KE, Wilker PR, Reiter PL, et al. Antibiotic treatment of Escherichia coli O157 infection and the risk of hemolytic uremic syndrome, Minnesota. Pediatr Infect Dis J 2012;31(1):37–41.

124. Wong CS, Jelacic S, Habeeb RL, et al. The risk of the hemolytic-uremic syndrome after antibiotic treatment of Escherichia coli O157:H7 infections. N Engl J Med 2000;342(26):1930–6.

125. Safdar N, Said A, Gangnon RE, et al. Risk of hemolytic uremic syndrome after antibiotic treatment of Escherichia coli O157:H7 enteritis: a meta-analysis. JAMA 2002;288(8):996–1001.

126. Buchholz U, Bernard H, Werber D, et al. German outbreak of Escherichia coli O104:H4 associated with sprouts. N Engl J Med 2011;365(19):1763–70.

127. Beneke J, Sartison A, Kielstein JT, et al. Clinical and laboratory consequences of platelet transfusion in shiga toxin-mediated hemolytic uremic syndrome. Transfus Med Rev 2017;31(1):51–5.

128. Balestracci A, Martin SM, Toledo I, et al. Impact of platelet transfusions in children with post-diarrheal hemolytic uremic syndrome. Pediatr Nephrol 2013; 28(6):919–25.

129. Menne J, Nitschke M, Stingele R, et al. Validation of treatment strategies for enterohaemorrhagic Escherichia coli O104:H4 induced haemolytic uraemic syndrome: case-control study. BMJ 2012;345:e4565.

130. Keenswijk W, Raes A, De Clerck M, et al. Is plasma exchange efficacious in shiga toxin-associated hemolytic uremic syndrome? A Narrative Review of Current Evidence. Ther Apher Dial 2019;23(2):118–25.

131. Yan K, Desai K, Gullapalli L, et al. Epidemiology of atypical hemolytic uremic syndrome: a systematic literature review. Clin Epidemiol 2020;12:295–305.

132. Dragon-Durey MA, Sethi SK, Bagga A, et al. Clinical features of anti-factor H autoantibody-associated hemolytic uremic syndrome. J Am Soc Nephrol 2010;21(12):2180–7.

133. Besbas N, Gulhan B, Soylemezoglu O, et al. Turkish pediatric atypical hemolytic uremic syndrome registry: initial analysis of 146 patients. BMC Nephrol 2017; 18(1):6.

134. Brocklebank V, Johnson S, Sheerin TP, et al. Factor H autoantibody is associated with atypical hemolytic uremic syndrome in children in the United Kingdom and Ireland. Kidney Int 2017;92(5):1261–71.

135. Fremeaux-Bacchi V, Fakhouri F, Garnier A, et al. Genetics and outcome of atypical hemolytic uremic syndrome: a nationwide French series comparing children and adults. Clin J Am Soc Nephrol 2013;8(4):554–62.

136. Diamante Chiodini B, Davin JC, Corazza F, et al. Eculizumab in anti-factor h antibodies associated with atypical hemolytic uremic syndrome. Pediatrics 2014; 133(6):e1764–8.

137. Gulleroglu K, Fidan K, Hancer VS, et al. Neurologic involvement in atypical hemolytic uremic syndrome and successful treatment with eculizumab. Pediatr Nephrol 2013;28(5):827–30.

138. Salem G, Flynn JM, Cataland SR. Profound neurological injury in a patient with atypical hemolytic uremic syndrome. Ann Hematol 2013;92(4):557–8.

139. Formeck C, Swiatecka-Urban A. Extra-renal manifestations of atypical hemolytic uremic syndrome. Pediatr Nephrol 2019;34(8):1337–48.

140. Yoshida Y, Kato H, Ikeda Y, et al. Pathogenesis of atypical hemolytic uremic syndrome. J Atheroscler Thromb 2019;26(2):99–110.

141. Feitz WJC, van de Kar N, Orth-Holler D, et al. The genetics of atypical hemolytic uremic syndrome. Med Genet 2018;30(4):400–9.

142. Kavanagh D, Goodship TH, Richards A. Atypical haemolytic uraemic syndrome. Br Med Bull 2006;77-78:5–22.

143. Caprioli J, Noris M, Brioschi S, et al. Genetics of HUS: the impact of MCP, CFH, and IF mutations on clinical presentation, response to treatment, and outcome. Blood 2006;108(4):1267–79.

144. Goodship TH, Cook HT, Fakhouri F, et al. Atypical hemolytic uremic syndrome and C3 glomerulopathy: conclusions from a "Kidney Disease: Improving Global Outcomes" (KDIGO) Controversies Conference. Kidney Int 2017;91(3):539–51.

145. Azoulay E, Knoebl P, Garnacho-Montero J, et al. Expert statements on the standard of care in critically ill adult patients with atypical hemolytic uremic syndrome. Chest 2017;152(2):424–34.

146. Chatzikonstantinou T, Gavriilaki M, Anagnostopoulos A, et al. An update in drug-induced thrombotic microangiopathy. Front Med (Lausanne) 2020;7:212.

147. Noris M, Bresin E, Mele C, et al. Genetic atypical hemolytic-uremic syndrome. In: Adam MP, Ardinger HH, Pagon RA, et al, editors. GeneReviews®. Seattle (WA): University of Washington, Seattle; 1993-2022.

148. Magro CM, Momtahen S, Mulvey JJ, et al. Role of the skin biopsy in the diagnosis of atypical hemolytic uremic syndrome. Am J Dermatopathol 2015;37(5): 349–56, quiz: 357-349].

149. Legendre CM, Licht C, Muus P, et al. Terminal complement inhibitor eculizumab in atypical hemolytic-uremic syndrome. N Engl J Med 2013;368(23):2169–81.

150. Licht C, Greenbaum LA, Muus P, et al. Efficacy and safety of eculizumab in atypical hemolytic uremic syndrome from 2-year extensions of phase 2 studies. Kidney Int 2015;87(5):1061–73.

151. Greenbaum LA, Fila M, Ardissino G, et al. Eculizumab is a safe and effective treatment in pediatric patients with atypical hemolytic uremic syndrome. Kidney Int 2016;89(3):701–11.

152. Fakhouri F, Hourmant M, Campistol JM, et al. Terminal complement inhibitor eculizumab in adult patients with atypical hemolytic uremic syndrome: a single-arm, open-label trial. Am J Kidney Dis 2016;68(1):84–93.

153. Cataland SR, Wu HM. How I treat: the clinical differentiation and initial treatment of adult patients with atypical hemolytic uremic syndrome. Blood 2014;123(16): 2478–84.

154. Vacca VM Jr. Acquired autoimmune thrombotic thrombocytopenic purpura. Nursing 2019;49(1):22–9.

155. Page EE, Kremer Hovinga JA, Terrell DR, et al. Thrombotic thrombocytopenic purpura: diagnostic criteria, clinical features, and long-term outcomes from 1995 through 2015. Blood Adv 2017;1(10):590–600.

156. Reese JA, Muthurajah DS, Kremer Hovinga JA, et al. Children and adults with thrombotic thrombocytopenic purpura associated with severe, acquired Adamts13 deficiency: comparison of incidence, demographic and clinical features. Pediatr Blood Cancer 2013;60(10):1676–82.

157. Scully M, Yarranton H, Liesner R, et al. Regional UK TTP registry: correlation with laboratory ADAMTS 13 analysis and clinical features. Br J Haematol 2008; 142(5):819–26.

158. Tsai HM. Pathophysiology of thrombotic thrombocytopenic purpura. Int J Hematol 2010;91(1):1–19.

159. Kremer Hovinga JA, Vesely SK, Terrell DR, et al. Survival and relapse in patients with thrombotic thrombocytopenic purpura. Blood 2010;115(8):1500–11 [quiz: 1662].

160. Jamme M, Rondeau E. The PLASMIC score for thrombotic thrombocytopenic purpura. Lancet Haematol 2017;4(4):e148–9.

161. Paydary K, Banwell E, Tong J, et al. Diagnostic accuracy of the PLASMIC score in patients with suspected thrombotic thrombocytopenic purpura: a systematic review and meta-analysis. Transfusion 2020;60(9):2047–57.

162. Zheng XL, Vesely SK, Cataland SR, et al. ISTH guidelines for treatment of thrombotic thrombocytopenic purpura. J Thromb Haemost 2020;18(10):2496–502.

163. Goshua G, Sinha P, Hendrickson JE, et al. Cost effectiveness of caplacizumab in acquired thrombotic thrombocytopenic purpura. Blood 2021;137(7):969–76.

164. Swisher KK, Terrell DR, Vesely SK, et al. Clinical outcomes after platelet transfusions in patients with thrombotic thrombocytopenic purpura. Transfusion 2009; 49(5):873–87.

165. Lim W, Vesely SK, George JN. The role of rituximab in the management of patients with acquired thrombotic thrombocytopenic purpura. Blood 2015; 125(10):1526–31.

166. Padden MO. HELLP syndrome: recognition and perinatal management. Am Fam Physician 1999;60(3):829–36, 839.

167. Fakhouri F, Vercel C, Fremeaux-Bacchi V. Obstetric nephrology: AKI and thrombotic microangiopathies in pregnancy. Clin J Am Soc Nephrol 2012;7(12): 2100–6.

168. Dashe JS, Ramin SM, Cunningham FG. The long-term consequences of thrombotic microangiopathy (thrombotic thrombocytopenic purpura and hemolytic uremic syndrome) in pregnancy. Obstet Gynecol 1998;91(5 Pt 1):662–8.

169. Fakhouri F, Scully M, Provot F, et al. Management of thrombotic microangiopathy in pregnancy and postpartum: report from an international working group. Blood 2020;136(19):2103–17.

170. Carbillon L, Boujenah J. Edema associated with low plasma protein level and any gestational hypertension as warning signs of HELLP syndrome. J Matern Fetal Neonatal Med 2021;1–4. https://doi.org/10.1080/14767058.2021.1949444.

171. Sibai BM, Ramadan MK, Usta I, et al. Maternal morbidity and mortality in 442 pregnancies with hemolysis, elevated liver enzymes, and low platelets (HELLP syndrome). Am J Obstet Gynecol 1993;169(4):1000–6.

172. Haram K, Mortensen JH, Nagy B. Genetic aspects of preeclampsia and the HELLP syndrome. J Pregnancy 2014;2014:910751.

173. Chen J, Khalil RA. Chapter four - matrix metalloproteinases in normal pregnancy and preeclampsia. In: Khalil RA, editor. Progress in molecular biology and translational science, Vol 148. San Diego (CA): Academic Press; 2017. p. 87–165.

174. Zeisler H, Llurba E, Chantraine F, et al. Predictive Value of the sFlt-1:PlGF ratio in women with suspected preeclampsia. N Engl J Med 2016;374(1):13–22.

175. Lamarca B. Endothelial dysfunction. An important mediator in the pathophysiology of hypertension during pre-eclampsia. Minerva Ginecol 2012;64(4):309–20.

176. Vaught AJ, Gavriilaki E, Hueppchen N, et al. Direct evidence of complement activation in HELLP syndrome: a link to atypical hemolytic uremic syndrome. Exp Hematol 2016;44(5):390–8.

177. Crovetto F, Borsa N, Acaia B, et al. The genetics of the alternative pathway of complement in the pathogenesis of HELLP syndrome. J Matern Fetal Neonatal Med 2012;25(11):2322–5.

178. Bazzan M, Todros T, Tedeschi S, et al. Genetic and molecular evidence for complement dysregulation in patients with HELLP syndrome. Thromb Res 2020;196:167–74.

179. Reese JA, Peck JD, Deschamps DR, et al. Platelet counts during pregnancy. N Engl J Med 2018;379(1):32–43.

180. Cines DB, Levine LD. Thrombocytopenia in pregnancy. Hematoly Am Soc Hematol Educ Program 2017;2017(1):144–51.

181. Caillon H, Tardif C, Dumontet E, et al. Evaluation of sFlt-1/PlGF ratio for predicting and improving clinical management of pre-eclampsia: experience in a specialized perinatal care center. Ann Lab Med 2018;38(2):95–101.

182. Verlohren S, Herraiz I, Lapaire O, et al. New gestational phase-specific cutoff values for the use of the soluble fms-like tyrosine kinase-1/placental growth factor ratio as a diagnostic test for preeclampsia. Hypertension 2014;63(2):346–52.

183. Sibai BM. Diagnosis, controversies, and management of the syndrome of hemolysis, elevated liver enzymes, and low platelet count. Obstet Gynecol 2004;103(5 Pt 1):981–91.

184. Hypertension in pregnancy. Report of the American College of obstetricians and gynecologists' task force on hypertension in pregnancy. Obstet Gynecol 2013;122(5):1122–31.

185. Barton JR, Sibai BM. Hepatic imaging in HELLP syndrome (hemolysis, elevated liver enzymes, and low platelet count). Am J Obstet Gynecol 1996;174(6):1820–5 [discussion: 1825-1827].

Zebras Seize the Day
Rare Causes of Status Epilepticus Across the Continuum of Critical Care

Dana Harrar, MD, PhD[a], Lileth Mondok, MD[b], Samuel Adams, MD[b], Raquel Farias-Moeller, MD[b],*

KEYWORDS

- Status epilepticus • Epileptic encephalopathy • Autoimmune encephalopathy
- New-onset refractory status epilepticus • Febrile infection-related epilepsy syndrome

KEY POINTS

- Status epilepticus (SE) is a common neurologic emergency associated with a high risk of morbidity and mortality.
- The effective management of SE hinges on stabilization and treatment, as well as on identifying and treating the underlying etiology.
- Genetic and metabolic disorders are important etiologies of SE, especially in neonates and children.
- Autoimmune and other inflammatory causes of SE have been identified in recent years, emerging as important contributors to the burden of SE seen in pediatric and adult intensive care units

INTRODUCTION

Status epilepticus (SE) is a common neurologic emergency associated with a high risk of morbidity and mortality. Convulsive SE (CSE) affects approximately 17 to 23 of 100,000 children[1] and 9 to 40 of 100,000 adults[2] in the United States and Europe each year. CSE is associated with a mortality of 3% to 5% in children[3] and up to 30% in adults.[2] Survivors often have cognitive and other neurologic sequelae.[2,3]

Early and effective treatment may halt the evolution of SE. However, not all patients will respond to first- and second-line antiseizure medications (ASMs). When this happens, the patient is generally considered to be in refractory SE. A large pediatric series suggests that this occurs in as many as one-fifth of episodes of SE.[4] Super-refractory SE (SRSE) occurs when SE continues or recurs 24 hours or more after the initiation of

---

[a] Division of Neurology, Department of Neurology and Pediatrics, Children's National Hospital, George Washington University, 111 Michigan Ave NW, Washington, DC 20010, USA; [b] Department of Neurology and Pediatrics, Division of Child Neurology, Children's Wisconsin, Medical College of Wisconsin, 999 N 92nd St, Wauwatosa, WI 53226, USA
* Corresponding author.
E-mail address: rfarias@mcw.edu

Crit Care Clin 38 (2022) 349–373
https://doi.org/10.1016/j.ccc.2021.11.006
criticalcare.theclinics.com
0749-0704/22/© 2021 Elsevier Inc. All rights reserved.

anesthetic therapy for seizure control and includes seizures that recur upon the reduction or withdrawal of anesthesia. A study in adults estimates that 15% of patients hospitalized for SE develop SRSE,[5] while in a series of 602 children with CSE, approximately 7% developed SRSE.[6]

The management of SE in the intensive care unit (ICU) centers on stabilization and treatment, as well as identifying and treating the underlying etiology. Numerous etiologies of SE are amenable to treatment, including certain genetic and metabolic disorders, autoimmune encephalitis and other inflammatory disorders, intracranial infections, and toxic/metabolic derangements. This article highlights rare but important causes of SE in the ICU across the continuum of care from neonates to adults.

DISCUSSION
Rare Genetic and Metabolic Causes of Status Epilepticus

Variants in over 120 genes have been associated with an increased risk of SE,[7] primarily in infants and children, although patients with genetic epilepsies may survive into adulthood and present to adult ICUs with SE. This section reviews select genetic and metabolic epilepsies that manifest early in life and that may first present with SE requiring admission to the neonatal or pediatric ICU.

Early infantile epileptic encephalopathy

Early infantile epileptic encephalopathy (EIEE), also known as Ohtahara syndrome, typically presents in the first 3 months of life with seizures and SE. Encephalopathy, severe developmental delay, and an abnormal neurologic examination may precede the onset of seizures. Tonic seizures predominate, although focal, atonic, myoclonic, and generalized tonic-clonic seizures can also be seen. Electroencephalogram (EEG) typically shows spontaneous burst suppression.[8]

The genetic etiologies of EIEE are diverse and include variants associated with structural brain abnormalities (e.g., variants in *ARX* associated with lissencephaly, variants in *PKNP* associated with microcephaly, variants in *SPTAN1* associated with global atrophy, and others).[9,10] EIEE can also result from functional, rather than structural, abnormalities.[7] For example, variants in *KCNQ2*, which encodes a central nervous system (CNS) voltage-gated potassium channel, can cause diverse epilepsy syndromes in neonates and infants, including EIEE. Diagnosis of a variant in *KCNQ2* as the etiology of EIEE can help guide treatment, with ASMs that act on sodium channels, such as carbamazepine, oxcarbazepine, and/or phenytoin, providing the greatest benefit.[11] Similarly, pathogenic variants in *STXBP1* account for 10% to 15% of EIEE cases and are associated with impaired neurotransmitter release.[12] Commonly used ASMs include phenobarbital, valproate, and vigabatrin, with over 20% of patients requiring multiple ASMs and over 25% refractory to therapy. As illustrated by these 2 representative examples, identification of the underlying genetic etiology can impact the choice of ASMs used for management, suggesting that genetic testing should be considered for all neonates presenting with EIEE of unknown etiology.

Pyridoxine-dependent epilepsy

Pyridoxine-dependent epilepsy (PDE) and related disorders, including pyridoxal-5'-phosphate (P5P) deficiency and folinic acid-responsive seizures (FARS), can also present in the neonatal period with refractory seizures and SE. PDE is caused by homozygous variants in *ALDH7A1*.[13] These result in the accumulation of metabolic intermediates that bind and inactivate P5P, the bioactive form of pyridoxine, and an important cofactor for numerous enzymatic reactions, including the conversion of glutamate to the inhibitory neurotransmitter γ-aminobutyric acid (GABA).

PDE should be considered in any neonate or infant with intractable seizures of unknown etiology, especially in the setting of a preceding encephalopathy. There is typically a progressive worsening of clinical and EEG abnormalities over an abbreviated time frame, including development of spontaneous burst suppression or hypsarrhythmia.

PDE often responds rapidly to treatment with pyridoxine administered as a 100 mg intravenous (IV) infusion repeated every 5 minutes up to a total dose of 500 mg. Of note, respiratory distress or arrest is possible with infusion of pyridoxine. A maintenance dose of 15 to 30 mg/k/d (maximum 200 mg/d) should then be started. Diagnostic markers for pyridoxine deficiency should be sent irrespective of the response to pyridoxine trial, and if a patient does not respond to IV pyridoxine, a trial of oral P5P and folinic acid is recommended to capture those patients with P5P deficiency and FARS.

Glycine encephalopathy

Glycine encephalopathy, formerly known as nonketotic hyperglycinemia, classically presents in the neonatal period with hypotonia, lethargy, apnea, and other signs of brainstem dysfunction.[14] There may be a history of excessive fetal hiccups. Prognosis is generally poor, with many patients not surviving the neonatal period.

Variants in genes encoding components of the glycine cleavage system, a mitochondrial multienzyme system, give rise to glycine encephalopathy. Symptoms arise because of the buildup of glycine, which is the major inhibitory neurotransmitter in the brainstem, as well as a co-agonist at the excitatory N-methyl-D-aspartate (NMDA) receptor. Cerebrospinal fluid (CSF) glycine and CSF/plasma glycine ratio are typically elevated, and the EEG often shows spontaneous burst suppression early in the disease course (**Fig. 1**). Molecular genetic testing is the preferred method for diagnostic confirmation, as up to 80% of patients have pathogenic variants in *GLDC*, and another 15% have pathogenic variants in *AMT*, both of which encode components of the glycine cleavage system. Magnetic resonance imaging (MRI) findings include nonspecific white matter changes, which can progress to spongy/cystic degeneration, while MR spectroscopy may reveal an abnormal glycine peak.

Treatment for glycine encephalopathy is aimed at reducing glycine levels. Sodium benzoate at high doses (250–750 mg/kg/d) reduces glycine concentrations and is of benefit in variant, but not classic, forms of glycine encephalopathy. Dextromethorphan acts as an antagonist at NMDA receptors and at a dose of 3 to 10 mg/kg/d has been shown to impact seizure control, with limited evidence for beneficial effects on long-term development. Ketamine, another NMDA receptor antagonist, may help to ameliorate the profound hypotonia and apnea seen in the classic form of glycine encephalopathy; however, long-term outcomes typically still include intractable epilepsy and severe developmental delay. In contrast, when used as part of early treatment in variant forms of glycine encephalopathy, outcomes may be more favorable. Seizure treatment with valproate should be avoided, as it can interfere with residual glycine cleavage system activity.

Metabolic disorders that may present in the neonatal period with seizures and/or SE are further outlined in **Table 1**.

POLG-related disorders

The *POLG* gene encodes the mitochondrial DNA polymerase responsible for replication of the mitochondrial genome.[15–18] Numerous syndromes can arise from pathogenic variants in this gene, with onset ranging from infancy to late adulthood. The syndrome most likely to be encountered in the critical care setting is

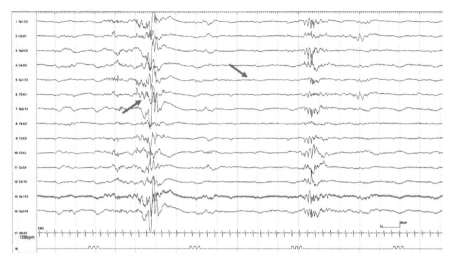

Fig. 1. Glycine encephalopathy. This neonatal EEG shows a burst suppression pattern with bursts of sharply contoured mixed-frequency activity (*red arrows*) alternating with periods of diffuse suppression (*blue arrow*). Glycine levels were elevated, and a disease-causing homozygous pathogenic variant in *GLDC* was detected. Settings: low-frequency filter (LFF) 1 Hz, high-frequency filter (HFF): 70 Hz. (*Reproduced with permission from* Davila-Williams D, Pearl PL, Pathognomonic EEG patterns in critically ill children and neonates. In Sansevere AJ, Harrar DB, editors. Atlas of pediatric and neonatal ICU EEG, New York: Demos Medical Publishing. Copyright Springer Publishing Company, LLC.; 2021. p. 387.)

Alpers-Huttenlocher syndrome (AHS), which typically presents with refractory epilepsy, psychomotor regression, and hepatopathy. Laboratory evidence supportive of the diagnosis includes elevated serum, CSF, and urine lactate. MRI findings of central atrophy with ex vacuo ventriculomegaly and an N-acetyl aspartate (NAA) peak on MR spectroscopy are also supportive of the diagnosis.

The epilepsy in patients with *POLG* variants can be explosive in onset and can first present as refractory SE. EEG findings may include rhythmic high-amplitude delta with superimposed spikes and polyspikes (RHADS), which are pathognomonic for this disorder (**Fig. 2**). Epileptiform abnormalities and slowing in the occipital regions are also common.

Valproate, although commonly used in the treatment of SE, is absolutely contraindicated in suspected or proven POLG disorders, as it can precipitate liver dysfunction including hepatitis, transaminitis, and hepatic failure. There are otherwise no specific ASMs indicated for epilepsy in patients with *POLG* variants; rather, a combination including benzodiazepines is often required. The ketogenic diet has been trialed, with benefit in seizure control, but little effect on overall outcome.

Mitochondrial encephalomyopathy, lactic acidosis, and stroke-like episodes (MELAS)

Mitochondrial encephalomyopathy, lactic acidosis, and stroke-like episodes (MELAS) comprise a rare disorder that typically begins in childhood.[19,20] Clinical diagnostic criteria include stroke-like episodes before age 40, encephalopathy with seizures, headaches with vomiting, and cortical blindness. Diagnostic markers include elevations of serum and CSF lactate and pyruvate. MRI during a stroke-like episode typically shows T2 hyperintensity that crosses vascular territories, while MR spectroscopy often reveals a lactate peak.

Table 1
Metabolic epilepsies that may present with seizures and status epilepticus in the neonate[51]

Diagnosis	Clinical Seizure Type[a]	EEG Findings[a]	Treatment
Disorders of vitamin metabolism			
PDE	Focal, atonic, myoclonic, infantile spasms, subclinical	Slowing, focal, multifocal, or generalized epileptiform discharges, generalized bursts of high-voltage delta with intermixed spikes and sharp waves and periods of asynchronous attenuation, burst suppression, infantile spasms	100 mg IV pyridoxine (repeat up to 500 mg) 50–200 mg/d (30 mg/kg/d) oral pyridoxine
P5P responsive epileptic encephalopathy	Same as PDE	Same as PDE	30 mg/kg/d pyridoxal-5′-phosphate
FARS	Myoclonic, tonic	Burst suppression	3–5 mg/kg/d (max 10–30 mg/kg/d) folinic acid
Holocarboxylase synthetase deficiency	Generalized tonic, focal motor, multifocal myoclonic	Burst suppression, multifocal spikes	10–20 mg/d biotin
Aminoacidopathies			
Glycine encephalopathy	Myoclonic, spasms	Burst suppression, hypsarrhythmia	Sodium benzoate, dextromethorphan, carnitine supplementation, ketamine
GABA transaminase deficiency	Focal, generalized tonic clonic, absence, myoclonic	Burst suppression, hypsarrhythmia, multifocal spikes, generalized spike wave, diffuse background slowing, slow spike wave	Flumazenil
MSUD	Focal and generalized	Diffuse slowing, loss of reactivity to auditory stimuli, comb-like rhythm	Dietary restriction of branched chain amino acids

(continued on next page)

Table 1
(continued)

Diagnosis	Clinical Seizure Type[a]	EEG Findings[a]	Treatment
Urea cycle disorders			
CPS, OTC*, AS, ASL, N-ACGS deficiency	Seizures on day of life 1–5, generalized tonic clonic, nonconvulsive status epilepticus	Low voltage diffuse slowing, multifocal epileptiform discharges, sustained monorhythmic theta activity, burst suppression (in citrullinemia)	Dialysis, ammonia scavengers, arginine supplementation, reversal of catabolic state Avoid valproic acid
Organic acidurias			
Propionic acidemia (PA) Isovaleric acidemia (IA) Methylmalonic acidemia (MA)	Focal motor, generalized tonic, myoclonic, atypical absence, spasms	PA: background disorganization with frontotemporal and occipital slow wave activity, fast central spikes, burst suppression IA: dysmaturity during sleep MA: multifocal spike wave discharges, depressed or slow background activity, lack of sleep spindles	PA: dietary protein restriction, carnitine supplementation, nitrogen-modulating drugs IA: low-protein, low-leucine diet, glycine and carnitine supplementation MA: dietary protein restriction, carnitine supplementation, nitrogen-modulating drugs
Peroxisomal disorders			
Zellweger syndrome (ZS) Neonatal adrenoleukodystrophy (NALD)	ZS: focal motor, myoclonic, spasms NALD: tonic, clonic, myoclonic, epileptic spasms	ZS: infrequent bilateral independent multifocal spikes, hypsarrhythmia, prolonged runs of vertex negative spikes NALD: high voltage slowing, polymorphic delta activity, multifocal paroxysmal discharges, burst suppression, hypsarrhythmia	ZS: Cholic acid[52] NALD: docosahexaenoic acid, dietary restriction of phytanic acid

Purine/pyrimidine metabolism

Adenylosuccinate lyase deficiency	Focal, myoclonic, generalized tonic clonic, spasms	Nonspecific	D-ribose, conventional ASMs, ketogenic diet[53]

Storage disorders

Gaucher disease type 2&3 (GD) Niemann-Pick type C (NPC)	GD: myoclonic NPC: focal or generalized, gelastic cataplexy[54]	GD2: photosensitive polyspikes, multifocal spike and wave, high voltage sharp waves in sleep[55] GD3: background slowing[56] NPC: nonspecific	GD: enzyme replacement therapy for visceral manifestations (ineffective for CNS manifestations)[57] NPC: Miglustat, avoid carbamazepine and vigabatrin[58]

Other

Molybdenum cofactor deficiency and sulfite oxidase deficiency	Focal, generalized, myoclonic	Multifocal spikes, burst suppression	Cyclic pyranopterin monophosphate[59]
PDH deficiency	Myoclonic, infantile spasms	Hypsarrhythmia, multifocal slow spike and wave	Ketogenic diet
GLUT 1	Focal, generalized tonic clonic, myoclonic, atonic, tonic, infantile spasms, atypical absence	Interictal epileptiform discharges in the posterior quadrants, 3 Hz spike and wave discharges with some variability in morphology and amplitude, background slowing	Ketogenic diet

Abbreviations: ASL, argininosuccinate lyase; AS, argininosuccinate synthetase; CPS, carbamoyl phosphate synthetase; FARS, folinic acid responsive seizures; GABA, gamma aminobutyric acid; GD, Gaucher's disease type 2&3; GLUT 1, glucose transporter 1 deficiency; IA, isovaleric acidemia; MA, methylmalonic acidemia; MSUD, maple syrup urine disease; N-ACGS, N-acetylglutamate synthetase; NALD, neonatal adrenoleukodystrophy; NPC, Niemann-Pick type C; OTC, ornithine transcarbamylase; P5P, Pyridoxal-5′-phosphate; PA, propionic acidemia, PDE, pyridoxine dependent epilepsy; PDH, pyruvate dehydrogenase; ZS, zellweger syndrome.

[a] at any age.

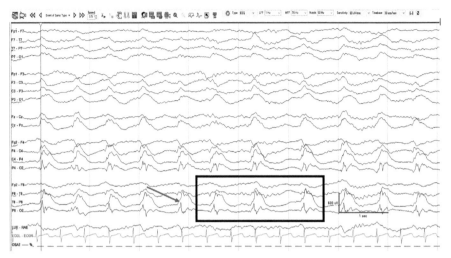

Fig. 2. Rhythmic high-amplitude delta with superimposed spikes and polyspikes (RHADS). A 5-year-old girl with recurrent SE and Alpers syndrome. EEG shows RHADS over the right posterior quadrant. The black box highlights high-amplitude rhythmic delta. The blue arrow points to a superimposed spike. Settings: LFF 1 Hz, HFF 70 Hz. (*Reproduced with permission from* Davila-Williams D, Pearl PL. Pathognomonic EEG patterns in critically ill children and neonates. In Sansevere AJ, Harrar DB, editors. Atlas of pediatric and neonatal ICU EEG, New York: Demos Medical Publishing. Copyright Springer Publishing Company, LLC; 2021. p. 391.)

SE is common, with all patients in some cohorts having experienced at least 1 episode of SE, and seizures can be triggered by, or provoke, a stroke-like episode. Over 90% of patients develop epilepsy, and unfortunately, ASM choices are limited because of the high potential for mitochondrial toxicity (e.g., valproate should be avoided in patients with suspected or confirmed MELAS).

Treatment for acute stroke-like episodes is based on expert consensus and open-label pilot studies. A loading dose of L-arginine at 0.5 g/kg followed by a continuous infusion of the same dose per day for 3 to 5 days is typically recommended. The concomitant use of citrulline for acute attacks, as well as daily oral arginine to prevent recurrence of attacks, has also been reported.

Special note
Epilepsia partialis continua (EPC) is a rare SE syndrome characterized by recurrent focal seizures with retained awareness (**Fig. 3**A) that can be seen in patients with a variety of disorders (**Table 2**), including POLG-related disorders and MELAS. Initially described as a variant of focal motor SE, broader definitions now include sensory variants referred to as aura continua.[21] Seizures recur over hours, days, or even years, and discrete episodes must last a minimum of 60 minutes to qualify for a diagnosis of EPC. EPC persists in sleep, and postictal weakness (Todd paralysis) is common. Notably, surface EEG is normal in up to 20% of patients, as abnormal cortical activity from the relatively small pool of neurons responsible for generating EPC may not be detectable via scalp electrodes (**Fig. 3**B). Treatment depends on addressing the underlying etiology of the EPC, as it is otherwise resistant to pharmacotherapy. Benzodiazepines can interrupt EPC but are a poor long-term option. Various advanced

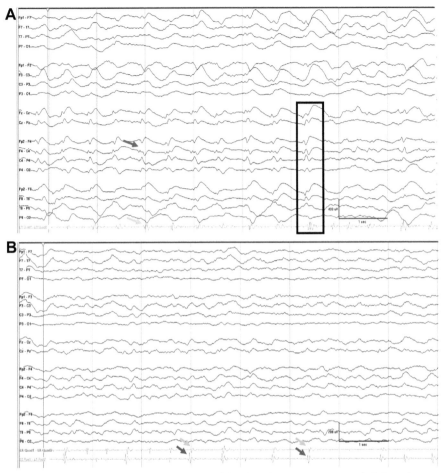

Fig. 3. Epilepsia partialis continua. A 9-year-old girl with Rasmussen encephalitis and repetitive left leg myoclonic jerks. (*A*) EEG shows 2 Hz lateralized periodic discharges maximal over the right parasagittal (*red arrow*) and midline regions. The blue arrow shows the electromyographic (EMG) potential of the left quadriceps muscle. The black box shows the relationship between the 2 potentials, with the EEG discharge preceding the EMG response. (*B*) EEG from the same patient as in Fig. 3A. The green arrow shows the EMG potential of the left quadriceps, and the blue arrow shows the EMG potential of the left foot. In contrast to Fig. 3A, neither EMG potential is preceded by a detectable EEG discharge. Settings: LFF 1 Hz, HFF 70 Hz. (*Reproduced with permission from Davila-Williams D, Pearl PL. Pathognomonic EEG patterns in critically ill children and neonates. In Sansevere AJ, Harrar DB, editors. Atlas of pediatric and neonatal ICU EEG. New York: Demos Medical Publishing. Copyright Springer Publishing Company, LLC; 2021. p. 401, 403.)*

therapeutic options have been trialed in small cohorts, including vagal nerve stimulation, transcranial magnetic stimulation, and neocortical stimulation.[21]

AUTOIMMUNE AND INFLAMMATORY ETIOLOGIES OF STATUS EPILEPTICUS

In addition to genetic and metabolic etiologies, autoimmune and other inflammatory causes of SE have been identified in recent years, emerging as important contributors

Table 2
Etiologies of epilepsia partialis continua[60]

Autoimmune disorders	Limbic encephalitis
	Multiple sclerosis
	Paraneoplastic encephalitis
	Sjogren syndrome
Brain malformations	Focal cortical dysplasia
	Hemimegalencephaly
Cerebrovascular disorders	Cavernoma
	Stroke
Infectious/inflammatory	*Bartonella henselae*
	Creutzfeldt-Jakob disease
	Herpes simplex encephalitis
	Human immunodeficiency virus/acquired immunodeficiency syndrome
	Japanese encephalitis
	Neurocysticercosis
	Rasmussen encephalitis
	Subacute sclerosing panencephalitis
	Tick-borne encephalitis
	Tuberculosis
Metabolic derangements	Hepatic encephalopathy
	Hypocalcemia
	Nonketotic hyperglycemia
	Toxemia gravidarum
	Renal failure
Mitochondrial disorders	*ADCK3* pathogenic gene variants
	Alpers disease
	Leigh syndrome
	MELAS
	Myoclonic epilepsy with ragged red fibers
	NADH-coenzyme Q reductase deficiency
Oncologic disease	Dysembryoplastic neuroepithelial tumors
	Glioma
	Gliomatosis cerebri
	Hemangioma and hemangioblastoma
	Lymphoma
	Meningioma
	Metastases
Trauma	Subdural hematoma
Other	Neuronal ceroid lipofuscinosis
	Menkes disease
	Methylmalonic acidemia with homocystinuria

to the burden of SE, including refractory and super-refractory SE, seen in both pediatric and adult ICUs. This includes the various autoimmune encephalitides, novel forms of which continue to be identified, and the rarer entities of new-onset refractory SE (NORSE) and febrile infection-related epilepsy syndrome (FIRES), which, in many cases, are thought to have an inflammatory etiology.

Autoimmune Encephalitis

Autoimmune encephalitis (AE) is caused by antibodies directed against neuronal cell surface or intracellular antigens. The clinical presentation is highly variable, and new-onset seizures are frequently seen. In a subset of patients, the clinical course is complicated by SE, and indeed, AE is increasingly recognized as an important cause of SE in both children and adults. In a single-center study of 570 consecutive adults with SE, 2.5% had an autoimmune cause.[22] AE is also the most frequently identified cause of NORSE. In a multicenter retrospective review of 130 patients with NORSE without an identified cause at 48 hours, 37% were ultimately found to have an autoimmune etiology, with anti-NMDA receptor encephalitis being the most common.[23]

Clinical and diagnostic features

Seizures and SE are often preceded by cognitive decline, behavioral changes, and movement disorders, and a preceding fever or presumed viral illness is common. Anti-NMDA receptor encephalitis can also manifest with autonomic instability.[24]

First-tier diagnostic evaluation for SE includes brain MRI, CSF analysis, and EEG monitoring. In patients with AE, T2/fluid-attenuated inversion recovery (FLAIR) hyperintensities may be seen in the limbic areas on MRI, although brain MRI is normal in over 50% of patients.[25] CSF analysis may show lymphocytic pleocytosis and other signs of CNS inflammation (i.e., oligoclonal bands or elevated immunoglobulin G [IgG] synthesis index). Infectious testing should be negative.

Definitive diagnosis of AE is made when an autoantibody is identified in CSF or serum; however, waiting for the results of such tests can lead to delays in diagnosis. Therefore, expert consensus criteria for a diagnosis of possible AE in adults were developed in 2016[26] (**Box 1**), with a pediatric-specific approach derived from these criteria in 2020.[27]

Given the need to identify AE as early as possible to optimize treatment and outcomes, models have also been developed to predict neuronal antibody positivity in epilepsy. The Antibody Prevalence in Epilepsy (APE) score was developed in 2017[28] to determine the prevalence of neuronal autoantibodies among adults with epilepsy of unknown etiology (**Table 3**). An APE score of 4 or more has a sensitivity of 82.6% and a specificity of 82.0% for detecting a neuronal antibody in cryptogenic SE.

Neuronal antibodies

Antibodies responsible for AE can target neuronal surface proteins, including synaptic receptors (e.g., NMDA and AMPA [alpha-amino-3-hydroxy-5-methyl-4-isoxazole propionic acid] receptors) or other cell surface molecules (e.g., LGI1 [leucine-rich glioma inactivated 1] and CASPR2 [contactin-associated protein like 2])[26] (**Table 4**). Autoantibodies can also target intracellular antigens (e.g., anti-Hu, anti-Ma). AE caused by autoantibodies to intracellular antigens is often accompanied by an underlying malignancy and tends to be less responsive to immune therapy than AE caused by cell surface proteins.

Box 1
Criteria for diagnosis of possible autoimmune encephalitis in adults[26]

1. Subacute onset (ie, over less than 3 months) of working memory deficits, altered mental status, or psychiatric symptoms

2. At least 1 of the following: new focal CNS findings, seizures not explained by a pre-existing disorder, CSF pleocytosis, and/or MRI features suggestive of encephalitis

3. Reasonable exclusion of alternative causes

Table 3
Antibody prevalence in epilepsy score[28]

Clinical Feature	Score
New-onset seizures or rapidly progressive mental status changes over 1–6 weeks	1
Neuropsychiatric changes	1
Autonomic dysfunction	1
Viral prodrome	2
Facial dyskinesias or faciobrachial dystonic movements	2
Seizures refractory to ≥2 ASMs	2
CSF findings consistent with inflammation	2
MRI with medial temporal T2/FLAIR signal changes	2
Malignancy	2
Total	15

Abbreviations: ASM, antiseizure medication; FLAIR, Fluid-attenuated inversion recovery.

Anti-NMDA receptor encephalitis is the most common of the autoimmune encephalitides in children and adults and is characterized by a well-defined syndrome of subacute neuropsychiatric symptoms. Antibodies target the GluN1 subunit of the NMDA receptor.[29] Seizures in this cohort are reported in up to 50% of patients, with SE occurring in 25% of patients.[30] An underlying tumor is uncommon in children younger than 12 years old but can be seen in up to 58% of women older than 18 years of age.[31]

Electroencephalogram and seizure characteristics

Continuous EEG monitoring is important for the optimal management of SE and has also been used in AE to gauge the degree of encephalopathy. Despite attempts to

Table 4
Autoantibodies associated with seizures

Cell-surface Receptors and Ilon Channels	Intracellular
NMDA-R	GAD65
AMPA-R	Amphiphysin
CASPR2	CRMP5
LGI1	Anti-Ta/Ma2
GABA$_A$-R GABA$_B$-R	GFAP
AchR ganglionic	ANNA Types 1 (anti-Hu), 2 (anti-Ri), 3
mGluR1	Purkinje Cell Cytoplasmic Types 1, 2 (anti-Yo)
N-Type & P/Q-Type Calcium Channel	
DPPX	

Abbreviations: AchR, acetylcholine receptor; AMPA-R, α-Amino-3-hydroxy-5-methyl-4-isoxazole-propionic acid receptor; ANNA, antineuronal nuclear antibodies; CASPR2, contactin-associated protein-like 2; CRMP5, collapsin response-mediator protein-5; DPPX, dipeptidyl-peptidase–like protein; GABA, gamma aminobutyric acid; GAD65, glutamic acid decarboxylase 65-kilodalton isoform; GFAP, glial fibrillary acidic protein; LGI1, leucine-rich glioma inactivated 1; mGLUR1, metabotropic glutamate receptor 1; NMDA-R, N-methyl ᴅ-aspartate receptor.

identify EEG features specific to AE, EEG findings remain heterogenous and nonspecific, with the possible exception of the extreme delta brush pattern of rhythmic delta, with superimposed beta frequency activity seen in anti-NMDA receptor encephalitis.[32]

Treatment

Early immunotherapy in AE improves outcomes,[33] and often, the decision to proceed with immune therapy must be made before results of antibody testing are available. Once common infectious etiologies have been excluded, empiric treatment with IV steroids (e.g., methylprednisolone 30 mg/kg/d, maximum 1 g, for 5 days), IV immunoglobulin (2 g/kg over 2–5 days), and/or plasmapheresis (5–7 sessions) should commence. Other acute treatments may include rituximab or cyclophosphamide. Tumor removal, if present, should be considered. Successful immunotherapy may result in improvement in seizure control and halt clinical progression but may not reverse the full spectrum of symptoms in the acute phase.[34]

New-Onset Refractory Status Epilepticus and Febrile Infection-Related Epilepsy Syndrome

NORSE is a rare clinical presentation of SE. In this condition, a patient without epilepsy or other neurologic disorder develops NORSE without a clear acute or active structural, toxic, or metabolic cause.[35] A paradigm of NORSE is the broad investigative process that must be performed to fulfill a crucial part of its definition: *the lack of a clear acute or active structural, toxic, or metabolic cause.* That process usually takes up to 72 hours.[35] Eventually, the etiology is identified in approximately 50% of adult patients with NORSE: most commonly, paraneoplastic, autoimmune, or other forms of encephalitis are found. In the remainder, the term cryptogenic NORSE is used.[36]

FIRES, a subcategory of NORSE, occurs when fever precedes NORSE by 1 to 14 days. Fever may or may not be present at the onset of SE.[35] FIRES was historically conceptualized as a pediatric-specific condition; however, age restrictions have been eliminated.[35] In contrast to NORSE, an etiology for FIRES is seldom identified; however, this may reflect the historic definition of FIRES, in which a lack of an etiology was a diagnostic criterion.[37]

Epidemiology and incidence

An accurate determination of the incidence of NORSE and FIRES has been stymied by the historic use of multiple terms to describe these conditions,[37] leading a group of investigators to propose consensus definitions in 2017.[35] Despite this, it is known that NORSE and FIRES are uncommon, and most often occur in previously healthy young adults and school-aged children.

Clinical presentation

In all patients with FIRES, fever precedes seizure onset by 1–14 days,[35] although at seizure onset, fever is absent in about half.[38] The prodromal illness in both FIRES and NORSE is usually banal and typically includes respiratory and/or gastrointestinal symptoms. Seizures may initially be brief and infrequent[37] but within a matter of hours to days increase in frequency up to hundreds of seizures per day.[36] Most patients require continuous infusions of anesthetic agents for seizure control.

Seizures are usually described as focal to bilateral, as well as myoclonic with facial and oro-buccal involvement.[36] EEG may show focal, generalized, or more often, bilateral multifocal interictal epileptiform discharges.[23,38,39] EEG patterns described in a case series of children with FIRES included: brief and relatively infrequent seizures at onset, with gradual evolution to SE; seizures beginning with prolonged focal fast activity followed by gradual appearance of rhythmic spike/wave complexes (**Fig. 4**); and

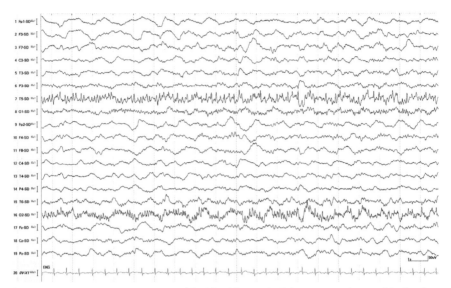

Fig. 4. Seizures in FIRES. A 6-year-old girl with FIRES. Seizure onset is notable for low-amplitude focal fast activity (*red arrow*; onset not shown), which evolved to well-formed rhythmic spike and wave complexes (not shown). Settings: LFF 1 Hz, HFF 70 Hz. (Reproduced with permission from Stredny CM, Farias-Moeller R, Febrile infection-related epilepsy syndrome (FIRES). In Sansevere AJ, Harrar DB, editors. Atlas of pediatric and neonatal ICU EEG. New York: Demos Medical Publishing. Copyright Springer Publishing Company, LLC; 2021. p. 502.)

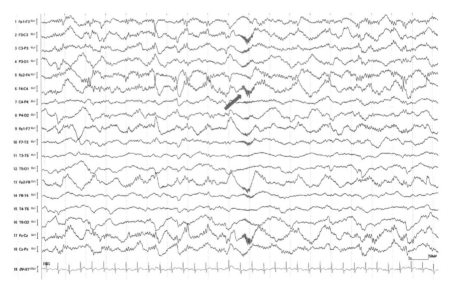

Fig. 5. Delta brush. A 6-year-old girl with FIRES. EEG shows beta frequency waves superimposed on a delta wave (*red arrow*). Settings: LFF 1 Hz, HFF 70 Hz. (*Reproduced with permission from* Stredny CM, Farias-Moeller R, Febrile Infection-related epilepsy syndrome (FIRES). In Sansevere AJ, Harrar DB, editors. Atlas of pediatric and neonatal ICU EEG. New York: Demos Medical Publishing. Copyright Springer Publishing Company, LLC; 2021. p. 501.)

Table 5
Diagnostic work-up for new-onset refractory status epilepticus and febrile infection-related epilepsy syndrome[61]

Screen	Disease/Agent Tested

Initial work-up	Recommended in most or all patients:
	• Whole blood/serum: complete blood cell count (CBC), bacterial and fungal cultures, RPR-VDRL, HIV-1/2 immunoassay with confirmatory viral load if appropriate
	• Serum: immunoglobulin G (IgG) and immunoglobulin M (IgM) testing (acute and convalescent) for *Chlamydia pneumoniae, Bartonella henselae, Mycoplasma pneumoniae, Coxiella burnetii, Shigella* species, and *Chlamydia psittaci*
	• Nares or nasopharyngeal swab (the latter preferred): respiratory viral panel; SARS-CoV2 PCR
	• CSF:
	  ○ Cell counts, protein, and glucose, bacterial and fungal stains and cultures
	  ○ PCR for HIV, PCR for HSV1, HSV2, VZV, EBV, M. Tb; consider WNV, VDRL, encephalitis panel
	  ○ PCR for *C pneumoniae* and *psittaci, Bartonella henslae, Mycoplasma pneumoniae, Coxiella burnetti,* and *Shigella* species
	  ○ Autoimmune epilepsy panel (see section 2)
	  ○ Consider metagenomics for any nonhuman nucleic acid material
	  ○ Consider cytokine profile (section 7)
	  ○ Consider cytology and flow cytometry
	Recommended in immunocompromised patients:
	• Serum: IgG *Cryptococcus* species, IgM and IgG *Histoplasma capsulatum,* IgG *Toxoplasma gondii*
	• Sputum: M. Tb Gene Xpert
	• CSF: eosinophils, silver stain for CNS fungi, PCR for JC virus, CMV, EBV, HHV6, EEE, enterovirus, influenza A/B, HIV, WNV, parvovirus. *Listeria* Ab, measles (rubeola)
	• Stool: adenovirus PCR, enterovirus PCR
	Recommended if geographic/seasonal/occupational risk of exposure:
	• Serum buffy coat and peripheral smear
	• Lyme EIA with IgM and IgG reflex
	• Hepatitis C immunoassay and viral load if appropriate
	• Send further serum and CSF samples to CDC DVBD Arbovirus Diagnostic Laboratory, CSF and serum rickettsial disease panel, flavivirus panel, bunyavirus panel
	• Serum testing for *Acanthamoeba* spp., *Balamuthia mandrillaris,* and *Baylisascaris procyonis*
	• Other
	• Consider CSF metagenomics for any infectious genetic material

Autoimmune/ paraneoplastic	Recommended: • Serum and CSF paraneoplastic and autoimmune epilepsy antibody panel-to include antibodies to: LGI-1, CASPR2, Ma1, Ma2/TaDPPX, GAD65, NMDA, AMPA, GABA-B, GABA-A, glycine receptor, Tr, amphiphysin, CV-2/CRMP-5, Neurexin-3alpha, adenylate kinase, antineuronal nuclear antibody types 1/2/3 (Hu, Yo and Ri), Purkinje cell cytoplasmic antibody types 1,2, GFAP- alpha, anti-SOX1, N-type calcium Ab, PQ-type calcium channel, Acetylcholine receptor (muscle) binding Ab, Ach-R ganglionic neuronal Ab, AQP4, MOG Ab, IgLON5 Ab, D2R Ab

(continued on next page)

Table 5 *(continued)*	
Screen	**Disease/Agent Tested**
	• Additional serologic studies-serum (likely not pathogenic but hint toward an autoimmune etiology) ANA (detection and identification), ANCA, antithyroid antibodies (antithryoglobulin, anti-TPO), antiendomysial, ESR, CRP, SPEP, IFE, RA, ACE., cold and warm agglutinins, tests for MAS/HLH (serum triglycerides and sIL2-r, ferritin) • Suggestion: store extra frozen CSF and serum for possible further autoimmune testing in a research laboratory

Neoplastic	Recommended:
	    Computed tomography (CT) chest/abdomen/pelvis, pelvic or scrotal ultrasound, mammogram, CSF cytology, flow cytometry, cancer serum markers. Pelvic MRI. Whole-body positron emission tomography (PET)-CT if previous tests are not conclusive
	Optional:
	    Bone marrow biopsy

Metabolic	Recommended:
	    Whole-blood/serum: blood urea nitrogen (BUN)/Cr, lactate dehydrogenase (LDH), liver function tests, electrolytes, Ca/Mg/ Phos, ammonia
	    Urine: Porphyria screen (spot urine), urinalysis with microscopic urinalysis
	Consider:
	    Vitamin B1 level, B12 level, homocysteine, folate, lactate, pyruvate, creatine kinase, troponin; tests for mitochondrial disorder (lactate, pyruvate, MR spectroscopy, muscle biopsy)

Toxicologic	Recommended:
	    Benzodiazepines, amphetamines, cocaine, fentanyl, alcohol, ecstasy, heavy metals, synthetic cannabinoids, bath salts
	Consider:
	    Extended opiate and overdose panel, LSD, heroin, PCP, marijuana

Genetic	Consider: Obtain genetics consult, if possible Genetic screens for mitochondrial disorders (*MERRF, MELAS, POLG1, SURF1, MT-ATP6*) and VLCFA screen, ceruloplasmin and 24-h urine copper, mendeliome, or exome sequencing (also look for gene polymorphisms in *IL1B, IL6, IL10, TNF-alpha, HMBG1, TLR4, IL1RN, SCN1A* and *SCN2A*), mitochondrial genome sequencing and deletion/duplication array
Cytokine assay	Serum and CSF: cytokine assay for quantitative measure of IL-1β, IL-1Ra, IL-2, IL-4, IL-5, IL-6, IL-10, IL-12, IL-17, granulocyte- macrophage colony stimulating factor, tumor necrosis factor-α, HMGB1, CCL2, CXCL8, CXCL9, CXCL10, CXCL11

Published with permission from the NORSE Institute. See http://www.norseinstitute.org for additional information, tables, and future updates. Table 5 reflects latest update (September 2020.).

beta delta complexes resembling the delta brush seen in NMDAR encephalitis[40] (**Fig. 5**).

MRI of the brain is obligatory to rule out a structural etiology of SE. In 70% of adults with NORSE, the MRI shows abnormalities in the limbic and/or neocortical areas, with basal ganglia and peri-insular involvement also reported.[36] The initial MRI is normal in almost two-thirds of pediatric patients with FIRES[36]; however, abnormalities in the temporal lobe and basal ganglia, as well as cortical edema and insular/peri-insular changes, have been described.[36]

Pathophysiology

FIRES is thought to be an immune-inflammatory condition,[36] with at least a subset of patients having intrathecal overproduction of proinflammatory cytokines and chemokines.[41] It is possible that inflammatory mediators released during systemic infection activate the innate immune system, triggering a neuroinflammatory cascade that promotes epileptogenesis. Refractory seizures, in turn, contribute to ongoing immune system activation, thereby perpetuating the cycle. Once neuroinflammation has ensued and a hyperexcitable milieu is established, the cycle continues because of changes in ion channels, alterations in neurotransmitter reuptake and release, modifications in receptor trafficking, and deficient astrocyte buffering.[36]

Diagnostic work-up

There is no confirmatory test for NORSE or FIRES. Rather, the diagnosis is made after exclusion of obvious causes of refractory SE. As such, the investigative process must be broad and comprehensive. The NORSE Institute (norseinstitute.org) provides guidance regarding a tiered diagnostic evaluation (**Table 5**).

Seizure management

Seizures in NORSE and FIRES are typically refractory to traditional ASMs, and at least one-third of patients require multiple continuous infusions to control seizures.[23] Use of the ketogenic diet has been described in several case series of patients with FIRES,[42] and expert consensus recommendations are to initiate the ketogenic diet within the first week, if safe to do so.[43] Cannabidiol has also been described as potentially effective in a multicenter series of 7 patients with FIRES.[44] Other retrospective series have described the use of lidocaine and hypothermia.[36]

Inflammatory control

Various anti-inflammatory agents, including IV steroids, immunoglobulins, and plasmapheresis, have been used for NORSE and FIRES with mixed results. The use of second-line immune modulators such as cyclophosphamide, rituximab, and tacrolimus has also been reported, with adults tending to be more responsive than children.[36]

More recently, the use of targeted immunomodulators, including anakinra and tocilizumab, has been described. Anakinra is a recombinant human interleukin 1 receptor antagonist (IL1RA) that reduced seizures in a subset of patients with FIRES.[45] Tocilizumab, an interleukin 6 (IL-6) antagonist, was reported effective in 6 of 7 patients with NORSE, 2 of whom had serious adverse effects.[46] It has also been used in a patient with FIRES refractory to anakinra, with resultant seizure cessation.[47]

Intrathecal dexamethasone was trialed in 6 patients with FIRES with improved seizure control and no adverse effects.[48]

Complications

Patients with NORSE and FIRES have prolonged ICU stays and exposure to medications that are associated with significant adverse effects. For example, continuous infusions are associated with longer mechanical ventilation days and higher rates of complications, including paralytic ileus and cardiorespiratory depression. Paralytic ileus is particularly problematic, as it impedes enteral medication administration and feeding, and this is of particular concern when considering ketogenic diet initiation.

Given exposure to multiple medications, including ASMs, patients with NORSE and FIRES are also at risk for hypersensitivity reactions and drug exanthems.

Outcomes

Outcomes for NORSE and FIRES are poor, with mortality rates of 12% and 16% to 27% in children[38] and adults,[36] respectively. Those who survive often experience serious neurologic sequelae such as cognitive impairment and refractory epilepsy,[36] with adults in particular experiencing a significant loss of independence.[49]

RARE TOXIC AND METABOLIC ETIOLOGIES OF STATUS EPILEPTICUS

In contrast to entities like NORSE and FIRES, electrolyte and other metabolic derangements are common in critically ill children and adults and can cause acute symptomatic seizures[50] as detailed in **Table 6**. Medications that can lower the seizure threshold are outlined in **Table 7** (**Fig. 6**).

Table 6 Toxic and metabolic etiologies of status epilepticus	
Condition	**Mechanism**
Hypercalcemia[62,63]	• Reduces neuronal membrane excitability • Infrequently associated with seizures • Associated with hypertensive encephalopathy and vasoconstriction, which may, in turn, be associated with seizures
Hypoglycemia[64,65]	• Glutamate and Ca^{++}-induced intracellular dysfunction • Commonly associated with seizures and SE • Imaging abnormalities less often recognized: potentially transient diffusion restriction in the cerebral cortex, basal ganglia, splenium of the corpus callosum, hippocampus, internal capsule, and cerebral white matter, as well as in the parietooccipital regions in neonates
Hyperammonemia[66]	• Impairs inhibitory neurotransmission and decreases astrocyte buffering, thus creating a hyperexcitable environment • Common precipitants: liver disease, medications, infections, and gastrointestinal bleeding • Rare disorders: urea cycle defects and organic acidemias
Copper accumulation[67]	• Increased intracellular copper leads to oxidative stress and free radical formation and mitochondrial dysfunction (independent of oxidative stress); this results in cell death in hepatic and brain tissue and other organs • Common manifestations: extrapyramidal dysfunction and cognitive/behavioral problems • SE, while rare, may occur at various stages of the disease and responds favorably to ASMs
Acute intermittent porphyria[68]	• Accumulation of delta-aminolevulinic acid may cause propagation of free radicals within the nervous system, compete for GABA-binding sites, and impair mitochondrial function with secondary inability to maintain axonal integrity • Radiologic features: high nonenhancing MRI-T2 signal in the occipital or frontoparietal cortices • Carbamazepine and phenytoin should be avoided • Treatment is with IV hemin

Table 7
Medications used in the intensive care unit that are associated with seizures[69]

Medication	Impact on Electroencephalogram
Antidepressants (highest risk: bupropion, maprotiline, tricyclics)	Epileptiform discharges with therapeutic doses, burst suppression with bupropion overdose
Antipsychotics	Epileptiform discharges with high doses
Baclofen	Generalized periodic discharges, burst suppression with overdose
Cephalosporins	Generalized periodic discharges
Ifosfamide	Slowing, intermittent rhythmic delta activity, epileptiform discharges, generalized periodic discharges
Lithium	Slowing, increased fast activity, epileptiform discharges and generalized periodic discharges with overdose
Penicillin	Epileptiform discharges, background slowing, triphasic waves[70]

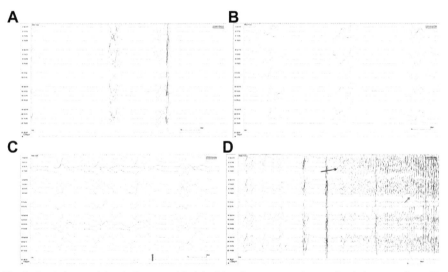

Fig. 6. Baclofen toxicity. A 12-year-old girl with seizures secondary to baclofen overdose. (*A*, *B*) EEG initially showed a burst suppression pattern. (*C*) As the baclofen washed out, EEG was notable for diffuse slowing and intermittent discontinuity (discontinuity indicated by *red arrow*). Settings: LFF 1 Hz, HFF 70 Hz. (*D*) EEG also showed generalized convulsive seizures with a focal lead-in (*black arrow*) followed by spike-wave discharges (*red arrow*). (*Reproduced with permission from* [A-C] Harrar DB, Carpenter JL. Encephalopathy, coma patterns, and other abnormalities of the EEG background in critically ill children. In Sansevere AJ, Harrar DB, Atlas of pediatric and neonatal ICU EEG. New York: Demos Medical Publishing. Copyright Springer Publishing Company, LLC; 2021. p. 79–80; [D] Galan F, Jayakar A. Seizures in critically ill children. In Sansevere AJ, Harrar DB, editors. Atlas of pediatric and neonatal ICU EEG. New York: Demos Medical Publishing. Copyright Springer Publishing Company, LLC; 2021. p. 128.)

RARE INFECTIOUS ETIOLOGIES OF STATUS EPILEPTICUS

Infectious encephalitis is also a common cause of SE. Although many bacterial and viral etiologies are well known, rarer infectious causes of SE may prove more challenging to diagnose. **Table 8** lists rare and emerging causes of infectious encephalitis and SE.

Table 8 Rare infectious etiologies associated with status epilepticus	
Murine typhus[71]	• Zoonotic infection caused by *Rickettsia typhi*, carried by rodents and arthropods • Typically associated with fever, headache, chills, and myalgias followed by rash • Neurologic manifestations include aseptic meningitis, papilledema, cranial nerve palsies, and other focal neurologic deficits • SE is rare • Preferred treatment is doxycycline
Neurosyphilis - Jarisch-Herxheimer reaction[72]	• Thought to involve the lipoprotein-mediated stimulation of macrophages, which in turn produce tumor necrosis factor; this aberrant production of cytokines then initiates an epileptogenic process • Pupillary abnormalities, such as a tonic pupil, should raise suspicion for neurosyphilis
Jamestown Canyon virus[73]	• Arbovirus-associated infection • Emerging endemic etiology of encephalitis in the northeastern United States and Quebec • Most infections occur in adults during the summer months • May be asymptomatic, although may also present with a meningoencephalitis
Powassan virus[74]	• Tick-borne flavivirus endemic to North America from spring to fall • Fever, encephalopathy, seizures, focal neurologic deficits, rash, and gastrointestinal symptoms are common • Treatment is supportive • Reported fatality rate of 10%–15% with residual neurologic deficits in 50% of survivors

SUMMARY

SE is a common neurologic emergency associated with high morbidity and mortality. Management of SE depends on stabilization and treatment as well as on identifying and treating the underlying etiology. Numerous etiologies of SE are amenable to treatment, which may, in turn, halt the evolution of SE.

CLINICS CARE POINTS

- Identification of the underlying genetic etiology can impact the choice of antiseizure medications used for the management of epilepticus, suggesting that genetic testing should be considered, especially for neonates presenting with early infantile epileptic encephalopathy.

- Pyridoxine-dependent epilepsy should be considered in any neonate or infant with intractable seizures of unknown etiology, and this responds rapidly to treatment with pyridoxine (vitamin B6).

- Rhythmic high-amplitude delta with superimposed spikes and polyspikes (RHADS) on EEG is pathognomonic for POLG-related disorders. Valproate can precipitate liver dysfunction, including hepatitis, transaminitis, and severe acute hepatic failure in patients with POLG-related disorders, and is therefore absolutely contraindicated.

- Seizures and SE are common in mitochondrial encephalomyopathy, stroke-like episodes, and lactic acidosis, and as with POLG-related disorders, valproate should be avoided.

- Autoimmune encephalitis is increasingly recognized as an important cause of SE in children and adults and should be considered in a patient who presents with subacute onset of working memory deficits, altered mental status, or psychiatric symptoms, as well as new focal CNS findings, seizures not explained by a pre-existing disorder, CSF pleocytosis, and/or MRI features suggestive of encephalitis.

- Early immunotherapy in AE improves outcome, and often, the decision to proceed with immune therapy must be made before results of antibody testing are available. Once diagnosis of possible AE has been entertained and common infectious etiologies excluded, empiric treatment with IV steroids, IV immunoglobulin, and/or plasmapheresis should begin.

- NORSE and FIRES are rare clinical presentations of SE that warrant an extensive diagnostic work-up for etiology.

- Toxic and metabolic derangements, including medications, can cause SE and should be considered in the differential diagnosis of SE of unclear etiology. They can also contribute to worsening of SE in a patient with SE from another primary etiology.

DISCLOSURE

D. Harrar receives royalties from Sansevere AJ, Harrar DB. Atlas of pediatric and neonatal ICU EEG, New York: Demos Medical Publishing. Copyright Springer Publishing, LLC; 2021. The remaining authors have nothing to disclose.

REFERENCES

1. Newton CR. Epidemiology of status epilepticus in children. Dev Med Child Neurol 2021. https://doi.org/10.1111/dmcn.14946.
2. Ascoli M, Ferlazzo E, Gasparini S, et al. Epidemiology and outcomes of status epilepticus. Int J Gen Med 2021;14:2965–73.
3. Chin RFM. The outcomes of childhood convulsive status epilepticus. Epilepsy Behav EB 2019;101(Pt B):106286. https://doi.org/10.1016/j.yebeh.2019.04.039.
4. Chin RFM, Neville BGR, Peckham C, et al. Treatment of community-onset, childhood convulsive status epilepticus: a prospective, population-based study. Lancet Neurol 2008;7(8):696–703. https://doi.org/10.1016/S1474-4422(08)70141-8.
5. Shorvon S, Ferlisi M. The treatment of super-refractory status epilepticus: a critical review of available therapies and a clinical treatment protocol. Brain J Neurol 2011;134(Pt 10):2802–18. https://doi.org/10.1093/brain/awr215.
6. Kravljanac R, Djuric M, Jankovic B, et al. Etiology, clinical course and response to the treatment of status epilepticus in children: a 16-year single-center experience based on 602 episodes of status epilepticus. Eur J Paediatr Neurol 2015;19(5):584–90. https://doi.org/10.1016/j.ejpn.2015.05.007.
7. Bhatnagar M, Shorvon S. Genetic mutations associated with status epilepticus. Epilepsy Behav EB 2015;49:104–10. https://doi.org/10.1016/j.yebeh.2015.04.013.
8. Cross JH, Guerrini R. The epileptic encephalopathies. Handb Clin Neurol 2013;111:619–26.
9. Parrini E, Ramazzotti A, Dobyns WB, et al. Periventricular heterotopia: phenotypic heterogeneity and correlation with Filamin A mutations. Brain J Neurol 2006;129(Pt 7):1892–906.

10. Parrini E, Conti V, Dobyns WB, et al. Genetic basis of brain malformations. Mol Syndromol 2016;7(4):220–33.

11. Pisano T, Numis AL, Heavin SB, et al. Early and effective treatment of KCNQ2 encephalopathy. Epilepsia 2015;56(5):685–91.

12. Khaikin Y, Mercimek-Andrews S. STXBP1 encephalopathy with epilepsy. In: Adam MP, Ardinger HH, Pagon RA, et al, editors. GeneReviews. Seattle: University of Washington; 1993. Available at: http://www.ncbi.nlm.nih.gov/books/NBK396561/. Accessed July 16, 2021.

13. Coughlin CR, Tseng LA, Abdenur JE, et al. Consensus guidelines for the diagnosis and management of pyridoxine-dependent epilepsy due to α-aminoadipic semialdehyde dehydrogenase deficiency. J Inherit Metab Dis 2021;44(1):178–92.

14. Van Hove JL, Coughlin C, Swanson M, et al. Nonketotic hyperglycinemia. In: Adam MP, Ardinger HH, Pagon RA, et al, editors. GeneReviews. Seattle: University of Washington; 1993. Available at: http://www.ncbi.nlm.nih.gov/books/NBK1357/. Accessed July 27, 2021.

15. Rahman S, Copeland WC. POLG-related disorders and their neurological manifestations. Nat Rev Neurol 2019;15(1):40–52.

16. Saneto RP, Cohen BH, Copeland WC, et al. Alpers-Huttenlocher syndrome. Pediatr Neurol 2013;48(3):167–78.

17. Wolf NI, Rahman S, Schmitt B, et al. Status epilepticus in children with Alpers' disease caused by POLG1 mutations: EEG and MRI features. Epilepsia 2009;50(6):1596–607.

18. Specchio N, Pietrafusa N, Calabrese C, et al. POLG1-Related epilepsy: review of diagnostic and therapeutic findings. Brain Sci 2020;10(11):E768.

19. Lee HN, Eom S, Kim SH, et al. Epilepsy characteristics and clinical outcome in patients with mitochondrial encephalomyopathy, lactic acidosis, and stroke-like episodes (MELAS). Pediatr Neurol 2016;64:59–65.

20. Koenig MK, Emrick L, Karaa A, et al. Recommendations for the management of strokelike episodes in patients with mitochondrial encephalomyopathy, lactic acidosis, and strokelike episodes. JAMA Neurol 2016;73(5):591–4.

21. Mameniškienė R, Wolf P. Epilepsia partialis continua: a review. Seizure 2017;44:74–80.

22. Spatola M, Novy J, Du Pasquier R, et al. Status epilepticus of inflammatory etiology: a cohort study. Neurology 2015;85(5):464–70.

23. Gaspard N, Foreman BP, Alvarez V, et al. New-onset refractory status epilepticus: etiology, clinical features, and outcome. Neurology 2015;85(18):1604–13.

24. Dalmau J, Graus F. Antibody-mediated encephalitis. N Engl J Med 2018;378(9):840–51.

25. Hacohen Y, Wright S, Waters P, et al. Paediatric autoimmune encephalopathies: clinical features, laboratory investigations and outcomes in patients with or without antibodies to known central nervous system autoantigens. J Neurol Neurosurg Psychiatr 2013;84(7):748–55.

26. Graus F, Titulaer MJ, Balu R, et al. A clinical approach to diagnosis of autoimmune encephalitis. Lancet Neurol 2016;15(4):391–404.

27. Cellucci T, Van Mater H, Graus F, et al. Clinical approach to the diagnosis of autoimmune encephalitis in the pediatric patient. Neurol Neuroimmunol Neuroinflamm 2020;7(2):e663.

28. Dubey D, Alqallaf A, Hays R, et al. Neurological autoantibody prevalence in epilepsy of unknown etiology. JAMA Neurol 2017;74(4):397–402.

29. Dalmau J, Lancaster E, Martinez-Hernandez E, et al. Clinical experience and laboratory investigations in patients with anti-NMDAR encephalitis. Lancet Neurol 2011;10(1):63–74.
30. Liu X, Yan B, Wang R, et al. Seizure outcomes in patients with anti-NMDAR encephalitis: a follow-up study. Epilepsia 2017;58(12):2104–11.
31. Titulaer MJ, McCracken L, Gabilondo I, et al. Treatment and prognostic factors for long-term outcome in patients with anti-NMDA receptor encephalitis: an observational cohort study. Lancet Neurol 2013;12(2):157–65.
32. Schmitt SE, Pargeon K, Frechette ES, et al. Extreme delta brush: a unique EEG pattern in adults with anti-NMDA receptor encephalitis. Neurology 2012;79(11):1094–100.
33. Byrne S, Walsh C, Hacohen Y, et al. Earlier treatment of NMDAR antibody encephalitis in children results in a better outcome. Neurol Neuroimmunol Neuroinflammation 2015;2(4):e130.
34. Linnoila J, Pittock SJ. Autoantibody-associated central nervous system neurologic disorders. Semin Neurol 2016;36(4):382–96.
35. Hirsch LJ, Gaspard N, van Baalen A, et al. Proposed consensus definitions for new-onset refractory status epilepticus (NORSE), febrile infection-related epilepsy syndrome (FIRES), and related conditions. Epilepsia 2018;59(4):739–44.
36. Specchio N, Pietrafusa N. New-onset refractory status epilepticus and febrile infection-related epilepsy syndrome. Dev Med Child Neurol 2020;62(8):897–905.
37. Sculier C, Gaspard N. New onset refractory status epilepticus (NORSE). Seizure 2019;68:72–8.
38. Kramer U, Chi C-S, Lin K-L, et al. Febrile infection-related epilepsy syndrome (FIRES): pathogenesis, treatment, and outcome: a multicenter study on 77 children. Epilepsia 2011;52(11):1956–65.
39. Mikaeloff Y, Jambaqué I, Hertz-Pannier L, et al. Devastating epileptic encephalopathy in school-aged children (DESC): a pseudo encephalitis. Epilepsy Res 2006;69(1):67–79.
40. Farias-Moeller R, Bartolini L, Staso K, et al. Early ictal and interictal patterns in FIRES: the sparks before the blaze. Epilepsia 2017;58(8):1340–8.
41. Kothur K, Bandodkar S, Wienholt L, et al. Etiology is the key determinant of neuroinflammation in epilepsy: elevation of cerebrospinal fluid cytokines and chemokines in febrile infection-related epilepsy syndrome and febrile status epilepticus. Epilepsia 2019;60(8):1678–88. https://doi.org/10.1111/epi.16275.
42. Nabbout R, Mazzuca M, Hubert P, et al. Efficacy of ketogenic diet in severe refractory status epilepticus initiating fever induced refractory epileptic encephalopathy in school age children (FIRES). Epilepsia 2010;51(10):2033–7.
43. Koh S, Wirrell E, Vezzani A, et al. Proposal to optimize evaluation and treatment of febrile infection-related epilepsy syndrome (FIRES): a report from FIRES workshop. Epilepsia Open 2021;6(1):62–72.
44. Gofshteyn JS, Wilfong A, Devinsky O, et al. Cannabidiol as a potential treatment for febrile infection-related epilepsy syndrome (FIRES) in the acute and chronic phases. J Child Neurol 2017;32(1):35–40.
45. Lai Y-C, Muscal E, Wells E, et al. Anakinra usage in febrile infection related epilepsy syndrome: an international cohort. Ann Clin Transl Neurol 2020;7(12):2467–74.
46. Jun J-S, Lee S-T, Kim R, et al. Tocilizumab treatment for new onset refractory status epilepticus. Ann Neurol 2018;84(6):940–5.
47. Stredny CM, Case S, Sansevere AJ, et al. Interleukin-6 blockade with tocilizumab in anakinra-refractory febrile infection-related epilepsy syndrome (FIRES). Child

Neurol Open 2020;7. https://doi.org/10.1177/2329048X20979253. 2329048X20979253.

48. Horino A, Kuki I, Inoue T, et al. Intrathecal dexamethasone therapy for febrile infection-related epilepsy syndrome. Ann Clin Transl Neurol 2021;8(3):645–55.

49. Nass RD, Taube J, Bauer T, et al. Permanent loss of independence in adult febrile-infection-related epilepsy syndrome survivors: an underestimated and unsolved challenge. Eur J Neurol 2021. https://doi.org/10.1111/ene.14958.

50. Nardone R, Brigo F, Trinka E. Acute symptomatic seizures caused by electrolyte disturbances. J Clin Neurol Seoul Korea 2016;12(1):21–33.

51. Davila-Williams D, Pearl PL. Pathognomonic EEG patterns in critically ill children and neonates. In: Sansevere A, Harrar D, editors. Atlas of pediatric and neonatal ICU EEG. 1st edition. New York: Demos Medical Publishing; 2021. p. 373–409.

52. Berendse K, Klouwer FCC, Koot BGP, et al. Cholic acid therapy in Zellweger spectrum disorders. J Inherit Metab Dis 2016;39(6):859–68.

53. Jurecka A, Zikanova M, Kmoch S, et al. Adenylosuccinate lyase deficiency. J Inherit Metab Dis 2015;38(2):231–42.

54. Alobaidy H. Recent advances in the diagnosis and treatment of Niemann-Pick disease type C in children: a guide to early diagnosis for the general pediatrician. Int J Pediatr 2015;2015:816593.

55. Pearl PL. Inherited metabolic epilepsies. In: Swaiman KF, Ashwal S, Ferriero D, et al, editors. Swaiman's pediatric neurology: principles and practice. New York: Elsevier; 2017. p. 594–9.

56. Poffenberger CN, Inati S, Tayebi N, et al. EEG abnormalities in patients with chronic neuronopathic Gaucher disease: a retrospective review. Mol Genet Metab 2020;131(3):358–63.

57. Roshan Lal T, Seehra GK, Steward AM, et al. The natural history of type 2 Gaucher disease in the 21st century: a retrospective study. Neurology 2020; 95(15):e2119–30.

58. Geberhiwot T, Moro A, Dardis A, et al. Consensus clinical management guidelines for Niemann-Pick disease type C. Orphanet J Rare Dis 2018;13(1):50.

59. Schwahn BC, Van Spronsen FJ, Belaidi AA, et al. Efficacy and safety of cyclic pyranopterin monophosphate substitution in severe molybdenum cofactor deficiency type A: a prospective cohort study. Lancet Lond Engl 2015;386(10007): 1955–63.

60. Andrews A. Status epilepticus and POLG-1. In: Sansevere A, Harrar D, editors. Atlas of pediatric and neonatal ICU EEG. 1st edition. New York: Demos Medical Publishing; 2021. p. 544–8.

61. Stredny C, Farias-Moeller R. Febrile infection-related epilepsy syndrome (FIRES). In: Sansevere A, Harrar D, editors. Atlas of pediatric and neonatal ICU EEG. 1st edition. New York: Demos Medical Publishing; 2021. p. 498–506.

62. Juvarra G, Bettoni L, Olivieri MF, et al. Hypercalcemic encephalopathy in the course of hyperthyroidism. Eur Neurol 1985;24(2):121–7.

63. Chen T-H, Huang C-C, Chang Y-Y, et al. Vasoconstriction as the etiology of hypercalcemia-induced seizures. Epilepsia 2004;45(5):551–4.

64. Kang EG, Jeon SJ, Choi SS, et al. Diffusion MR imaging of hypoglycemic encephalopathy. AJNR Am J Neuroradiol 2010;31(3):559–64.

65. Kim SY, Goo HW, Lim KH, et al. Neonatal hypoglycaemic encephalopathy: diffusion-weighted imaging and proton MR spectroscopy. Pediatr Radiol 2006; 36(2):144–8.

66. Rangroo Thrane V, Thrane AS, Wang F, et al. Ammonia triggers neuronal disinhi-bition and seizures by impairing astrocyte potassium buffering. Nat Med 2013; 19(12):1643–8.
67. Prashanth LK, Sinha S, Taly AB, et al. Spectrum of epilepsy in Wilson's disease with electroencephalographic, MR imaging and pathological correlates. J Neurol Sci 2010;291(1–2):44–51.
68. O'Malley R, Rao G, Stein P, et al. Porphyria: often discussed but too often missed. Pract Neurol 2018;18(5):352–8.
69. Harrar D, Carpenter JL. Encephalopathy, coma patterns, and other abnormalities of the EEG background in critically ill children. In: Sansevere A, Harrar D, editors. Atlas of pediatric and neonatal ICU EEG. 1st edition. New York: Demos Medical Publishing; 2021. p. 33–81.
70. Bhattacharyya S, Darby RR, Raibagkar P, et al. Antibiotic-associated encepha-lopathy. Neurology 2016;86(10):963–71.
71. Stephens BE, Thi M, Alkhateb R, et al. Case report: fulminant murine typhus pre-senting with status epilepticus and multi-organ failure: an autopsy case and a re-view of the neurologic presentations of murine typhus. Am J Trop Med Hyg 2018; 99(2):306–9.
72. Rissardo JP, Caprara ALF, Silveira JOF. Generalized convulsive status epilepticus secondary to Jarisch-Herxheimer reaction in neurosyphilis: a case Report and Literature review. Neurologist 2019;24(1):29–32.
73. Solomon IH, Ganesh VS, Yu G, et al. Fatal case of chronic Jamestown Canyon virus encephalitis diagnosed by metagenomic sequencing in patient receiving rit-uximab. Emerg Infect Dis 2021;27(1). https://doi.org/10.3201/eid2701.203448.
74. Piantadosi A, Rubin DB, McQuillen DP, et al. Emerging cases of powassan virus encephalitis in New England: clinical presentation, imaging, and review of the literature. Clin Infect Dis Off Publ Infect Dis Soc Am 2016;62(6):707–13.

Primary Causes of Hypertensive Crisis

Scott K. Van Why, MD*, Cynthia G. Pan, MD

KEYWORDS

- Hypertensive crisis • Infancy • Childhood • Adult • Cause • Evaluation

KEY POINTS

- Hypertensive crisis is a rare medical presentation that deserves prompt evaluation and treatment.
- The cause of hypertensive crisis is usually able to be identified.
- Principal causes of hypertensive crisis vary significantly according to age, divided into infancy, childhood, and adult groups.
- A directed diagnostic approach typically will rapidly identify the cause of hypertensive crisis.

INTRODUCTION

Hypertensive crisis is a rare condition and is defined as a sudden and abrupt elevation in blood pressure that poses the threat of rapid-onset end-organ damage. Hypertensive urgency occurs when a patient has mild or no symptoms, whereas a hypertensive emergency is when severe symptoms and end-organ damage are present.

Acute severe hypertension in children is considered when a validated blood pressure is far above the 99th percentile for age, as defined in the 2017 American Academy of Pediatrics clinical practice guidelines for management of hypertension in children and adolescents.[1] In children, the individualized assessment of risk for end-organ damage more often dictates the urgency of treatment to lower blood pressure rather than the actual blood pressure measurement. In adults, the American Heart Association and America College of Cardiology set forth guidelines for hypertension in 2017 in which a hypertensive crisis is defined by a blood pressure measure greater than 180 mm Hg systolic and greater than 120 mm Hg diastolic. In these guidelines, the differentiation between a hypertensive crisis being urgent or emergent is also defined by

Department of Pediatrics, Medical College of Wisconsin, 999 North 92nd Street, Suite C510, Milwaukee, WI 53226, USA
* Corresponding author.
E-mail address: svanwhy@mcw.edu

Crit Care Clin 38 (2022) 375–391
https://doi.org/10.1016/j.ccc.2021.11.016
0749-0704/22/© 2021 Elsevier Inc. All rights reserved.

absence or presence of end-organ damage.[2,3] A detailed history and physical examination will help guide the assessment for cause and urgency of management.

PRESENTATION
Symptoms of Hypertensive Crisis and Associated Diseases

Chronic severe hypertension is silent in most cases, but acute severe hypertension can present with symptoms related to high blood pressure that also provide clues to the cause of the hypertension. Eliciting symptoms related to acute hypertension that could indicate end-organ damage in a hypertensive emergency is critical in the initial assessment and management. A summary of common and uncommon symptoms is provided in **Table 1**. Presentations of hypertensive crisis can include severe headache, vision changes, mental status changes, or seizure. Patients may have atypical chest pain, respiratory distress from pulmonary edema, abdominal pain, or vomiting accompanying severely high blood pressure. Diplopia or altered vision, focal paresthesia, or obtundation may be signs of an impending neurologic crisis. All these

Table 1	
Presentations in hypertension	
• History	*Hypertension-related symptoms:* Headache, dizziness, blurry vision, altered mental status, chest pain, palpitations, abdominal pain, vomiting
	Cause-related symptoms: Hematuria, joint pain or swelling, generalized edema, rash, cardiac/respiratory issues, voiding problems
	Past history: Prematurity and related complications, intensive care unit stay and related complications, urinary issues, including previous urinary tract infection
	Social history: Drug and supplement history
	Family history: Renal issues or blood pressure problems
• Physical examination	• Accurate method: Auscultatory
	• Appropriate size cuff
	○ The bladder length 80% of the midarm circumference
	○ The bladder width at least 40%
	• All extremity blood pressure measurements
	• Findings in symptomatic hypertension
	○ Focal neurologic findings
	○ Mental status changes
	○ Papilledema
	○ Gallop cardiac rhythm on auscultation
	• Other findings
	○ Constitutional: Syndromic features
	○ Fundus: Retinal hemorrhage, arterial narrowing
	○ Skin: Rash, purpura, café-au-lait macules
	○ Swelling: Periorbital or extremity
	○ Cardiac: Femoral radial pulse lag, murmur
	○ Abdominal mass, bruit
	• Occasional findings
	○ Coloboma
	○ Ear tag/pit
	○ Webbed neck
	○ Genital abnormality

Box 1
Causes of severe infantile hypertension

Infantile hypertension
  Neonatal
  • Vascular
    ○ Thrombotic/thromboembolic: umbilical artery catheter-associated or renal vein thrombosis
    ○ Aortic coarctation
    ○ Renal artery stenosis, congenital or acquired
  • Congenital urinary tract malformations (obstructive lesions)
  • Polycystic kidney disease
  Later infancy
  • Prematurity associated
    ○ History of thrombotic/thromboembolic renal insult
    ○ Renal artery stenosis, congenital or acquired
    ○ Immature kidneys, history of renal insults: Acute kidney injury, nephrotoxins
  • Congenital urinary tract malformations (obstructive lesions)
  • Polycystic kidney disease
  • Aortic coarctation
  • Tumors: Nephroblastoma, neuroblastoma
  • Glomerulopathy
    ○ Congenital infection
    ○ Congenital/infantile nephrotic syndrome, familial FSGS, Denys-Drash syndrome
    ○ Atypical HUS

---

symptoms should be considered emergent in any age group and need immediate attention.[4,5]

Symptoms related to potential cause should be sought. Renal causes of hypertension are high in the differential diagnosis in all children and vary according to age. Potential causes for each age group, described in later sections and in **Boxes 1** and **2**, guide the symptoms to be elicited and the focus of the physical examination. Severe hypertension in neonates is uncommon but may present with symptoms of heart failure, gross hematuria, or abdominal mass. In later infancy, the presentation may be similar to that in neonates, but more commonly consists of nonspecific symptoms of poor growth, weight loss, or fussiness. Childhood and adolescent severe hypertension may present with symptoms of gross hematuria, swelling, rash, joint complaints, dyspnea, or diarrhea, depending on the more common causes in this age group. Edema would suggest glomerular pathology or renal failure. Urinary symptoms with the presentation of hypertension in childhood suggest a urologic abnormality not previously discovered. In later childhood and adolescence, the risk of recreational drug use increases, so symptoms of lethargy, irritability, anorexia, and poor school performance are relevant. Episodic palpitation or flushing may be symptoms from rare catecholamine-secreting tumors or hyperthyroidism.

In adults, symptoms of severe hypertension are often absent, but like children, symptoms should be ascertained to assess potential target organ damage. Atypical chest pain, headache, dyspnea, lightheadedness, and epistaxis may be associated symptoms.[2] Rare and unique to adults are diseases with specific symptoms, such as the dermatopathy of scleroderma that when diffuse and rapidly progressive precedes scleroderma renal crisis. Acute aortic dissection (AAD), depending on its location, may present with severe chest pain, back pain, or abdominal pain. In rare cases of nongenetic sporadic pheochromocytoma, the combination of palpitations,

Box 2
Causes of severe childhood and adult hypertension

Childhood and adult hypertension
  Common causes
  • Parenchymal renal disease
    ○ Acute and chronic glomerulonephritis
      ■ Postinfectious glomerulonephritis
      ■ Systemic vasculitis with renal involvement (SLE, HSP, ANCA vasculitis, scleroderma)
      ■ Primary, idiopathic (IgA nephropathy, focal segmental glomerulosclerosis, crescentic glomerulonephritis)
    ○ Hemolytic uremic syndrome
    ○ Hereditary cystic kidney disease: polycystic kidney disease, medullary cystic kidney disease, nephronophthisis
    ○ Sickle cell disease
    ○ Interstitial nephritis
  • End-stage kidney disease of unknown cause
  • Congenital urinary tract malformations: Obstructive or cystic dysplasia, either isolated or syndromic
  • Scarred kidney: Congenital Ask-Upmark kidney or acquired from renal injury (eg, pyelonephritis)
  • Drug-induced: Therapeutic and recreational
  • Preeclampsia
  Less common and rare causes
  • Vascular/renal artery stenosis
    ○ Aortic coarctation or dissection
    ○ Fibromuscular dysplasia
    ○ Syndromic: Williams syndrome, neurofibromatosis, Turner syndrome, middle aortic syndrome
    ○ Tumor-associated extrinsic compression: Wilms tumor, neuroblastoma, lymphoma
    ○ Large vessel vasculitis: Takayasu, moyamoya, polyarteritis nodosa
    ○ Trauma-associated perirenal hematoma
  • Neoplasia: Wilms tumor, neuroblastoma, pheochromocytoma, infiltrative lymphoma
  • Persistent or late-onset hypertension from perinatal renal insult, prematurity associated
  • Neurologic
    ○ High intracranial pressure from head trauma, intracranial tumor, or pseudotumor cerebri
    ○ Brainstem tumor mimicking catecholamine-secreting tumor (presents with paroxysmal hypertension and neurologic signs)
    ○ Secondary to seizure
    ○ Peripheral neuropathies: Guillain-Barré, poliomyelitis
  • Monogenic
    ○ Liddle syndrome
    ○ Von Hippel-Lindau syndrome (may present with brainstem hemangioblastoma and neurologic hypertension and/or with pheochromocytoma)
    ○ Hyperaldosteronism: Familial and glucocorticoid remediable
    ○ Congenital adrenal hyperplasia
    ○ Gordon syndrome: pseudohypoaldosteronism
    ○ Apparent mineralocorticoid excess
  • Dysautonomia
  • Endocrine
    ○ Thyroid disease
    ○ Cushing syndrome
    ○ Catecholamine-secreting tumors (pheochromocytoma)
    ○ Hypercalcemia: Vitamin D intoxication, hyperparathyroidism, malignancy associated

Abbreviations: HSP, Henoch-Schonlein purpura; MCKD, multicystic dysplastic kidney; SLE, systemic lupus erythematosus.

headache, and diaphoresis with paroxysmal hypertension is highly predictive of disease. Preeclampsia in pregnancy at greater than 20 weeks' gestation can present with headache, visual disturbance, and abdominal pain.

Adult practice guidelines bring attention to specific clinical situations of acute ischemic stroke, AAD, acute kidney injury, and acute heart failure as events that require different approaches to hypertension management. Therefore, the specific presenting symptoms of these conditions are important to recognize early because management is dictated by diagnosis.[6]

Physical Examination

Accurate blood pressure measurement is fundamental in identifying hypertension. Manual, auscultatory blood pressure is the most accurate, and normative data are based on this method of blood pressure measurement. In infants and those in whom Korotkoff sounds are not well heard, Doppler can be used to measure blood pressure accurately, but only systolic readings are obtained by this method. An oscillatory method may not be accurate but is useful as a screening tool if done with a device calibrated for pediatric use. In an emergency setting, a manual blood pressure measurement may not initially be feasible. A well-calibrated oscillatory device can be used for initial screening and frequent monitoring and then validated with auscultatory method at the earliest opportunity. In large registries of adult hospitalized patients, oscillometric blood pressure measurement underestimates intra-arterial blood pressure readings by as much as 50/30; this method is discouraged when managing hypertensive emergencies.[2]

Blood pressure measurement should be done on the right arm, unless there is known atypical anatomy that can confound that assessment. If blood pressure is found to be elevated, 4-extremity readings should be obtained to evaluate for vascular anomalies, in particular, aortic coarctation, which might further be suggested by the presence of a heart murmur. Lower-extremity blood pressure is typically equal or higher than upper-extremity blood pressure. A right upper-extremity blood pressure greater than 10 mm Hg above that of lower-extremity blood pressure is a strong indication of aortic coarctation.

Other pertinent physical examination information is critical in determining the urgency of the situation as well as the cause. Abnormal fundoscopic findings, such as papilledema and retinal hemorrhages, focal neurologic deficits or encephalopathy indicate acute hypertensive emergency and the need for immediate therapeutic intervention along with prompt evaluation to identify the cause. Similar to symptoms, the physical findings can speak to both effects of hypertension and the potential cause. The presence of a gallop rhythm and rales on auscultation, along with edema, suggests volume overload as a cause of severe symptomatic hypertension, possibly from underlying glomerulonephritis. Alternately, hypertensive cardiomyopathy may produce similar findings. Edema, rash, and arthritis would suggest hypertension secondary to renal involvement from autoimmune disease. Diminished lower-extremity pulses with discrepancy between upper- and lower-extremity blood pressures, along with a heart murmur, points to coarctation of the aorta or aortic dissection. Abdominal or flank bruit may be present with renal artery stenosis (RAS). Cushingoid features, ambiguous genitalia, or features of hyperthyroidism can direct evaluation to endocrine causes. Physical examination findings associated with genetic syndromes that can have hypertension caused by abnormal renal or vascular development include coloboma, lens dislocation, ear tags, brachial cysts, café-au-lait spots, or webbed neck.

CAUSES

The preponderance of severe hypertension in adulthood is seen in those with an established diagnosis of primary hypertension, formerly called "essential hypertension," and hypertension secondary to diabetic nephropathy. Although the prevalence of primary hypertension is increasing in childhood, it does not cause hypertensive crisis during childhood. The cause of hypertensive crisis in children and adolescents usually is secondary to an identifiable cause and is most often from renal disease. Disease processes that cause severe hypertension in childhood typically manifest at different ages, with the major differences being between infants and older children.

Infantile Hypertension

Neonatal
Causes of severe hypertension in infancy can be separated into neonatal forms and those identified in later infancy (see **Box 1**). During the neonatal period, the causes are typically identified in the context of prenatal fetal imaging, premature birth, or perinatal stress. The principal causes in this age group can be separated into abnormalities in either the vasculature or the renal architecture. With premature birth, vital signs are routinely monitored so hypertension is readily identified in this group. In apparently healthy term neonates, blood pressure is not routinely assessed, so hypertension is often not identified unless symptoms or signs dictate measuring blood pressure, such as development of gross hematuria, presentation in extremis from severe hypertension, or palpation of an intra-abdominal mass.

The most common cause of hypertension in the sick or premature neonate is vascular, with the preponderance being secondary to having had an umbilical artery catheter (UAC) for vascular access. Although rarely identifiable by any imaging study, presumably these infants sustain a focal thromboembolic insult to a kidney that then drives elevated blood pressure. This cause of hypertension can be severe but tends not to last indefinitely. Often antihypertensive treatment of this cause can be discontinued during later infancy or early childhood. However, significant hypertension can then recur later in childhood and may be severe. Less commonly, having had a UAC is associated with being found to have renal artery stenosis (RAS) later during infancy or early childhood, presumably acquired from focal injury to the ostium of the renal artery that then progresses to ostial stenosis.

Renal vein thrombosis occurs in infants subjected to perinatal stress or volume depletion but can occur spontaneously in an otherwise healthy infant. The combination of gross hematuria, hypertension, and low-platelet count should alert the clinician to this possibility. Doppler study of the renal veins typically identifies a significant thrombus, and at times associated diminished global renal perfusion.

Congenital vascular abnormalities that cause hypertension in the neonate include congenital RAS and aortic coarctation. The former is a difficult diagnosis to establish during infancy. Aortic coarctation, however, is readily identified with 4-extremity blood pressure measurement and confirmation with echocardiography.

With the routine use of prenatal fetal ultrasound, most renal structural anomalies causing severe neonatal hypertension are identified before birth. These are broadly categorized as congenital abnormalities of the kidneys and urinary tract (CAKUT) and include cystic kidney disease and abnormalities of drainage of the urinary tract. Although many forms of CAKUT do not cause hypertension, those associated with urinary tract obstruction are more likely to have hypertension. This includes any form of bladder outlet obstruction, such as posterior urethral valves in male infants, neurogenic bladder, or ureteral obstruction, most often at the ureteropelvic junction. A multicystic dysplastic kidney, a more common renal anomaly, can on occasion cause hypertension, but usually not unless associated with ureteral obstruction.

Polycystic kidney disease (PKD) manifesting in infancy is rare, but almost always is associated with severe hypertension. In this context, the kidneys typically are readily palpable and found on ultrasound study to be massively enlarged with cysts. The cause may be either autosomal recessive (ARPKD) or infantile-onset autosomal dominant (ADPKD). Imaging, including finding associated liver abnormalities in ARPKD, may differentiate between the 2 diagnoses. However, ARPKD and ADPKD at times may not be able to be differentiated solely on imaging findings or family history. In that instance, genetic testing can be helpful, especially for providing a diagnosis of ARPKD.

Later infancy

Most of the causes of hypertension in the neonatal period may also present during later infancy. Hypertension in later infancy is not found incidentally, but rather is often diagnosed owing to associated symptoms or signs. This is because blood pressure measurement is not commonly performed in otherwise healthy-appearing infants, with primary care practice guidelines recommending that routine measurement of blood pressure begin at age 3 years. In addition, there is additional skill required to take an accurate blood pressure measurement in infants.

Several of the causes of hypertension associated with premature birth may persist or may not become manifest until later infancy. These include intrarenal thrombotic and thromboembolic insults to the kidney that may not have caused hypertension earlier in the neonatal course but become manifest later in infancy. In addition, even without any evident risk factor for a thrombotic or thromboembolic cause, premature birth alone, especially severely premature birth, is associated with early-onset hypertension, as early as later infancy. The cause in this scenario is thought to be from incompletely developed, immature kidneys at birth becoming complicated by events during the early neonatal course after birth. Events predisposing to later-onset hypertension include subclinical insults to the kidneys, such as from multiple nephrotoxins and transient hypotensive events, causing occult acute kidney injury.

Congenital vascular and renal architecture abnormalities that cause hypertension, detailed in the section above, may present later in infancy as symptomatic hypertension, or when blood pressure is measured at an urgent care visit for an unrelated acute illness. PKD, especially ARPKD in which progression often manifests as rapidly enlarging kidneys during infancy, may be found by palpation of an abdominal mass. Blood pressure when then measured typically is severely elevated.

Rare causes of severe hypertension in infancy include intra-abdominal tumors, found by palpation of a mass or on imaging for abdominal symptoms. The 2 most likely in this age group are nephroblastoma (also referred to as Wilms tumor) and neuroblastoma. Both tumors may cause hypertension by compromising the renal vasculature. Neuroblastoma also can cause hypertension by obstructing the urinary tract, depending on location and size of the tumor, or by secreting catecholamines.

Rarely, glomerulopathies become manifest in infancy and can cause severe hypertension. These include those secondary to congenital infection, such as syphilis and cytomegalovirus. Congenital or infantile nephrotic syndrome, such as from familial focal segmental glomerulosclerosis (FSGS) or the glomerulopathy of Denys-Drash syndrome, often have hypertension as a manifestation. Atypical nontoxigenic hemolytic uremic syndrome (HUS) with accompanying glomerulopathy is rare but can present in infancy with anemia and thrombocytopenia, renal insufficiency, and hypertension. The lack of a diarrheal prodrome is a hallmark of the disease.

Childhood Hypertension

Box 2 outlines common and less common causes of hypertensive crisis that present during childhood. Several of the diseases that cause hypertension during childhood may be present during infancy but may not progress to cause severe hypertension until later in the course of the disease. Examples of these include hereditary cystic kidney diseases, such as PKD, medullary cystic kidney disease, nephronophthisis, or any form of CAKUT with an obstructive lesion. CAKUT that can cause hypertension may become apparent in childhood in those who have been diagnosed with a syndrome that has significantly increased risk of associated urinary tract or renal anomalies. These include Turner syndrome, branchio-oto-renal syndrome, and coloboma-renal syndrome. Renal injury sustained early in life, in either the setting of premature birth, perinatal complications, or early pyelonephritis with associated later development of renal scarring, may not manifest hypertension until later in childhood.

Common causes

The younger the child, the more likely there is an identifiable cause of secondary hypertension. Acute and symptomatic hypertension in childhood is most likely to be secondary to glomerular disease. Acute postinfectious glomerulonephritis is the most common cause of nephritis in childhood and often presents with symptomatic hypertension when gross hematuria is not the heralding symptom. Patients with systemic vasculitis with renal involvement, including lupus, immunoglobulin A (IgA) vasculitis, and antineutrophil cytoplasmic antibody (ANCA) -positive vasculitis, often have significant hypertension as a prominent feature at presentation and during flares of the disease. HUS, both toxigenic and atypical forms, routinely have associated hypertension during the episode that can accelerate to hypertensive crisis.

Patients with crescentic glomerulonephritis, whether idiopathic or secondary to other identifiable nephropathy, often have severe hypertension at presentation. Primary idiopathic forms of glomerulonephritis, such as IgA nephropathy and FSGS,

---

Box 3
Common drugs inducing hypertension

- Therapeutic drugs
  - Immunosuppressants
    - Corticosteroids
    - Calcineurin inhibitors: Tacrolimus, cyclosporine A
  - Oral contraceptives
  - Ephedrine
  - Nonsteroidal anti-inflammatory analgesics
  - Stimulant medication for attention-deficit/hyperactivity disorder: Amphetamines, methylphenidate

- Recreational drugs
  - Cocaine
  - Amphetamines, methamphetamines, methylphenidate
  - Phencyclidine

- Other
  - Nicotine
  - Ethanol
  - Caffeine
  - Yohimbine
  - Ephedra

may be indolent and not have hypertension at presentation. However, if severe and therapy for the primary process is not effective, hypertension then becomes a nearly uniform feature and may progress to crisis levels.

Early-onset hypertension in patients with sickle cell disease is often asymptomatic in childhood. However, when associated with overt sickle cell nephropathy, with significant proteinuria and development of renal insufficiency, hypertension manifested during adolescence may progress to severe, symptomatic hypertension. The predisposition to hypertension in those with sickle cell disease appears to be secondary to endothelial cell dysfunction.

Drug-induced hypertension is common in childhood and adolescence. Usual agents that cause hypertension include several classes of therapeutic medications, recreational drugs, and other agents, including supplements (**Box 3**). Most of these agents cause hypertension by enhancing vasoconstriction. Any child or adolescent presenting in hypertensive crisis, who does not have evident renal disease on initial testing and is not on a prescribed medication known to cause hypertension, should be evaluated for the possibility of other drug-induced hypertension.

Less common causes

Although less common than renal parenchymal causes of hypertension, vascular causes of hypertension should always be considered in a child with severe hypertension. A child with a vascular cause of hypertension often presents with asymptomatic and severe hypertension with no evident renal disease based on urinalysis or blood tests. For example, because the hypertension has been longstanding, those with aortic coarctation or RAS typically present with incidentally found severe hypertension that is asymptomatic. RAS can be idiopathic, such as with fibromuscular dysplasia, or syndromic. Any child with a diagnosis of Williams syndrome, Turner syndrome, or neurofibromatosis should be routinely screened for hypertension, because aortic coarctation (Williams and Turner syndrome) or renal artery stenotic lesions associated with these syndromes are typically asymptomatic and can become manifest as severe hypertension at any time during childhood.

Renal vascular stenosis or compromise can be acquired acutely and in that setting more often presents as symptomatic hypertension. Tumor compression of renal vasculature from Wilms tumor, abdominal neuroblastoma, or lymphoma can cause severe acute hypertension. Large-vessel vasculitis, such as Takayasu arteritis or moyamoya disease, may be occult but then present with neurologic symptoms and severe hypertension.

Neurologic injury or disease often has associated elevation in blood pressure and in cases of increased intracranial pressure is also associated with bradycardia. Typically, the elevated blood pressure is acute and transient, not resulting in established hypertension. Increased intracranial pressure from head trauma, intracranial tumor, or pseudotumor cerebri can cause high blood pressure, which if present speaks to the severity of the intracranial pressure and need for acute intervention for the primary problem. Other intracranial tumors, such as isolated or syndromic hemangioblastomas of the brainstem, may cause paroxysmal or sustained severe hypertension in the absence of increased intracranial pressure. Von Hippel-Lindau syndrome, caused by pathogenic variants in the *VHL* gene, can lead to both hemangioblastomas as well as pheochromocytoma, and if the hypertension from a hemangioblastoma is episodic, the blood pressure fluctuations may mimic those caused by pheochromocytoma. Peripheral neuropathies, such as from Guillain-Barré syndrome or poliomyelitis, not uncommonly have hypertension from autonomic dysfunction in the acute phase of the disease. Hypertension in this setting typically resolves with recovery from the illness, but in some cases can persist.

Blood pressure is often elevated during seizure activity and does not require antihypertensive treatment or specific evaluation if seizure alone is clearly the cause of the elevated blood pressure. However, because hypertensive crisis caused by several underlying diseases, such as acute glomerulonephritis, may present with new-onset seizure, it must always be considered whether the finding of elevated blood pressure is the cause or effect of the seizure. If the latter, blood pressure usually returns to normal rapidly after the seizure resolves. However, if blood pressure remains severely elevated with resolution of seizure activity, that the hypertension caused the seizure then becomes much more likely. In that instance, treatment of and evaluation for the underlying cause of symptomatic hypertension are imperative. The posterior reversible encephalopathy syndrome consists of headache, seizures, alterations in consciousness and vision secondary to severe hypertension with associated vasogenic changes in the distribution of the posterior cerebral circulation (typically the parieto-occipital lobe) on MRI. Normalization of blood pressure typically results in resolution of seizures and vasogenic edema on MRI.

Rare causes
Neoplastic diseases, separate from those that cause compromise of the major renal vasculature, can directly cause hypertension. Nephroblastoma or lymphoma may cause hypertension by direct infiltration of normal renal parenchyma. Neuroblastoma can cause hypertension through elaboration of excessive catecholamines, which is often symptomatic at presentation.

Although well known to cause elevated blood pressure, endocrine causes of hypertension are rare in childhood (see **Box 2**). Other than catecholamine-secreting tumors, endocrine causes of hypertension do not typically present with severe hypertension as the principal feature. More often, high blood pressure is found when being evaluated for other signs or symptoms attributable to the underlying endocrine disorder.

Monogenic forms of hypertension (see **Box 2**) are exceedingly rare and considered only when renal disease or other identifiable causes of secondary hypertension have been ruled out. Most monogenic forms of hypertension do not cause or present with hypertensive crisis. Exceptions include Liddle syndrome, which may be silent and unrecognized until presenting in hypertensive crisis, as well as von Hippel-Lindau syndrome, discussed above. A unifying feature of most monogenic forms of hypertension is that the causative single-gene pathogenic variant effects enhanced renal sodium resorption, leading to volume expansion with resultant hypertension. A clue that a monogenic cause of hypertension might be present is that on screening tests abnormalities in blood potassium, either low or high, may be found because several of the gene variants in this group of disorders affect mineralocorticoid pathways.

Adult Hypertension

Common causes
Primary hypertension is the most common underlying cause of hypertensive crisis in adulthood. What distinguishes treating adults from children is that most adults are already receiving antihypertensive treatment. Acute acceleration to hypertensive crisis is often associated with poor medical adherence, dietary sodium indiscretion, use of over-the-counter drugs such as pseudoephedrine or nonsteroidal anti-inflammatory drugs, use of recreational drugs, or corticosteroids, and rarely, it may signal the onset of a secondary cause.

Rare causes

Almost all the potential causes of severe hypertension during childhood and adolescence (see **Box 2**) may also be the cause of severe hypertension in adults. However, in progressing through adulthood, the childhood causes become rarer, especially some of the tumors of childhood, such as nephroblastoma, and the congenital causes are usually identified before adulthood. Other less-common causes of severe hypertension, essentially not seen during childhood, then come into play. Each of the additional entities discussed later that cause hypertensive crisis in adults, just as those in childhood, require prompt identification and treatment.

Scleroderma is an autoimmune disease characterized by vasculopathy, fibrosis, and inflammation of the skin and internal organs, including the kidney. Although sclerodermal renal disease is more often a slow, mildly progressive kidney disease, sclerodermal renal crisis (SRC) is a rare and potentially life-threatening condition that occurs in those who experience an early, rapid progression of diffuse cutaneous disease within the first 3 to 5 years of symptoms.[7] Treatment with glucocorticoid steroids for scleroderma is a risk factor for development of SRC. In most patients with SRC, presentation is characterized by an acute symptomatic increase in blood pressure with increased creatinine, oliguria, and in ~50% patients, there are signs of microangiopathic hemolytic anemia. Acute increase in serum creatinine in the absence of hypertension is also recognized but remains controversial as a sole criterion for SRC. Kidney biopsy may be needed to differentiate SRC from other kidney diseases that may cause severe hypertension. Early detection and treatment of SRC along with rapid control of blood pressure in established SRC may have favorable impact on outcome.

Acute aortic dissection is a rare, life-threatening condition. Commonly classified using the Stanford system, type A involves the ascending aorta with or without involvement of the descending aorta, whereas type B involves only the descending aorta.[8] Common symptoms include acute, severe chest pain, or back pain in type B lesions. Abdominal pain is a symptom of mesenteric ischemia. Syncope from hypotension can be a presenting symptom, but when hypertension is present, one of the major goals of medical management is rapid control of systolic blood pressure to less than 100 mm Hg and controlling tachycardia. Chronic, long-standing hypertension is a major risk factor for AAD, along with aortic aneurysm, male gender, advanced age, and smoking. Aortic dissection can also affect younger patients with genetic connective tissue disorders, such as Marfan, Loeys-Dietz, or Ehlers-Danlos. Bicuspid aortic valve may also give rise to AAD, and risk increases with age. Diagnosis based on physical findings can be difficult, as signs of pulse deficit or murmur of aortic regurgitation may be absent. Symptoms from AAD can mimic myocardial infraction or pulmonary embolism, so evaluation for these diagnoses may delay diagnosis. Therefore, a high index of suspicion for AAD is necessary. Transthoracic echocardiography, transesophageal echocardiography, computed tomographic (CT) scan with contrast, and MRI have high sensitivity and specificity to make the diagnosis. Given the surgical urgency of AAD, CT scan with contrast is likely to be the best imaging, as it typically is the fastest of these studies to complete.

Sympathetic overactivity leading to adult hypertensive crisis can be seen in conditions associated with autonomic dysfunction, such as Guillain-Barré syndrome and spinal cord injury, ingestion of tyramine-containing foods when on monoamine oxidase inhibitors, and withdrawal of medications such as clonidine and beta-blockers. Tumors that secrete excessive catecholamines, both hereditary and sporadic pheochromocytoma, account for less than 1% of hypertensive crises in adults. Hereditary forms of pheochromocytoma typically present in younger adults less than 40 years of age, whereas sporadic cases occur in those greater than 40 years of age.[9]

Pheochromocytomas/paragangliomas may present with the classic triad of inter-mittent (although possibly sustained) hypertension, palpitations, and diaphoresis. Flushing, anxiety-like panic attacks, and polyuria may also be present. The average age of onset in children is 11 to 13 years. The "rule of 10" is a helpful mnemonic to remember that 10% of pheochromocytomas are malignant, 10% are bilateral, 10% are extra-adrenal, and 10% are familial. Pheochromocytomas arise in the adrenal gland, whereas paragangliomas often arise in extra-adrenal neural crest–derived sites in the chest, abdomen, or pelvis. Pheochromocytomas secrete epinephrine and norepinephrine, whereas paragangliomas may secrete norepinephrine and dopamine. Most are sporadic, but some may be associated with recognizable syndromes (MEN 2A and MEN 2B, von Hippel-Lindau, neurofibromatosis type 1, Carney-Stratakis) or pathogenic gene variants (SDHB, TMEM127, MAX, HIF2A).

Preeclampsia accounts for most peripartum morbidity and mortality and is a condition in pregnant women greater than 20 weeks' gestation who present with acute hypertensive crisis.[10,11] Major risk factors include obesity, chronic hypertension, family history, diabetes, prior history of preeclampsia, and antiphospholipid antibody syndrome. Presentation with blood pressure $\geq$140/90, when the mother was normotensive before 20 weeks' gestation, along with proteinuria, should alert clinicians to act immediately so as to prevent progression to eclampsia (seizures), HELLP syndrome, acute kidney injury, pulmonary edema, and placental abruption. It is now recognized that proteinuria may be absent in preeclampsia. In such patients, criteria for diagnosis include severe features such as blood pressure $\geq$160/110 in the presence of thrombocytopenia, elevated liver function tests, serum creatinine greater than 1.1 (or doubling of creatinine), oliguria, pulmonary edema, or new-onset cerebral symptoms or visual disturbances. The risk of mortality is high in patients with preeclampsia before 32 weeks' gestation, estimated to be 20-fold in comparison to those at full term. In cases of severe hypertension, patients should be attended to urgently and in a critical care setting.

EVALUATION

In all patients found to have severe hypertension, the initial approach is garnering a thorough history and physical examination. Not only does this direct the practitioner to investigations likely to be fruitful in identifying the cause but also it identifies those in whom investigation must move promptly, as in those with hypertensive crisis. The younger the patient, the more likely an identifiable cause of secondary hypertension is present, to the point where in infancy nearly all affected patients have a cause found.

Table 2	
Investigation of infantile hypertension	
Test	**Potential Causes Identified**
Renal ultrasound with Doppler	Cystic kidney disease and CAKUT
	Major renal vessel thrombosis
	Intra-abdominal or retroperitoneal tumor
Urinalysis	Congenital/infantile glomerulopathy
Complete blood count	Major intrarenal thrombus
	Atypical hemolytic uremic syndrome
Blood creatinine and electrolytes	Acute or chronic kidney disease
	Monogenic or endocrine cause of hypertension

Investigation of Infantile Hypertension

Because the causes of hypertension in infancy are limited, the scope of studies needed to define the cause is similarly limited (**Table 2**). Foremost in this population is renal imaging, specifically, renal ultrasound with Doppler investigation of the major vessels. Cystic kidney disease and CAKUT are readily identified on ultrasound. In addition, neonatal or infantile solid tumors that lead to hypertension are typically seen on renal ultrasound.

Doppler ultrasonography is primarily intended to exclude thrombus in a major renal vessel, especially in the main renal vein; rarely, a major renal artery thrombus is found. Doppler study of the renal arteries has low sensitivity for identifying RAS, either acquired or congenital.[12] Thus, if not positively identified on Doppler ultrasonography, RAS is not excluded. A clue to the possibility of unilateral RAS on the ultrasound is significant size discrepancy between the kidneys, which otherwise have normal architecture and echogenicity. If other entities are ruled out and RAS is suspected, an angiographic study is required to provide the diagnosis. Direct, invasive angiography to evaluate for RAS carries significant risk in early infancy, so typically is deferred until late infancy or later, depending on the severity of hypertension and ability to control the hypertension with medication. Oftentimes then the first step to evaluate for RAS is via noninvasive methods, such as CT or MRI. As image resolution of the vasculature

Table 3
Investigation of severe hypertension in child, adolescent, or adult

Tests	Potential Causes Identified
Urinalysis Blood creatinine and electrolytes Complete blood count	Glomerulonephritis (GN) Preeclampsia Cystic kidney disease and CAKUT Monogenic hypertension
C3 and C4 complement levels ANA, anti-dsDNA ANCA, anti-RNA polymerase antibodies	Postinfectious GN Lupus nephritis ANCA-associated GN Sclerodermal renal crisis (adults)
Renal ultrasound	Cystic kidney disease CAKUT Acquired obstructive nephropathy
Blood and urine metanephrines	Catecholamine-secreting tumors
Urine drug investigation	Unreported medical or recreational drug use
T4, TSH, plasma renin, aldosterone, cortisol	Endocrine causes of hypertension Monogenic causes of hypertension
Echocardiogram	Aortic coarctation Left ventricular hypertrophy from long-standing severe hypertension Acute aortic dissection
Noninvasive angiography (CT angiogram or MRI/MRA)	Renovascular disease Acute aortic dissection
Renal nuclear scan	Renal scar from previous injury, pyelonephritis
Genetic analysis	Monogenic cause (eg, Liddle syndrome)
Kidney biopsy	Glomerulopathies Interstitial nephritis

using either of these methods improves with the age of the infant, the timing of performing the study is commonly determined by a nephrologist in consultation with an imaging specialist, with the same consideration of whether the study is urgent based on ability to control the infant's hypertension with medication.

Urinalysis should be performed on a sample obtained by bag collection, which helps avoid a false positive result for blood from catheterization. The lack of blood or protein on the urinalysis effectively rules out a rare congenital or acquired glomerulopathy of infancy. Complete blood count should also be performed, as thrombocytopenia may herald an occult major thrombus, such as a renal vein thrombus, or a microangiopathy affecting the kidneys, such as a rare atypical HUS. Finally, renal function should be assessed by measuring blood electrolytes and creatinine levels.

Investigation of Severe, Symptomatic Childhood and Adult Hypertension

Children who present with symptomatic hypertension are likely to have acute glomerular disease, whether the symptoms be from the hypertension (eg, headache, visual disturbance, seizure, or other neurologic symptoms) or from the underlying disease causing the hypertension (eg, constitutional symptoms, joint symptoms, skin lesions, gross hematuria, or edema). The initial investigation should be prompt and focus on causes of acute glomerular disease (**Table 3**). Initial testing should include blood and urine tests to screen for acute glomerulopathy. Urinalysis showing blood and/or protein in the urine likely indicates underlying glomerular disease. Urine microscopy showing red blood cell (RBC) casts confirms glomerulonephritis, although the lack of RBC casts does not exclude glomerulonephritis.[13] A complete metabolic panel may reveal renal insufficiency (high blood urea nitrogen and creatinine), suggesting a renal cause for the hypertension. Low blood albumin may indicate nephrotic-range proteinuria or may be secondary to inflammation from underlying systemic vasculitis. Complete blood count is also indicated at presentation. Anemia along with low-platelet count raises the possibility of HUS but may alternately indicate hematologic involvement from systemic lupus erythematosus, in which case leukopenia often is an accompanying feature.

If there is clear evidence on the initial blood and urine tests that acute glomerulopathy is the cause of the hypertension, then renal imaging is not needed. In that instance, further investigation with serologic studies to determine the precise cause of the glomerulopathy is indicated. If the pattern does not fit HUS, then additional testing should include C3 and C4 blood complement levels along with an ANA panel and ANCA.

However, if the urinalysis and blood creatinine are normal, other nonrenal causes of severe and symptomatic hypertension need to be pursued (see **Table 3**). If neurologic symptoms are a prominent feature of the presentation and brain imaging is unremarkable, drug ingestion needs to be considered. Urine toxicology screening can rapidly identify common agents, such as cocaine and amphetamines, that cause symptomatic hypertension, but cannot identify a variety of other recreational drugs that can cause severe hypertension. If drug ingestion is suspected and urine toxicology screening is not informative, the urine sample should also be sent for a comprehensive drug investigation, often via liquid chromatography-mass spectrometry. This investigation takes much longer to complete, but if not considered and sent during the acute presentation, the window to identify this temporary cause of acute symptomatic hypertension may then be missed.

If acute glomerulopathy or toxic ingestion appears to be ruled out, renal imaging is then indicated, because other forms of parenchymal renal disease may present as severe hypertension at any age, and on occasion have associated symptoms. Renal ultrasound in this setting readily identifies congenital urinary tract abnormalities as well as cystic kidney diseases that may present primarily with hypertension, including severe hypertension.

Investigation for Rare Causes of Severe Childhood and Adult Hypertension

If the blood creatinine and urinalysis are normal on initial screening and renal ultrasound is normal, an abnormality in blood electrolytes on the chemistry panel may suggest other causes for the significant hypertension. Low blood potassium is commonly seen when RAS is present, as the hypertension is secondary to prominent activation of the renin-angiotensin system. In addition, several of the monogenic causes of hypertension have associated abnormality of blood potassium, especially those with low-potassium level from hyperaldosteronism (see **Table 3**).

If the hypertension is severe at presentation and the more common causes of secondary hypertension have been ruled out with the initial investigations as above, the possibility of an underlying renovascular cause then needs to be explored. Aortic coarctation should always be considered and can be ruled out on examination using 4-extremity blood pressure measurements. As discussed in the preceding section, the first step to evaluate for a possible RAS is with a noninvasive abdominal CT or MR angiogram.

Nuclear scans may identify isolated renal vascular or focal parenchymal disease as the cause of hypertension. Radionucleotide renal perfusion scan can identify an area of segmental poor renal perfusion indicative of a scar from a previous renal insult, such as from an episode of pyelonephritis or an occult segmental renal infarction as may occur from thromboembolism or secondary to vasculitis. Unilateral poor global perfusion of a kidney on a captopril renal perfusion scan indicates unilateral RAS. The need to use a captopril renal scan to identify likely RAS has waned, as the resolution of the renal vasculature imaging on CT and MR angiography has improved substantially, thus usually obviating a nuclear scan to assess for this entity.

An echocardiogram can serve two roles in the evaluation of a severely hypertensive patient. First, echocardiography has high sensitivity in identifying aortic abnormalities, such as dissection, and in confirming aortic coarctation in a patient who has strong evidence for coarctation based on discrepant arm and leg blood pressure values. Second, an echocardiogram can give some sense of duration of hypertension in those who present with symptomatic or severe hypertension. Finding significant left ventricular hypertrophy (LVH) on echocardiogram indicates end-organ effect from hypertension that is not acute and may have been occult and longstanding. If LVH is present on echocardiogram and initial studies have not found one of the more common causes of hypertension, it then becomes imperative to pursue further diagnostic studies, including those for rare forms of hypertension.

Rare causes of hypertension are pursued as symptoms suggest or if hypertension is significant and otherwise unexplained. Associated symptoms or signs of tachycardia and flushing suggest the possibility of a catecholamine-secreting tumor or thyroid disease. In that scenario, thyroid function tests or blood and urine catecholamine studies reveal the cause. CT or MRI (with or without PET imaging) may help localize the catecholamine-secreting tumor. If an endocrine cause other than thyroid disease is suspected (see **Box 2**) based on clinical presentation or blood electrolyte abnormality on screening studies, then blood renin, aldosterone, and cortisol levels are tested.

Monogenic forms of hypertension, because they are so rare, are not explored unless the clinical pattern does not fit that of primary hypertension; all other potential identifiable causes are ruled out, or if an abnormality on blood electrolytes, especially blood K level, consistent with a monogenic cause of hypertension is present. When considering a monogenic form of hypertension, blood renin and aldosterone levels are measured to start, because many of the single-gene variants that cause hypertension impact the aldosterone pathway. However, the most effective method to make a diagnosis of a monogenic form of hypertension is by genetic sequencing and analysis.

SUMMARY

Hypertensive crisis is rare and is defined as urgent when symptoms are absent or mild, and as emergent when symptoms of end-organ damage are present. Causes vary by age; history and physical examination can identify likely causes in many patients. In patients in whom a renal cause is suspected, renal imaging and serum investigations are often sufficient to identify the underlying cause. The evaluation of possible extrarenal causes is dictated by the presence of localizing signs or symptoms, or relevant exposure history. A stepwise approach, stratified by age, additional risk factors, and associated symptoms, can minimize unnecessary investigations and more rapidly identify a cause so as to initiate appropriate treatment.

CLINICS CARE POINTS

- Vascular or renal structural causes are the most common cause of hypertension during infancy, so the first step in evaluation should be renal imaging.
- Acute glomerulopathy is the most common cause of severe hypertension during childhood, so the first tests should include urinalysis and measure of renal function.
- In an older child presenting with neurologic manifestations and severe hypertension, if initial evaluation does not suggest a primary intracranial process or renal disease, drug ingestion should always be considered, and urine drug investigation sent at presentation.
- Adults presenting with hypertensive crisis usually have a history of preceding hypertension, often primary hypertension that has accelerated. If not, further investigation for underlying cause is warranted to include causes common in childhood or those causes unique to adulthood.

DISCLOSURE

The authors have nothing to disclose.

REFERENCES

1. Flynn JT, Kaelber DC, Baker-Smith CM, et al. Clinical practice guideline for screening and management of high blood pressure in children and adolescents. Pediatrics 2017;140(3):e20171904.
2. Peixoto AJ. Acute severe hypertension. N Engl J Med 2019;381:1843–52.
3. Whelton PK, Carey RM, Aronow WS, et al. 2017 ACC/AHA/AAPA/ABC/ACPM/ AGS/APhA/ASH/ASPC/NMA/PCNA guideline for the prevention, detection, evaluation, and management of high blood pressure in adults: a report of the American College of Cardiology/American Heart Association Task Force on Clinical Practice Guidelines for prevention, detection, evaluation, and management of high blood pressure in adults: a report of the American College of Cardiology/American Heart Association Task Force on Clinical Practice Guidelines. Hypertension 2018;71(6):e13–115.
4. Seeman T, Hamdani G, Mitsnefes M. Hypertensive crisis in children and adolescents. Pediatr Nephrol 2019;34:2523–37.
5. Van Why SK, Boydstun II, Gaudio KM, et al. Abdominal symptoms as presentation of hypertensive crisis. Am J Dis Child 1993;147:638–41.

6. Satheeshkumar A, Pena C, Nugent K. Current U.S. guideline-based management strategies for special clinical situations involving hypertensive crises: a narrative review of the literature. Cardiol Rev 2020. https://doi.org/10.1097/CRD. 0000000000000364.
7. Woodworth TG, Suliman YA, Li W, et al. Scleroderma renal crisis and renal involvement in systemic sclerosis. Nat Rev Nephrol 2016;12:678–91.
8. Gawinecka J, Schonrath F, vonEckardstein A. Acute aortic dissection: pathogenesis, risk factors and diagnosis. Swiss Med Wkly 2017;147:w14489.
9. Lenders JWM, Eisenhofer G, Mannelli M, et al. Phaeochromocytoma. Lancet. 2005;366:665–75.
10. Rana S, Lemoine E, Granger JP, et al. Preeclampsia: pathophysiology, challenges and perspectives. Circ Res 2019;124(7):1094–112.
11. Arulkumaran N, Lightstone L. Severe pre-eclampsia and hypertensive crises. Best Pract Res Clin Obstet Gynaecol 2013;27:877–84.
12. Trautmann A, Roebuck DJ, McLaren CA, et al. Non-invasive imaging cannot replace formal angiography in the diagnosis of renovascular hypertension. Pediatr Nephrol 2017;32(3):495–502.
13. Rasoulpour M, Banco L, Laut JM, et al. Inability of community-based laboratories to identify pathological casts in urine samples. Arch Pediatr Adolesc Med 1996; 150:1201–4.

Autoimmune Encephalitis: Distinguishing Features and Specific Therapies

Dominic O. Co, MD, PhD[a],*, Jennifer M. Kwon, MD[b]

KEYWORDS

- Autoimmune encephalitis • Diagnosis • Treatment • Critical care • Autoantibody
- Paraneoplastic • NMDA receptor encephalitis

KEY POINTS

- Early recognition of autoimmune encephalitis and treatment with immune suppression can improve long-term functional outcomes.
- Diagnostic workup should be obtained before instituting immune therapies that might cloud the results.
- Supportive treatment of patients with autoimmune encephalitis is similar to other critically ill patients.
- Early engagement of a multidisciplinary team including neurologists, psychiatrists, and experts in immune therapy is essential to efficient diagnosis and treatment of autoimmune encephalitis.
- Diagnosis, treatment, and monitoring of autoimmune encephalitis continues to evolve.

Autoimmune encephalitis is a rapidly progressive neurologic condition with significant morbidity and mortality, characterized by altered mental status that can often progress to autonomic instability and refractory seizures requiring care in the intensive care unit.[1] While infectious, especially viral, encephalitis is generally more common,[2] the last decade has seen increasing recognition of noninfectious, immune-mediated causes of encephalitis. The pathogenic mechanisms of immune-mediated encephalitis are diverse, ranging from encephalitis mediated by the innate immune system such as in febrile infection-related epilepsy syndromes (FIRES, reviewed elsewhere in this issue), to encephalitis dominated by T cell-mediated immunity triggered by onconeural antigens (typified by anti-Hu associated encephalitis), to encephalitis whose pathogenesis is dominated by autoantibody (autoAb)-mediated effects. Our discussion of "autoimmune encephalitis" (AE) will focus on autoAb-mediated encephalitis whereby

[a] Division of Allergy, Immunology and Rheumatology, Department of Pediatrics, University of Wisconsin – Madison, Clinical Science Center (CSC) H6/572, 600 Highland Avenue, Madison, WI 53792, USA; [b] Department of Neurology, University of Wisconsin – Madison, Medical Foundation Centennial Building (MFCB) 7138, 1685 Highland Avenue, Madison, WI 53705, USA
* Corresponding author.
E-mail address: doco@wisc.edu

Crit Care Clin 38 (2022) 393–412
https://doi.org/10.1016/j.ccc.2021.11.007
0749-0704/22/© 2021 Elsevier Inc. All rights reserved.
criticalcare.theclinics.com

the autoAb causes disease by interfering with the function of neuronal cell-surface or synaptic antigens (**Fig. 1**), such as in NMDA receptor encephalitis (NMDARe).

The incidence and prevalence of AE, estimated at 0.8 per 100,000 person-years and 13.7/100,000 persons, respectively, are comparable to infectious encephalitis (IE).[3,4] The medical impact of AE is higher,[5] as patients with AE have more relapses and repeated hospitalizations than those with IE, and incur higher costs and burdens of care. Mortality and morbidity are higher if patients are critically ill at presentation.[6–8]

Early treatment of AE with immunotherapy can improve these clinical outcomes; as such, AE needs to be recognized promptly.[9,10] Recognizing the challenges in making a definitive diagnosis of AE, criteria for "possible" AE in adults[9] and children[10] have been developed to identify patients who may benefit from early immunotherapy, while awaiting more definitive antibody confirmation from specialized laboratories (**Box 1**).

This review describes initial steps to identifying encephalitis in a critically ill patient and suggests a broad diagnostic workup that will help distinguish AE from other important diagnoses. After outlining a general approach to AE, selected specific AE clinical syndromes and their associated antibodies will be described, with the discussion of pathogenesis, and the rationale for initial first-line therapies and long-term

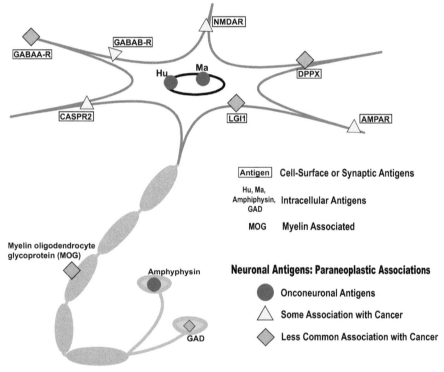

Fig. 1. Neuronal antigens associated with autoimmune encephalitis. AEs associated with antibodies to synaptic and cell-surface antigens (boxed labels) respond to immune therapy. AMPAR, α-amino-3-AE arhydroxy-5-methyl-4-isoxazolepropionic acid receptor; CASPR2, contactin-associated protein-like 2; D2R, dopamine 2 receptor; DPPX, dipeptidyl-peptidase–like protein 6; GABA$_A$-R, γ-aminobutyric acid type A receptor; GABA$_B$-R, γ-aminobutyric acid type b receptor; GAD, glutamic acid decarboxylase; LGI1, leucine-rich, glioma-inactivated 1; NMDAR, N-methyl-D-aspartate receptor.

Box 1

Diagnostic criteria for possible autoimmune encephalitis (AE)

Subacute onset (rapid progression of <3 months) of working memory deficits (short-term memory loss), altered mental status, or psychiatric symptoms

$\geq$ 1 of the following clinical or paraclinical features:
- New focal CNS findings
- Seizures not explained by a previously known seizure disorder or other condition
- Presence of inflammatory changes in CSF (CSF leukocytosis >5 cells/mm^3)
- MRI features suggestive of encephalitis (brain MRI hyperintense signal on T2/FLAIR sequences highly restricted to one or both medial temporal lobes (limbic encephalitis) or in multifocal areas involving gray matter, white matter or both compatible with demyelination or inflammation)

AE serology not available

Reasonable exclusion of alternative causes, including infectious

From Graus F, Titulaer MJ, Balu R, et al. A clinical approach to diagnosis of autoimmune encephalitis. Lancet Neurol. 2016;15(4):391-404. doi:10.1016/S1474-4422(15)00401-9; Reprinted with permission from Elsevier

---

management. Other noninfectious inflammatory central nervous system (CNS) disorders whose presentation could be confused with AE will be discussed briefly, as well.

INITIAL PRESENTATION OF AUTOIMMUNE ENCEPHALITIS AND DIAGNOSTIC EVALUATION

AE should be considered in the patient presenting with subacute onset, then the rapid progression of behavioral or personality changes, short-term memory loss, decreased or altered levels of consciousness, seizures, and abnormal movements. At this initial stage, infectious and immune-mediated causes, as well as toxic and metabolic causes of encephalopathy, should be considered. Criteria for "possible AE" (see **Box 1**) can facilitate earlier recognition and treatment of AE.[9] These criteria were developed for adults; criteria for children include caveats that mental status changes may occur more acutely and that early encephalitis may also present with cognitive difficulties, acute developmental regression, and movement disorders (excluding tics).[10]

A careful history can suggest whether AE is a strong consideration. AE is less likely if there are chronic mental status changes, which should raise concerns about neurodegenerative or dementing disorders. AE is also not typically hyperacute in presentation; in such cases, a vascular process should be considered.[11] AE can occur in those with a history of cancer, immunocompromise, use of immune checkpoint inhibitors, or recent history of encephalitis. While AE may present as vague behavioral changes, there may be more unusual symptoms pointing to AE, such as brief facial seizures, chorea, or new-onset psychosis.[9,11,12]

Initial investigations (**Box 2**) can support the diagnosis of encephalitis and distinguish infectious from other immune-mediated causes. Testing includes broad screening for toxic and metabolic etiologies of encephalopathy. If there is concern about raised intracranial pressure or focal neurologic findings, imaging (preferably with MRI) should be conducted before a lumbar puncture. Cerebrospinal fluid (CSF) and MRI findings may point to infectious etiologies, especially with a more acute presentation with fever. There can be an overlap between IE and AE with these studies. CSF can show pleocytosis in both IE and AE, though the presence of oligoclonal bands suggests AE.[9] MRI findings may not distinguish between IE and AE, but can

---

Box 2
Diagnostic evaluation of patients presenting with acute encephalopathy[1,9,11]

Blood testing
- Complete blood cell count and differential
- Complete metabolic profile, ammonia
- Erythrocyte sedimentation rate, C-reactive protein
- Infectious studies
  - Blood culture
  - Enterovirus and parechovirus PCR
  - Varicella-zoster antibody panel
  - Epstein–Barr virus (EBV) antibody panel; if positive, send EBV PCR in cerebrospinal fluid (CSF)
  - HIV-1 RNA
  - Lyme antibody with reflex Western blot; if positive, send Lyme antibody on CSF
  - Bartonella and West Nile virus antibody titers
  - Brucella antibody; if positive, send Brucella antibody titers in CSF
  - If appropriate season (May–October), add tick-borne PCR panel and Powassan virus antibody
- Autoimmune serologies
  - Antinuclear antibody (ANA) with reflex extractable nuclear antigen (ENA) antibody panel (anti-SS-A, anti-SS-B, anti-ribonucleoprotein [RNP], and anti-Smith antibodies) and anti–double-stranded DNA (dsDNA)
  - Complement C3, C4
  - MOG antibody testing if imaging shows white matter changes consistent with ADEM
  - Aquaporin 4 antibody testing if imaging and history suggest NMO spectrum disorder
  - Autoimmune encephalitis serum panel ("broader" scope is preferable and should include antibodies to GAD65, ANNA-1, ANNA-2, ANNA-3, PCA-1, PCA-2, PCA-Tr, amphiphysin, CRM-5 Ig, AGNA-1, N-methyl-D aspartate [NMDA] receptor, alpha-amino-3-hydroxy-5-methyl-4-isoxazolepropionic acid [AMPA] receptor, gamma-aminobutyric acid-B receptor)
- Set aside extra serum for future studies

Urine
- Consider urine toxicology studies
- Urinalysis, urine protein:creatinine ratio to assess for nephritis/systemic autoimmunity

Neuroimaging
- Magnetic resonance imaging (MRI) of brain with and without contrast
- Consider MR angiogram and MR venogram if there are concerns for stroke or raised intracranial pressure

Cerebrospinal fluid (CSF) studies
- Opening pressure
- Routine studies: cell count with differential, glucose, protein
- Infectious studies
- Bacterial culture and Gram stain
- Polymerase chain reaction (PCR) assays for varicella-zoster virus, herpes simplex virus
- In May through October, add West Nile virus IgM, arbovirus antibody
- Immune studies
- Oligoclonal bands
- Aquaporin 4 antibody
- Autoimmune encephalopathy panel ("broader" scope is preferable and should include antibodies to GAD65, VGKC, ANNA-1, ANNA-2, ANNA-3, PCA-1, PCA-2, PCA-Tr, amphiphysin, CRM-5 Ig, AGNA-1, N-methyl-D aspartate [NMDA] receptor, alpha-amino-3-hydroxy-5-methyl-4-isoxazolepropionic acid [AMPA] receptor, gamma-aminobutyric acid-B receptor)
- Set aside extra-CSF for future studies

Cancer screening
- Computed tomography (CT) chest, abdomen, and pelvis
- Mammogram/breast MRI
- Pelvic or testicular ultrasound
- Body positron emission tomography (PET) scan

direct investigations to other inflammatory disorders of the CNS, as when focal diffusion restriction suggests stroke from inflammatory angiitis. If MRI is normal despite clinical suspicion of AE, brain fluorodeoxyglucose positron emission tomography (FDG-PET) may show brain abnormalities before they are apparent on MRI; however, FDG-PET is not widely used and is nonspecific.[11]

EEG is often performed early in encephalitis evaluations. It can help identify seizures (including nonconvulsive seizures), show background changes indicating encephalopathy, and indicate a pure psychiatric presentation (wherein the EEG is normal.) Seizures are seen in encephalitis, but there are often other epileptiform discharges, lateralized periodic discharges, and slowing.[9–11] The appearance of seizures and the EEG findings are not usually specific enough to distinguish between IE and AE or the different etiologies of AE. One exception is the EEG pattern known as "extreme delta brush" noted in NMDARe.[9,11] While refractory seizures or status epilepticus are not common in either IE or AE, it is important to monitor for their occurrence to prevent additional morbidity.

In adults, cancer screening, including breast, chest, abdomen, and pelvic imaging, is part of the initial evaluation of AE (see **Box 2**). The common neoplasms associated with AE include small cell lung cancer (SCLC), thymic neoplasm, breast cancer, ovarian teratoma or carcinoma, and testicular teratoma.[11]

These early investigations (blood testing, MRI, lumbar puncture) should be complemented by sending serum and CSF autoimmune encephalitis panels for the identification of a specific antibody cause and definitive diagnosis of AE. But if clinical suspicion is high, immunotherapy is started as soon as possible, well before a specific antibody is identified.

SELECTED AUTOIMMUNE ENCEPHALITIS PHENOTYPES

Specific clinical syndromes have been associated with certain autoAb. Two patterns of encephalitis stand out. One is the rapid progression over days to weeks of psychiatric symptoms and abnormal movements seen in NMDARe. The other is the behavior changes, memory disturbances, and seizures referred to as limbic encephalitis (LE) that is associated with antibodies to proteins of the voltage-gated potassium channel (VGKC) complex and other neuronal antigens (**Table 1**). However, there is considerable overlap in presentation. For this reason, when AE is suspected, blood and CSF should be tested with a panel of autoAb rather than individual ones.

N-methyl-ᴅ-aspartate Receptor Antibody-associated Autoimmune Encephalitis

The most common form of AE is caused by autoAb directed against the NMDA receptor.[13] NMDARe was first described in 2005 in 4 young women presenting with acute psychiatric symptoms, seizures, memory loss, and encephalopathy associated with an ovarian teratoma. It has since been recognized in men and children without malignancy, sometimes following recovery from HSV (herpes simplex virus) encephalitis.[13,14] Overall, it is a disorder of younger individuals, with a median age of presentation of 21 years, mostly women.[15,16] Greater than 50% of women have an ovarian teratoma (but extragonadal teratomas are rare).[16]

Teenagers and adults present with a stereotypical progression of *psychosis* (hallucinations, paranoia, and delusions), *mood volatility*, and *sleep disturbances* (eg, insomnia, lethargy). Speech and memory difficulties, involuntary movements, and autonomic instability such as hypoventilation and cardiac dysrhythmia can follow. Children are more likely to present with seizures, abnormal movements, irritability, and sleep disturbance. Despite age-related differences initially, as time progresses, children and adults show a similar spectrum of symptoms.[13,14]

Table 1
Antibodies associated with autoimmune encephalitis[9,16]

Antigen	Patient Population	Clinical Presentation	Associated Disorders	Localization	Treatment Response
NMDAR	Children and young adults More females affected	Anti-NMDAR encephalitis presents in: • Children with seizures and dyskinesias • Adults with psychosis, behavior changes	Ovarian teratoma (up to 58% of young women); may follow HSV encephalitis	Synaptic receptor	Good response to immune treatments (see text)
LGI1	Older men	Limbic encephalitis, particularly, confusion, faciobrachial dystonic seizures, hyponatremia	Not associated with cancer; but population is at risk for cancer	Extracellular synaptic protein	Good response to immune treatments
CASPR2	Older men	Limbic encephalitis, particularly memory loss and peripheral neurologic hyperexcitability (Morvan syndrome)	Those presenting with Morvan syndrome are likely to have thymoma	Extracellular synaptic protein	Good response to immune treatments
GABA$_B$R	Adults, slight male predominance	Limbic encephalitis, prominent seizures	Associated with small-cell lung cancer (SCLC)	Synaptic receptor	Good response to immune treatments
GABA$_A$R	Children and adults	Seizures and status epilepticus common; confusion, behavioral changes	In children, associated with viral infections In adults, associated with thymoma	Synaptic receptor	Good response to immune treatments; including seizures
AMPAR	Adults; female predominance	Limbic encephalitis	SCLC	Synaptic receptor	Good response to immune treatments
DPPX	Older children and adults; male predominance	Limbic encephalitis, confusion, diarrhea, weight loss; sleep disturbances and CNS excitability	Not associated with cancer	Synaptic protein associated with Kv4.2 potassium channels	Good response to immune treatments

Antibody	Population	Clinical syndrome	Cancer association	Protein location	Treatment response
GAD65 (GAD)	Seen in children and adults; population depends on the clinical phenotype	Several different neurologic syndromes are associated with high GAD Ab titers (either in serum or CSF): stiff-person syndrome is the most common, also LE, refractory epilepsy, as paraneoplastic syndrome	Some presentations are associated with cancer; some presentations commonly associated with other autoAb	Intracellular protein	Limited response but adequate enough that many are on long-term immunosuppressant
MOG	Children and young adults	*NOT AE phenotype; acute disseminated encephalomyelitis, optic neuritis, transverse myelitis	Not associated with cancer	Myelin protein	Good response to immune treatments
Hu (ANNA-1)	Older adults with cancer (smoking history)	Limbic encephalitis; cerebellar degeneration, sensory neuronopathy	SCLC and other cancers	Intraneuronal protein, "classic" onconeuronal proteins	Poor response to immune treatments
Ma	Younger men (testicular cancer)	Limbic encephalitis; symptoms may develop over months; hyperphagia, excessive sleepiness	Testicular (men <50 y), non-SCLC, breast cancer		
Amphiphysin	Adults	Limbic encephalitis; stiff-person syndrome	SCLC		

The results of early clinical investigations tend to be nonspecific, with the exception of the electrographic EEG finding of "extreme delta brush."[9,11] Other EEG findings include focal or generalized slowing and interictal epileptiform discharges. CSF analysis may reveal a lymphocyte-predominant pleocytosis in 80% of patients that is typically mild (<100 cells/mm3); oligoclonal bands are typically present.[13,16] Brain MRI is abnormal in about 1/3 of those with NMDARe,[16,17] showing inflammatory changes in cortical or subcortical structures. Diagnosis is made by demonstrating NMDAR antibodies in the CSF. The presence of these antibodies in the serum is suggestive, although less specific.[13]

HSV encephalitis is thought to trigger NMDARe. Anyone presenting with encephalopathy or apparent relapse after HSV encephalitis should have CSF testing sent for an AE autoAb panel. If positive, most of the autoAb will be to NMDAR, though other AEs might be triggered by HSV infection.[13] The time between developing HSV encephalitis and NMDARe is shorter in children, who also tend to have a worse outcome.[13] In female patients, there should be a thorough evaluation for ovarian teratoma. These tumors may be the source of antigens eliciting autoimmunity.[16] In men or children, there is no obvious paraneoplastic association.

NMDARe generally causes cortical or subcortical inflammation, but some patients will develop white matter lesions.[17,18] About 5% of patients with NMDARe may concurrently or at another time develop neuromyelitis optica (NMO) or acute disseminated encephalomyelitis (ADEM), often associated with antibodies to aquaporin-4 or myelin oligodendrocyte glycoprotein (MOG), respectively. Identifying these antibodies may change treatment.[17]

Many patients with NMDARe are admitted to intensive care units for airway management, seizures, abnormal movements, dysautonomia, and depressed consciousness. Failure to respond within 4 weeks of treatment, or the presence of MRI abnormalities or CSF pleocytosis greater than 20 cell/mm3 are associated with poorer outcomes at a year after presentation.[15] Those with coexisting ADEM or NMO may experience a more complicated recovery.[17]

Leucine-rich Glioma Inactivated 1 Antibody-associated Autoimmune Encephalitis

The leucine-rich glioma inactivated 1 (LGI1) protein forms a complex with the presynaptic VGKC. Leucine-rich glioma inactivated 1 antibody-associated autoimmune encephalitis (LGI1-AE) is the second most common cause of AE in adults, more likely in men between the ages of 50 and 70 years.[19] It is rarely seen in children.[20] LGI1-AE usually presents as *LE*, and is the most common etiology of LE. Seizures occur in about 90% of patients with LGI1-AE and there may be multiple seizure types.[19] A characteristic seizure of brief facial grimacing and arm posturing, called *faciobrachial dystonic seizure (FBDS)* may be the initial symptom. Early immune treatment of FBDS may prevent cognitive decline and memory deficits.[21] The seizures often respond better to immune treatments than to anticonvulsants. In patients with initial cognitive dysfunction, seizures are often mistaken for myoclonic jerks, raising concerns of Creutzfeldt–Jakob disease.[19] Initial testing may show noninflammatory CSF, and MRIs may be normal or show limbic T2 hyperintensity. Hyponatremia is commonly seen. LGI1-AE is associated with cancer only 10% of the time. The LGI1 antibody can be detected in serum and CSF, but serum testing is recommended due to higher sensitivity.[19]

Contactin-associated Protein 2 Antibody-associated Autoimmune Encephalitis

Contactin-associated protein 2 (CASPR2) is another protein associated with the VGKC complex, and like LGI1-AE, contactin-associated protein 2 antibody-associated autoimmune encephalitis (CASPR2-AE) is similarly seen in older men.

While some develop LE, a greater proportion shows *peripheral nerve hyperexcitability causing persistent muscle activity (neuromyotonia) and neuropathic pain.*[19] Some develop *Morvan syndrome*, a syndrome of peripheral nerve hyperexcitability, dysautonomia, and encephalopathy.[21] CASPR2 antibody is not commonly associated with cancer, but 10% of the time there may be thymoma.[19,21] As with LGI1 Ab presentations, CSF and MRI findings may be normal or show mild abnormalities in CSF, and MRI may show bilateral mesial temporal changes. Identifying the antibody may require both serum and CSF testing.[19]

Gamma-aminobutyric Acid Type B Receptor Antibody-associated Autoimmune Encephalitis

Antibodies directed against gamma-aminobutyric acid type B receptor ($GABA_BR$) are another common cause of AE and frequently present as an LE with *prominent seizures,* often refractory to antiseizure medications. There may be *rapid onset of dementia* causing confusion with Creutzfeldt–Jakob disease,[22] and highlighting the importance of considering treatable causes. CSF studies may show nonspecific markers of AE, like mild pleocytosis and oligoclonal bands. MRI may be suggestive as well, but these studies may be normal. This is a disease of adults, and about half are associated with small-cell lung cancer.[22,23]

Gamma-aminobutyric Acid Type A Receptor Antibody-associated Autoimmune Encephalitis

AE due to $GABA_AR$ antibodies has been recently described in both children and adults. The presentation is one of a *rapidly progressive encephalopathy* whereby seizures are common, may be refractory to standard seizure medications, and respond to immune therapies. The presentation in children echoes the presentation of NMDARe in that there may be *movement disorders* and a history of prior viral encephalitis. In adults, there may be underlying cancer (often thymoma). MRI can show striking asymmetric cortical-subcortical lesions.[24]

DIFFERENTIAL DIAGNOSIS

Much of the evaluation discussed in **Box 2** is meant to rule out conditions other than AE that may be treated differently including IE, toxic/metabolic conditions, and systemic autoimmune diseases. In addition, other CNS autoimmune conditions may overlap somewhat with AE.

Acute disseminated encephalomyelitis (ADEM) primarily affects children and younger adults, who present with acute encephalopathy and multifocal neurologic signs and symptoms with characteristic MRI findings.[9,25] The encephalopathy can present as sluggishness or more active irritability and aggression. There may be neurologic findings of cerebellar ataxia, cranial neuropathy, hemiparesis, optic neuritis, and spinal cord dysfunction. Imaging is notable for bilateral, multifocal, poorly demarcated, and asymmetric changes in subcortical and central white matter, as well as thalami, basal ganglia, brainstem, and cortical grey-white junction. *These MRI changes, especially involving the white matter, distinguish ADEM from AE.* In contrast to AE, CSF protein and cell count are more likely to be elevated and to a greater degree.[25,26] ADEM is considered a postinfectious disorder and there is often a history of illness and fever before developing symptoms. Most cases respond to the same first-line treatments for AE, are typically monophasic, and do not require second-line therapy. However, some do have relapses and a more protracted course.[25,26]

A significant proportion of ADEM cases are associated with antibodies to MOG. The MOG antibody is associated with a wide range of demyelinating conditions including ADEM, brainstem encephalitis, optic neuritis, and transverse myelitis, and their treatment is similar to ADEM (and AE). There is some controversy about whether the presence of MOG antibodies is associated with more relapses and greater morbidity.[26-28]

Neuromyelitis optica spectrum disorders (NMOSD) are another set of autoimmune CNS diseases that present with an acute attack of optic neuritis with or without myelitis. A major distinction from AE is that patients with NMOSD are not encephalopathic and do not present with behavioral symptoms. Some NMOSD are associated with MOG antibodies but most are associated with aquaporin-4 (AQP4) antibodies which bind to AQP4 receptors on astrocytes leading to an astrocytopathy, and eventually, neuronal death. The hallmarks of AQP4 NMOSD are the limited response to standard first-line immune therapies and the recurrent attacks that result in cumulative deficits. Newer agents, such as eculizumab, offer improved efficacy.[29]

New-onset refractory status epilepticus (NORSE) and *febrile infection-related epilepsy syndrome (FIRES)* can also present with refractory seizures similar to AE, but without preceding behavioral changes. NORSE and FIRES have not consistently been associated with neuronal cell-surface autoAb.[30,31] Typical immune therapies directed against adaptive immune responses such as IVIG and rituximab are often ineffective, though treatment with innate immune therapies such as anakinra, an anti-IL-1 biologic, may induce rapid improvement.[32-34] This raises the question of if these are autoinflammatory rather than autoimmune conditions.

PATHOGENESIS

Understanding the pathogenesis of AE is helpful to understand the current treatment. AE begins through the breaking of immune tolerance to CNS antigens via unclear mechanisms. For the NMDARe, the best-studied AE, teratomas—especially those harboring neuronal tissue—have been found in many female patients.[15,35] It is hypothesized that teratomas elicit a tolerance-breaking antitumor response generating autoantibodies to NMDAR and other neuronal surface antigens. In patients with AE without a malignant trigger, preceding flu-like symptoms are also elicited from a subset of patients, suggesting an infectious trigger as the initial tolerance-breaking event. As discussed previously, preceding HSV encephalitis is associated with AE and is hypothesized to stimulate the development of neuronal autoAb.[36] Regardless of origin, these autoAb alter the function of cell surface receptors. They cause clustering and internalization of target antigens reducing cell surface expression or interfering with signaling.[37] (**Fig. 2**) Most treatments thus far aim to stop the aberrant immune response, and eliminate autoAb. In those with associated malignancy, treatment of the underlying malignancy may be curative.[38] However, some patients may still need immune-directed therapy. The remainder of this article will focus on those therapies (**Table 2**).

TREATMENT
First and Second-line Treatments

Table 1 summarizes the mechanisms and side effects of AE therapies. Commonly used immune therapies for autoimmune encephalopathy are grouped into first-line and second-line therapies. First-line therapies include steroids, intravenous immunoglobulin (IVIG), and plasma exchange (PLEX). Steroids have broad immune suppressive effects, but also have significant side effects. To avoid these, steroid-sparing agents such as IVIG and/or PLEX are often started concurrently. IVIG and PLEX

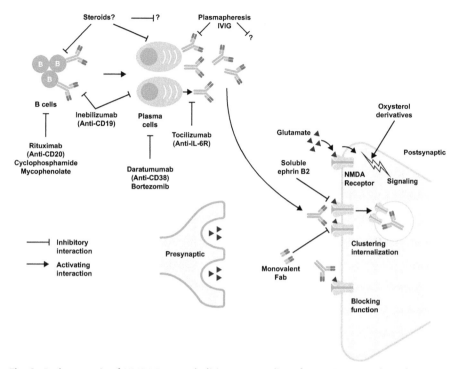

Fig. 2. Pathogenesis of NMDAR encephalitis as a paradigm for AE in general. Both current and emerging therapies are included at their putative sites of action.

may have similar mechanisms of action in blocking pathogenic antibodies. PLEX is thought to directly remove pathogenic antibody from systemic circulation. IVIG likely has multifactorial actions, including interference with pathogenic antibody effector mechanisms via competition for binding sites, negative signaling through Fc receptors, and activation of regulatory T cells.[39] There have been no randomized trials assessing the efficacy of first-line therapies, though several large series support their use. Still, about half or more patients with AE progress up the therapeutic ladder to second-line therapy.[15,40–42]

Second-line therapies including cyclophosphamide and rituximab are often started soon after first-line therapies, as an early institution of second-line therapies leads to better outcomes.[15,40–43] However, interpretation of these data is complicated as recovery from AE can be prolonged,[15,44] making it difficult to assess if patients thought to have "failed" first-line therapy would have recovered if given more time. Nevertheless, the goal of second-line therapies is to shut down production of the pathogenic antibody. Cyclophosphamide preferentially targets B and T lymphocytes, suppressing both humoral and cellular immunity. Cyclophosphamide can directly affect plasma cells, the main producers of antibodies, and thus have more immediate effects on antibody levels and clinical symptoms. Rituximab is a monoclonal antibody (mAb) to the CD20 cell surface marker, which is expressed on pre-B and mature B lymphocytes, but not plasma cells. As a result, in contrast to cyclophosphamide, the effects of rituximab may not be felt for 2 months, as it takes time for plasma cells to die; however, the effects of B cell depletion may continue for 6 months. Both cyclophosphamide and rituximab can cause profound immune suppression. Cyclophosphamide has broader

Table 2
Treatments for autoimmune encephalitis

Treatment	Putative Mechanism	Side Effects	Notes
First-Line Therapies			
Corticosteroids	Broad immune suppression	Bradycardia (mainly with pulse steroids) Hypertension Mood changes, psychosis Weight gain Cataracts Osteopenia Growth Failure (children)	High dose "pulse" steroid therapy (e.g., methylprednisolone 30 mg/kg) is often used at initiation of therapy. Intermittent pulse dosing versus daily dosing is also sometimes continued to avoid steroid side effects (including behavioral side effects).
Plasmapheresis	Removal of antibodies, immune complexes, and high molecular weight toxins	Removal of biological drugs (eg, IVIG) and drugs bound to plasma proteins Hypotension Anaphylactoid reactions Coagulopathy Electrolyte and calcium disturbances Complications associated with vascular access	
Intravenous immunoglobulin (IVIG)	Saturation and modulation of Fc receptors Modulation of dendritic cells Activation of regulatory T cells Inhibition of complement Neutralization of cytokines Neutralization of autoantibodies	Anaphylactoid reactions (especially in IgA-deficiency patients) Aseptic meningitis Hemolytic anemia Thromboembolic events Infection	A 2 g/kg dose given over 1-2 days is felt to be more efficacious than spreading the dose over 5 days.
Second-Line Therapies			
Cyclophosphamide	Alkylating agent Antiinflammatory effects of monocytes and lymphocytes	Opportunistic infections Cytopenias, especially B and T cell lymphopenia Hypogammaglobulinemia Hemorrhagic cystitis Infertility (correlates with cumulative dose)	Typically administered as monthly pulse therapy

Mycophenolate mofetil	Inhibition of B and T cells	Opportunistic infections Gastrointestinal toxicity Cytopenias	
Rituximab	Lysis of CD20+ B cells Decreased antibody production (delayed) Modulation of other B cell functions (antigen presentation, cytokine production)	Opportunistic infections B cell lymphopenia Hypogammaglobulinemia Anaphylactoid reactions (more common and severe than other biologics)	2 or 4 dose course administered over a month. B cells typically reconstitute after about 6 months, though both earlier reconstitution and persistent B lymphopenia can be seen.
Third-Line Therapies			
Tocilizumab	Binds IL-6 receptor and prevent IL-6 binding	Cytopenias Transaminitis Psoriasis	
Bortezomib	Inhibition of 26S proteasome causing apoptotic cell death of plasma cells and other cells with high protein production	Fatigue Gastrointestinal toxicity Cytopenias Peripheral neuropathy Fever	

side effects (hair thinning/loss, GI toxicity, hemorrhagic cystitis, etc.) related to its cytotoxic mechanism of action. A recent case report of successful treatment of NMDARe by the intrathecal administration of rituximab raises the question of if intrathecal therapy for rituximab or other agents may be able to limit systemic side effects.[45] Mycophenolate is another agent with similar immune effects to cyclophosphamide and used in similar situations but with fewer side effects; however, there are fewer reports of its use in AE.[46]

Third-line Treatments

IL-6 is a cytokine with broad effects on inflammation and the development of adaptive immunity.[47] IL-6 inhibition can decrease antibody production. A large retrospective study of 91 patients with seropositive and seronegative AE refractory to first and second-line therapies suggested more patients treated with tocilizumab (an anti-IL-6 receptor mAb) achieved significant improvement in comparison to patients treated with repeat dosing of rituximab or observation alone (~60% vs ~20% for the other 2 groups).[48] In addition, this improvement was relatively rapid, occurring within a month of starting treatment. Similar results were reported in a series of 3 pediatric patients with refractory AE.[49] These results suggest that IL-6 therapy may be useful in AE and may have fewer side effects than rituximab and cyclophosphamide.

Bortezomib is a proteasome inhibitor originally used in multiple myeloma, an oncologic disorder of plasma cells.[50] Proteasome inhibition results in the accumulation of misfolded proteins leading to apoptosis of plasma cells.[51] Case reports and a case series in children and young adults have reported response in refractory AE, often within a few weeks of initiation.[52–55] The timing of response makes it difficult to know if this is due to bortezomib or to late effects of rituximab.

TREATMENTS IN PRECLINICAL STAGES

Prevailing treatments putatively work by decreasing pathogenic antibodies. However, some of the most intriguing developments in treatment are methods that more directly target the effects of these autoantibodies.[56] As monovalent versions of autoAb do not cause the loss of synaptic NMDAR seen with natural NMDAR antibodies,[57] monovalent fragment antigen-binding (Fab) versions of autoantibodies may be able to prevent or treat NMDAR encephalitis (see **Fig. 2**, right). Indeed, recombinant monovalent Fab successfully treated an animal model of myasthenia gravis,[58] but this has not been tried in NMDARe models to our knowledge.

Another strategy to prevent the removal of NMDAR from the synaptic surface is to enlist other molecules that stabilize NMDAR's surface expression. Activation of ephrin B2 receptor by a soluble form of its ligand in vitro can prevent NMDAR internalization in a model of NMDARe.[59] Clinical symptoms could be treated by directly enhancing the signaling of affected receptors. For NMDAR, numerous agents have been found to selectively increase NMDAR signaling.[60] Oxysterol derivatives have been shown to partially prevent synaptic NMDAR loss as well as directly improve postsynaptic currents, correlating with the prevention of memory loss in a mouse model.[61] It will be exciting to see if these novel approaches will lead to clinically useful therapies.

GENERAL APPROACH TO MANAGEMENT

As with any critical illness, the early steps in management require stabilizing the patient while at the same time gathering diagnostic information needed to select a more definitive treatment. Treatment of AE is complicated by its heterogenous presentation and the need to initiate therapy before a definitive diagnosis is obtained, and when the differential diagnosis is broad. The need to institute treatment rapidly must be balanced by the need to obtain certain diagnostic tests before giving therapies that might confound the interpretation of those tests. In addition, attention must be paid to the response even to the initial supportive therapies, as sometimes this may offer clues to the diagnosis and best choice of management strategies. Early involvement and coordination of a multidisciplinary team including neurologists, psychiatrists, infectious disease specialists, and rheumatologists are critical in the optimal management of patients with AE.

Stabilization

The initial supportive management of seizures, ventilation, and autonomic dysfunction in patients with AE should be approached similar to other critically ill patients and is beyond the scope of this article. It is worth mentioning that the seizures can be difficult to treat, and that seizures not responding to the usual antiseizure treatments should prompt consideration of AE in the differential diagnosis. It can be tempting to initiate immune suppressive therapy early on before sufficient diagnostic information has been obtained, but this must be approached with caution. It is reasonable to initiate empiric antiinfectives (eg, acyclovir, broad-spectrum antibiotics) during the initial stabilization phase, but ideally only after appropriate cultures are drawn, especially from CSF. Similarly, basic workup should be completed before starting first-line immunotherapies such as steroids, IVIG, and plasmapheresis. For example, inflammatory markers including more specialized ones such as ferritin, von Willebrand factor antigen, C3, and C4 can be altered rapidly by immune therapy. Before administering steroids, the team should seek reassurance from the overall picture of clinical features and diagnostic studies that infection is a less likely underlying etiology. The team should also be careful to obtain any serologic testing for infection or autoimmune conditions before administration of IVIG or plasmapheresis, as IVIG is derived from pooled donor serum and therefore may lead to false-positive testing, while plasmapheresis removes antibodies from the blood and may cause false negative testing. Early consultation with infectious disease specialists and rheumatologists can help.

"Definitive" Treatment of Autoimmune Encephalitis

Immune suppressive therapy often must be initiated when only a provisional diagnosis based on a clinical impression is in hand. As soon as the risk or suspicion of more life-threatening etiologies has been reduced and AE remains high on the differential diagnosis, the patient should be treated with first-line therapies. Retrospective analyses have repeatedly supported early initiation of immune-modulatory therapy in predicting better outcomes.[15,41,43,62] This typically begins with pulse IV steroids (30 mg/kg up to a max of 1000 mg) of methylprednisolone or equivalent) daily for 3 to 5 days. Enteral dosing of steroids (2 mg/kg up to 60 mg of prednisone or equivalent daily) may be started after this. Dexamethasone is sometimes considered due to its better CNS penetration. Patients with AE may be more sensitive to the psychiatric side effects of steroids, so daily steroids are sometimes avoided in favor of intermittent IV pulse steroids. Depending on the severity of the presentation and initial response, plasmapheresis or IVIG can be given concurrently or soon after pulse steroids. If plasmapheresis is considered, it should be conducted before IVIG, as plasmapheresis will remove IVIG and its beneficial effects. The availability and appropriateness of plasmapheresis may vary depending on the center and the situation. For example, some centers may not be adequately equipped to perform plasmapheresis in young children, or there may be difficulty obtaining central venous access. As a result, IVIG is used more commonly. With IVIG, the authors would favor treatment with a single high dose of 2 g/

kg dose, as studies have suggested a trend to stronger immunomodulatory effects in other inflammatory conditions than when the dose is spread out over several days.[63–65] As it is a large fluid load, lengthening the duration of infusion could be considered if there are concerns about poor cardiac function.

Studies also support the early initiation of second-line therapies as being associated with a better prognosis.[41,43] This should be considered if there is no or partial response 2 to 4 weeks after first-line therapies, as second-line therapies address the underlying immune abnormality in a more definitive way, and it can take a long time to see improvement.[11] There is a relative paucity of data on third-line therapies, but the available data are encouraging.

Deciding when to escalate therapy is hampered by a lack of measures of disease activity. CSF antibody titers in NMDARe have been suggested to correlate with clinical improvement.[66,67] Clinical measures of improvement currently rely on the modified Rankin scale, a crude subjective measure of overall functioning originally developed for stroke outcomes, with scores ranging from 0 to 3.[68] More recently, the Clinical Assessment Scale for Autoimmune Encephalitis (CASE) was developed and measures severity in 9 domains with scores ranging from 0 to 27.[69] This provides a more granular assessment with scores more clearly defined. It still requires validation and may not apply as well to pediatric patients.

SUMMARY

Autoimmune encephalopathy is a challenging condition to define, let alone diagnose and treat. The diagnosis is largely a clinical one, especially in the early stages when treatment decisions must be made before definitive antibody testing has resulted, or in cases whereby the clinical course is convincing, but the antibody testing is negative (ie, "seronegative" cases). Involving a multidisciplinary team at the outset can help in stabilizing the patient while obtaining a comprehensive and accurate diagnostic workup in a timely fashion. That team continues to be important in helping devise the treatment plan and deciding when to escalate therapy or reconsider the diagnosis. There have been some exciting advances in the care of these patients, but there remains much work to be conducted to develop better treatments with less toxicity, as well as to measure the impact of those treatments.

DISCLOSURE

The authors have nothing to disclose.

CLINICS CARE POINTS

- Autoimmune encephalopathy can be associated with autonomic instability that requires critical care.
- Early immune therapy of autoimmune encephalitis is associated with improved outcomes.
- Autoimmune encephalitis is a clinical diagnosis for which engagement of a multidisciplinary team of neurologists, psychiatrists and experts in immune therapy can aid in workup and treatment.

REFERENCES

1. Venkatesan A, Tunkel AR, Bloch KC, et al. Case definitions, diagnostic algorithms, and priorities in encephalitis: consensus statement of the international encephalitis Consortium. Clin Infect Dis 2013;57(8):1114–28.

2. Venkatesan A, Benavides DR. Autoimmune encephalitis and its relation to infection. Curr Neurol Neurosci Rep 2015;15(3):3.

3. Gable M, Glaser C. Anti-N-Methyl-d-aspartate receptor encephalitis appearing as a new-onset psychosis: disease course in children and adolescents within the California encephalitis project. Pediatr Neurol 2017;72:25–30.

4. Dubey D, Pittock SJ, Kelly CR, et al. Autoimmune encephalitis epidemiology and a comparison to infectious encephalitis. Ann Neurol 2018;83(1):166–77.

5. Cohen J, Sotoca J, Gandhi S, et al. Autoimmune encephalitis: a costly condition. Neurology 2019;92(9):e964–72.

6. Mittal MK, Rabinstein AA, Hocker SE, et al. Autoimmune encephalitis in the ICU: analysis of phenotypes, serologic findings, and outcomes. Neurocrit Care 2016; 24(2):240–50.

7. McGetrick ME, Varughese NA, Miles DK, et al. Clinical features, treatment strategies, and outcomes in hospitalized children with immune-mediated encephalopathies. Pediatr Neurol 2020;116:20–6.

8. Thakur KT, Motta M, Asemota AO, et al. Predictors of outcome in acute encephalitis. Neurology 2013;81(9):793–800.

9. Graus F, Titulaer MJ, Balu R, et al. A clinical approach to diagnosis of autoimmune encephalitis. Lancet Neurol 2016;15(4):391–404.

10. Cellucci T, Van Mater H, Graus F, et al. Clinical approach to the diagnosis of autoimmune encephalitis in the pediatric patient. Neurol Neuroimmunol Neuroinflammation 2020;7(2). https://doi.org/10.1212/NXI.0000000000000663.

11. Abboud H, Probasco JC, Irani S, et al. Autoimmune encephalitis: proposed best practice recommendations for diagnosis and acute management. J Neurol Neurosurg Psychiatry 2021;92(7):757–68.

12. Co DO, Bordini BJ, Meyers AB, et al. Immune-mediated diseases of the central nervous system: a specificity-focused diagnostic paradigm. Pediatr Clin North Am 2017;64(1):57–90.

13. Dalmau J, Armangué T, Planagumà J, et al. An update on anti-NMDA receptor encephalitis for neurologists and psychiatrists: mechanisms and models. Lancet Neurol 2019;18(11):1045–57.

14. Florance-Ryan N, Dalmau J. Update on anti-N-methyl-D-aspartate receptor encephalitis in children and adolescents. Curr Opin Pediatr 2010;22(6):739–44.

15. Titulaer MJ, McCracken L, Gabilondo I, et al. Treatment and prognostic factors for long-term outcome in patients with anti-NMDA receptor encephalitis: an observational cohort study. Lancet Neurol 2013;12(2):157–65.

16. Dalmau J, Graus F. Antibody-mediated encephalitis. N Engl J Med 2018;378(9): 840–51.

17. Titulaer MJ, Höftberger R, Iizuka T, et al. Overlapping demyelinating syndromes and anti–N-methyl-D-aspartate receptor encephalitis. Ann Neurol 2014;75(3): 411–28.

18. Hacohen Y, Absoud M, Hemingway C, et al. NMDA receptor antibodies associated with distinct white matter syndromes. Neurol Neuroimmunol Neuroinflammation 2014;1(1). https://doi.org/10.1212/NXI.0000000000000002.

19. van Sonderen A, Petit-Pedrol M, Dalmau J, et al. The value of LGI1, Caspr2 and voltage-gated potassium channel antibodies in encephalitis. Nat Rev Neurol 2017;13(5):290–301.

20. López-Chiriboga AS, Klein C, Zekeridou A, et al. LGI1 and CASPR2 neurological autoimmunity in children. Ann Neurol 2018;84(3):473–80.

21. Binks SNM, Klein CJ, Waters P, et al. LGI1, CASPR2 and related antibodies: a molecular evolution of the phenotypes. J Neurol Neurosurg Psychiatry 2018;89(5): 526–34.

22. van Coevorden-Hameete MH, de Bruijn M, de Graaff E, et al. The expanded clinical spectrum of anti-GABABR encephalitis and added value of KCTD16 autoantibodies. Brain 2019;142(6):1631–43.

23. Lancaster E, Lai M, Peng X, et al. Antibodies to the GABAB receptor in limbic encephalitis with seizures: case series and characterisation of the antigen. Lancet Neurol 2010;9(1):67–76.

24. Spatola M, Petit-Pedrol M, Simabukuro MM, et al. Investigations in GABA(A) receptor antibody-associated encephalitis. Neurology 2017;88(11):1012–20.

25. Pohl D, Alper G, Van Haren K, et al. Acute disseminated encephalomyelitis: updates on an inflammatory CNS syndrome. Neurology 2016;87(9 Suppl 2):S38–45.

26. Santoro JD, Chitnis T. Diagnostic considerations in acute disseminated encephalomyelitis and the interface with MOG antibody. Neuropediatrics 2019;50(5): 273–9.

27. Reindl M, Jarius S, Rostasy K, et al. Myelin oligodendrocyte glycoprotein antibodies: how clinically useful are they? Curr Opin Neurol 2017;30(3):295–301.

28. Waters P, Fadda G, Woodhall M, et al. Serial anti-myelin oligodendrocyte glycoprotein antibody analyses and outcomes in children with demyelinating syndromes. JAMA Neurol 2020;77(1):82–93.

29. Brod SA. Review of approved NMO therapies based on mechanism of action, efficacy and long-term effects. Mult Scler Relat Disord 2020;46:102538.

30. Spatola M, Dalmau J. Seizures and risk of epilepsy in autoimmune and other inflammatory encephalitis. Curr Opin Neurol 2017;30(3):345–53.

31. Gaspard N, Hirsch LJ, Sculier C, et al. New-onset refractory status epilepticus (NORSE) and febrile infection-related epilepsy syndrome (FIRES): state of the art and perspectives. Epilepsia 2018;59(4):745–52.

32. DeSena AD, Do T, Schulert GS. Systemic autoinflammation with intractable epilepsy managed with interleukin-1 blockade. J Neuroinflammation 2018;15:38.

33. Kenney-Jung DL, Kahoud RJ, Vezzani A, et al. Super-refractory status epilepticus and febrile infection-related epilepsy syndrome treated with anakinra. Ann Neurol 2016;80(6):939–45.

34. Westbrook C, Subramaniam T, Seagren RM, et al. Febrile infection-related epilepsy syndrome treated successfully with anakinra in a 21-year-old woman. WMJ 2019;118(3):135–9.

35. Chefdeville A, Treilleux I, Mayeur M-E, et al. Immunopathological characterization of ovarian teratomas associated with anti-N-methyl-D-aspartate receptor encephalitis. Acta Neuropathol Commun 2019;7(1):38.

36. Armangue T, Leypoldt F, Dalmau J. Autoimmune encephalitis as differential diagnosis of infectious encephalitis. Curr Opin Neurol 2014;27(3):361–8.

37. Bien CG, Vincent A, Barnett MH, et al. Immunopathology of autoantibody-associated encephalitides: clues for pathogenesis. Brain J Neurol 2012;135(Pt 5):1622–38.

38. Thiyagarajan M, Sebastian A, Thomas DS, et al. Ovarian Teratoma and N-Methyl-D-aspartate receptor autoimmune encephalitis: insights into imaging diagnosis of teratoma and timing of surgery. J Clin Gynecol Obstet 2021;10(1):22–7.

39. Hartung H-P. Advances in the understanding of the mechanism of action of IVIg. J Neurol 2008;255(Suppl 3):3–6.

40. Suthar R, Saini AG, Sankhyan N, et al. Childhood anti-NMDA receptor encephalitis. Indian J Pediatr 2016;83(7):628–33.

41. Sartori S, Nosadini M, Cesaroni E, et al. Paediatric anti-N-methyl-d-aspartate receptor encephalitis: the first Italian multicenter case series. Eur J Paediatr Neurol 2015;19(4):453–63.
42. Kong S-S, Chen Y-J, Su I-C, et al. Immunotherapy for anti-NMDA receptor encephalitis: experience from a single center in Taiwan. Pediatr Neonatol 2019; 60(4):417–22.
43. Thompson J, Bi M, Murchison AG, et al. The importance of early immunotherapy in patients with faciobrachial dystonic seizures. Brain J Neurol 2018;141(2): 348–56.
44. Rutatangwa A, Mittal N, Francisco C, et al. Autoimmune encephalitis in children: a case series at a tertiary care center. J Child Neurol 2020;35(9):591–9.
45. Casares M, Skinner HJ, Gireesh ED, et al. Successful intrathecal rituximab administration in refractory nonteratoma anti–N-Methyl-D-Aspartate receptor encephalitis: a case report. J Neurosci Nurs 2019;51(4):194–7.
46. Stingl C, Cardinale K, Van Mater H. An update on the treatment of pediatric autoimmune encephalitis. Curr Treat Options Rheumatol 2018;4(1):14–28.
47. Tanaka T, Narazaki M, Kishimoto T. Interleukin (IL-6) immunotherapy. Cold Spring Harb Perspect Biol 2018;10(8):a028456.
48. Lee W-J, Lee S-T, Moon J, et al. Tocilizumab in autoimmune encephalitis refractory to rituximab: an institutional cohort study. Neurother J Am Soc Exp Neurother 2016;13(4):824–32.
49. Randell RL, Adams AV, Van Mater H. Tocilizumab in refractory autoimmune encephalitis: a series of pediatric cases. Pediatr Neurol 2018;86:66–8.
50. Segarra A, Arredondo KV, Jaramillo J, et al. Efficacy and safety of bortezomib in refractory lupus nephritis: a single-center experience. Lupus 2020;29(2):118–25.
51. Bryl E. B cells as target for immunotherapy in rheumatic diseases - current status. Immunol Lett 2021;236:12–9.
52. Cordani R, Micalizzi C, Giacomini T, et al. Bortezomib-responsive refractory anti-N-Methyl-d-Aspartate receptor encephalitis. Pediatr Neurol 2020;103:61–4.
53. Schroeder C, Back C, Koc Ü, et al. Breakthrough treatment with bortezomib for a patient with anti-NMDAR encephalitis. Clin Neurol Neurosurg 2018;172:24–6.
54. Lazzarin SM, Vabanesi M, Cecchetti G, et al. Refractory anti-NMDAR encephalitis successfully treated with bortezomib and associated movements disorders controlled with tramadol: a case report with literature review. J Neurol 2020; 267(8):2462–8.
55. Wang T, Wang B, Zeng Z, et al. Efficacy and safety of bortezomib in rituximab-resistant anti-N-methyl-d-aspartate receptor (anti-NMDAR) encephalitis as well as the clinical characteristics: an observational study. J Neuroimmunol 2021; 354:577527.
56. Sell J, Haselmann H, Hallermann S, et al. Autoimmune encephalitis: novel therapeutic targets at the preclinical level. Expert Opin Ther Targets 2021;25(1):37–47.
57. Hughes EG, Peng X, Gleichman AJ, et al. Cellular and synaptic mechanisms of anti-NMDA receptor encephalitis. J Neurosci 2010;30(17):5866–75.
58. Papanastasiou D, Poulas K, Kokla A, et al. Prevention of passively transferred experimental autoimmune myasthenia gravis by Fab fragments of monoclonal antibodies directed against the main immunogenic region of the acetylcholine receptor. J Neuroimmunol 2000;104(2):124–32.
59. Mikasova L, De Rossi P, Bouchet D, et al. Disrupted surface cross-talk between NMDA and Ephrin-B2 receptors in anti-NMDA encephalitis. Brain 2012;135(5): 1606–21.

60. Hackos DH, Hanson JE. Diverse modes of NMDA receptor positive allosteric modulation: mechanisms and consequences. Neuropharmacology 2017;112(Pt A):34–45.
61. Mannara F, Radosevic M, Planagumà J, et al. Allosteric modulation of NMDA receptors prevents the antibody effects of patients with anti-NMDAR encephalitis. Brain J Neurol 2020;143(9):2709–20.
62. Irani SR, Stagg CJ, Schott JM, et al. Faciobrachial dystonic seizures: the influence of immunotherapy on seizure control and prevention of cognitive impairment in a broadening phenotype. Brain J Neurol 2013;136(Pt 10):3151–62.
63. Newburger JW, Takahashi M, Beiser AS, et al. A single intravenous infusion of gamma globulin as compared with four infusions in the treatment of acute Kawasaki syndrome. N Engl J Med 1991;324(23):1633–9.
64. Durongpisitkul K, Gururaj VJ, Park JM, et al. The prevention of coronary artery aneurysm in Kawasaki disease: a meta-analysis on the efficacy of aspirin and immunoglobulin treatment. Pediatrics 1995;96(6):1057–61.
65. Terai M, Shulman ST. Prevalence of coronary artery abnormalities in Kawasaki disease is highly dependent on gamma globulin dose but independent of salicylate dose. J Pediatr 1997;131(6):888–93.
66. Dalmau J, Gleichman AJ, Hughes EG, et al. Anti-NMDA-receptor encephalitis: case series and analysis of the effects of antibodies. Lancet Neurol 2008;7(12):1091–8.
67. Gresa-Arribas N, Titulaer MJ, Torrents A, et al. Antibody titres at diagnosis and during follow-up of anti-NMDA receptor encephalitis: a retrospective study. Lancet Neurol 2014;13(2):167–77.
68. van Swieten JC, Koudstaal PJ, Visser MC, et al. Interobserver agreement for the assessment of handicap in stroke patients. Stroke 1988;19(5):604–7.
69. Lim J-A, Lee S-T, Moon J, et al. Development of the clinical assessment scale in autoimmune encephalitis. Ann Neurol 2019;85(3):352–8.

Rapid Onset of Neuromuscular Paralysis or Weakness

Robert Charles Tasker, MBBS, MD, FRCP[a,b],*

KEYWORDS

- Pediatric • Acute flaccid myelitis • Acute flaccid paralysis • Critical illness
- Intensive care • Neuromuscular respiratory failure • Weakness

KEY POINTS

- Across the lifespan, neonate to adult, the underlying reason for *rapid-onset* neuromuscular disease-related respiratory impairment varies: congenital neuromuscular disease in the neonatal period; progressive neuromuscular disorder of infancy through to adolescence; and, acute and acute-on-chronic neuromuscular disorder at any age.
- Typical mechanisms by which neuromuscular disorders lead to respiratory failure are a dysfunctional respiratory pump, loss of ability to maintain airway patency or airway control, and failure or loss of airway protective reflexes.
- In pediatric practice, the designation *rapid onset* is arbitrary because an underlying disease or inherited or congenital condition may have gone unnoticed until there is fulminant deterioration with respiratory failure.
- Three *respiratory* phenotypes should alert the clinician to unappreciated genetic neuromuscular disease: neonatal onset respiratory distress out of proportion to any lung pathologic condition; or a later onset with respiratory insufficiency and failure with predominantly diaphragmatic weakness; or bulbar motor dysfunction.

INTRODUCTION

The neurology of breathing is well characterized,[1] and this mechanism may be perturbed by several diseases that affect the cerebral hemispheres, brainstem, spinal cord, nerves, neuromuscular junction, or axial musculature.[2] When breathing is so deranged, intensive care unit (ICU) admission is typically needed for one of 3 reasons:

[a] Department of Anesthesiology, Critical Care and Pain Medicine, Boston Children's Hospital, 300 Longwood Avenue, Bader 627, Boston, MA 02115, USA; [b] Selwyn College, Cambridge University, UK
* Boston Children's Hospital, 300 Longwood Avenue, Bader 627, Boston, MA 02115.
E-mail address: Robert.tasker@childrens.harvard.edu
Twitter: @RobertCTasker (R.C.T.)

Crit Care Clin 38 (2022) 413–428
https://doi.org/10.1016/j.ccc.2021.11.011
0749-0704/22/© 2021 Elsevier Inc. All rights reserved.

1. The mechanics of the respiratory pump are dysfunctional, leading to respiratory failure
2. Loss of ability to maintain airway patency or airway control, again leading to respiratory failure
3. Failure or loss of airway protective reflexes, often resulting in aspiration and respiratory failure

Across the lifespan, neonate to adult, the underlying reason for neuromuscular disease-related respiratory impairment varies, for example, congenital neuromuscular disease in the newborn or neonatal period[3]; progressive neuromuscular disorder of infancy through to adolescence[4]; and acute and acute-on-chronic neuromuscular disorder at any age.[5]

The focus of this narrative review is the clinical differential diagnosis of disease involving the peripheral or lower motor neuron component of the neurology of breathing. Here, the peripheral nervous system (PNS) refers to the portion of the nervous system from the anterior horn cell through to the muscle and the sensory pathways back to the dorsal root ganglia. The clinical context of the review is limited to those PNS conditions with a time course often described as acute or of rapid onset, meaning within days to weeks. However, in pediatric and neonatal practice, the designation *rapid onset* is somewhat arbitrary because an underlying disease or inherited or congenital condition may have gone unnoticed until there is a fulminant deterioration with respiratory failure.

In the PNS diseases considered in this review, the diagnostic approach will involve a detailed clinical history, careful physical examination, and selected investigations. When the acquired conditions (**Table 1**) are excluded, there are also other inherited or genetic conditions to consider (see later sections). Here, 2 reports give some insight into the potential scale of this latter problem and the types of unsuspected conditions or rare disorders that occur in practice. Both studies were carried out in highly selected populations of cases with unexplained causes of neuromuscular respiratory failure in the ICU. First, at the older end of the age spectrum, there is a report of 85 adults (aged 20–88 years) with acute neuromuscular failure treated in a major referral center in the United States over a period of 7 years.[6] There were 47/85 patients (prevalence 55%, 95% confidence interval [95% CI] 45%–65%]) without a previously known neuromuscular condition, and the most frequent final diagnoses were Guillain-Barré syndrome (GBS) and amyotrophic lateral sclerosis (ALS). Of note, 8 of 12 patients with ALS were newly diagnosed at the time of presentation with acute respiratory failure. Overall, 10 of the 85 (or 47 undiagnosed) patients (prevalence 12%, 95% CI, 7%–20%) remained undiagnosed, and by the time of discharge, 2 patients had died, and 7 others suffered severe disability (2 of these patients died during follow-up between 3 and 12 months after discharge). Only 1 patient was independent at discharge and last follow-up.

The other report covers the youngest patients in the ICU, infants and children aged less than 2 years of age.[7] Over a period of 12 months in this national referral center in the United Kingdom, nerve conduction studies (NCS) and needle electromyography (EMG) were carried out in 147 patients in the ICU. In 33/147 patients (prevalence 22%, 95% CI, 16%–30%), the reason for referral was "unspecified neuromuscular abnormality," including diaphragmatic abnormality and unexplained failure to wean mechanical ventilation. In a further 23/147 patients (prevalence 16%, 95% CI, 11%–22%), the reason for referral was "bulbar palsy" or other airway abnormality, such as unexplained stridor.

Table 1
Framework for categorizing recognizable patterns of acquired neuromuscular disease with respiratory failure

Lesion	Causes	Notes
Anterior horn cell involved	Transverse myelitis and AFM *AFP viral:* Poliomyelitis, enterovirus (EV-71), Coxsackie, echoviruses, mumps, Japanese encephalitis *Vascular:* Anterior spinal artery infarction	See **Table 2** Polio: Fever, neck stiffness EV-A71: Hand, foot, and mouth disease Coxsackie: Myocarditis and/or hepatitis Mumps: Parotitis
Peripheral nerve and roots	Immune mediated: GBS	Prodrome of neck stiffness → autonomic signs, ascending weakness, myalgia, facial weakness (note: all conditions listed in this table are in a differential diagnosis of GBS)
	Acute intermittent porphyria	Intermittent exacerbations with abdominal pain, peripheral neuropathy, and central signs (seizures, cortical blindness, and coma)
	Nerve toxins: Heavy metals (lead or arsenic) poisoning, postdiphtheritic	Exposure → acute neuropathy, weakness, and hyperreflexia
	CIP (see CIM below)	Sepsis and pARDS-related weakness, distal areflexia and delayed weaning from mechanical ventilation
Neuromuscular junction	Presynaptic: Botulism; spider venom; paralytic shellfish poisoning; tick paralysis	Infantile botulism: Constipation → descending weakness, facial weakness
	Synaptic: Organophosphate poisoning	Exposure → ↑cholinergic activity, destroying central and peripheral acetylcholinesterase → muscarinic, nicotinic, and central signs with dyspnea, ↑secretions, sweating, salivation, tears, myositis, muscle twitching, cramps, weakness, seizures, and coma
	Postsynaptic: Autoimmune myasthenia gravis	Massive ACh-receptor blockade by antibodies prevents muscle contraction → quadriplegia with normal reflexes, ptosis, ophthalmoparesis, swallowing disorder, and respiratory failure

(continued on next page)

Table 1 (continued)		
Lesion	Causes	Notes
Muscle	CIM (see CIP above) and ICUAW	Necrotizing myopathy affecting type II fibers rich in myosin associated with ↑CPK; weakness is predominantly proximal

Abbreviations: ACh-receptor, acetylcholine receptor; AFM, acute flaccid myelitis; AFP, acute flaccid paralysis; CIM, critical illness myopathy; CIP, critical illness polyneuropathy; CPK, creatine phosphokinase; GBS, Guillain-Barré syndrome; ICUAW, intensive care unit-acquired weakness; pARDS, pediatric acute respiratory distress syndrome.

INITIAL APPROACH IN THE PATIENT WITH RECOGNIZABLE PATTERN OF ACQUIRED NEUROMUSCULAR DISEASE

The framework in **Table 1** helps categorize most patients at initial evaluation. In those with rapid onset of flaccid lower-extremity paralysis, the diagnostically informative details include answering questions such as:

1. *What are the reflexes like?* Are both right and left lower limbs symmetrically flaccid (ie, reduced tone)? In GBS there is a rapid, progressive, ascending, and symmetric pattern of weakness. The reflexes are reduced or absent. Patients can feel pain and paresthesia (sharp tingling sensation or pins and needles). There may be autonomic instability with sweating and tachycardia, as well as bladder dysfunction and paralytic ileus.
2. *Does anyone in the family have a diarrheal illness?* If so, there is a possibility of fecal-oral transmission of enterovirus (eg, poliovirus, or another enterovirus, such as EV-A71), or adenovirus infection. Alternatively, did the patient have any upper-respiratory tract symptoms, or do they have rhinorrhea that would point toward other viral cause? *Acute flaccid paralysis* (AFP) due to poliovirus may involve one or all 4 limbs. The legs are involved more than arms, and often there is asymmetry at presentation.
3. *Did the initial symptoms include pain and/or paresthesia followed by weakness of the affected limb?* If so, *acute flaccid myelitis* (AFM) is in the differential diagnosis. AFM is related to nonpolio enteroviruses (eg, EV-D68, EV-A71), adenoviruses, herpesviruses, and flaviviruses (eg, West Nile virus).
4. *Is bladder or bowel function affected?* In the setting of acute respiratory failure, transverse myelitis is something to consider. In this instance, expect motor deficit and a sensory level. Postinfectious myelitis is also in the differential, but it takes days to weeks for weakness to develop.

After history taking and the examination, investigations should be prioritized. In particular, if paraspinal infection and inflammation need to be excluded, urgent spinal imaging is required, with possible referral for neurosurgery. Lumbar puncture with examination of cerebrospinal fluid (CSF) comes next. If there is pleocytosis with elevated protein concentration, then the findings support the diagnosis of AFM or AFP rather than GBS. Electrodiagnostic testing with NCS and EMG is a specialist investigation and should be available in most centers, but access varies. In the United States, in regard to the focus of the current review, there is a 2020 pediatric practice guideline from the *American Association of Neuromuscular and Electrodiagnostic Medicine* that discusses current utility of these investigations in patients with polyneuropathy, inflammatory neuropathy, and neuromuscular junction (NMJ) disorders.[8]

The next step is often a multidisciplinary approach between teams of critical care, infectious disease, and neurology specialists. The diagnostic strategy involves considering the origin of the difficulty anatomically: anterior horn cell to peripheral nerve, NMJ, and muscle, and developing a management plan accordingly.

Anterior Horn Cell Disorders

Acute flaccid paralysis

In the United States, as of the 2020 *Council of State and Territorial Epidemiologists* report,[9] AFP is now considered a generalized "umbrella" term for multiple clinical entities, including paralytic poliomyelitis (see AFP), transverse myelitis, AFM, GBS, toxic neuropathy, and muscle disorders (see **Table 1**). Essentially, this grouping helps with case ascertainment of AFM, but the individual diagnoses remain important because each has their own differential diagnoses to consider.

A pragmatic case definition of AFP is "a clinical syndrome with rapid onset of weakness that frequently involves the respiratory and bulbar muscles." Whenever these criteria are met, and poliomyelitis is a possibility, thorough investigation and reporting of potential poliomyelitis are required. Two diagnostic stool samples, more than 24 hours apart, should be collected within 14 days of onset of paralysis and then processed in a World Health Organization–approved laboratory.[10] If poliomyelitis is confirmed, it may be caused by, for example, *wild poliovirus* (serotypes 1–3) or *vaccine-associated paralytic poliomyelitis*, and it will need full epidemiologic investigation. In the individual patient, disease progression with paralysis (with sensory preservation) is rapid, is asymmetrical, and involves proximal more than distal muscles.[11]

Other potential viral causes of AFP include Coxsackie and echoviruses, Japanese B encephalitis, Murray Valley encephalitis, St. Louis encephalitis, Russian Spring encephalitis, tick-borne viruses, and herpesvirus. These causes vary by geography with, for example, EV-A71 being the cause in parts of southeast Asia, and West Nile virus being a cause in the United States. Therefore, consider the following investigations for possible viral causes of AFP, as well as other conditions in the differential diagnosis[11,12]:

- Imaging with MRI of spine (and possibly brain)
- CSF sampling for differential cell counts, glucose, protein; microbiology and diagnostic polymerase chain reaction (PCR) testing for enteroviruses and other infectious diseases; and, for autoantibodies such as antimyelin oligodendrocyte glycoprotein (anti-MOG, see later discussion)
- Respiratory/nasopharyngeal secretion samples for viral PCR testing (eg, enterovirus)
- Peripheral neurophysiology with NCS if differentiation from GBS is needed, or botulism is suspected
- Studies for identification of possible metabolic disease (eg, acute hypokalemic periodic paralysis, thyrotoxic periodic paralysis, acute intermittent porphyria) and/or toxin exposures (eg, sporadic hypokalemic paralysis secondary to licorice, barium, cottonseed oil exposure)
- Investigations to exclude paralytic syndromes that mimic or are misdiagnosed as AFP, such as vitamin B_{12} deficiency, which may be exacerbated by chronic cycad poisoning from evergreens, cyanide toxicity from cassava ingestion, and lathyrism.

In regard to imaging in AFP, and what to expect, we have the benefit of old necropsy studies in children,[13,14] as well as more recent experimental neuropathology investigations.[15] These studies inform us about the distribution of poliovirus infection within the body and the evolution of poliomyelitis to destruction of anterior horn motor neurons in the spinal cord. Now consider the MRI findings in children during the 2013 outbreak of EV-A71 in Sydney, Australia.[16] All 4 children with the AFP phenotype showed brainstem abnormality, and 3 of 4 showed spinal cord abnormality with a pattern of inflammation involving the central gray matter as well as the anterior horns.

Acute flaccid myelitis

AFM is considered a subset within the "umbrella" term, AFP,[9] with central spinal cord lesions on MRI, a pattern of abnormality seen in poliomyelitis, nonpolio AFP,[16] and anti-MOG-associated myelitis.[17] Of note, the differentiation between transverse myelitis and AFM is not as straightforward as diagnosing one or the other. Transverse myelitis is an immune-mediated condition causing demyelination within spinal cord white matter.[18] However, different diagnostic labels do not mean that we are dealing with easily determined and discrete conditions. For example, when a patient with "myelitis" presents with flaccid weakness in at least 1 limb and MRI changes in gray matter (see later discussion; **Table 2**),[9] they are labeled as having AFM. Of particular relevance here is the CAPTURE (Collaboration About Pediatric Transverse myelitis: Understand, Reveal, Educate) cohort study, which identified 2 patterns of AFM based on MRI T2-hyperintense signal changes: a predominantly gray matter restricted form with signal changes in the anterior horns versus a mixed gray and white matter form of AFM.[19] These differences or overlap in conditions may be relevant to future understanding of nosology, pathophysiology, and potential response to new therapies.

At the present time, in the United States, the Centers for Disease Control and Prevention (CDC) surveillance definition of AFM includes the necessity for clinical and radiological features consistent with polio-like weakness and injury that favors the cervical spinal cord gray matter spanning over one or more vertebral segments.[20] Other potential causes, such as malignancy, vascular disease, or anatomic abnormality, should be excluded. **Table 2** covers the contemporary CDC case definition for case classification of AFM.[9]

AFM is now also recognized as a global disease[21] because, since 2012, the incidence of this severe paralytic disease appears to have been driven by world-regional epidemics of enterovirus (EV-D68) infection. The underlying pathophysiology

Table 2 Acute flaccid myelitis clinical case definition and criteria for classification based on spinal cord MRI[a]	
Clinical features with focus on rapidity of clinical development	Acute onset of flaccid weakness (ie, low muscle tone) of one or more limbs AND no clear alternative diagnosis (see **Table 1**)
MRI classification: exclude malignancy, vascular disease, or an anatomic abnormality that may explain gray matter findings, and focus on terms reporting spinal cord gray matter involvement of "central cord," "anterior myelitis," "poliomyelitis," or "anterior horn cells"	Confirmed Predominant gray matter involvement spanning one or more vertebral segments Presumed Indeterminant gray matter predominance Supported At least some gray matter involved spanning one or more vertebral segments

[a] See text; based on information available in Ref.[9]

of rapid-onset weakness and respiratory failure, hence admission to the ICU, is un-known, and it is presumed that there may be host genetic and immunologic factors, as well as viral and virus-induced inflammatory factors involved, but further research is needed.[22] There are no proven treatments for AFM apart from supportive respiratory care and rehabilitation.

Peripheral Nerve

Guillain-Barré syndrome

Acute inflammatory demyelinating polyneuropathy, or GBS, is not common in pediatric ICU practice,[5] and it is rare in the very young.[23] Progression to thoracic pump-related respiratory insufficiency will need mechanical ventilation support. Bulbar involvement may also require ICU management and intervention for airway protection.

GBS should be considered in any patient with rapidly progressive, symmetric limb weakness with or without sensory disturbances, hyporeflexia or areflexia, and disso-ciation in CSF albumin and cytology. All the conditions listed in **Table 1** are in the dif-ferential diagnosis of GBS. As far as searching for cause, the list of investigations is standard,[24] but added to it now should be the possibility of GBS associated with in-fections of Zika virus[25] or severe acute respiratory syndrome coronavirus 2.[26–28]

In regard to using NCS and EMG investigations in the diagnostic strategy of poten-tial pediatric GBS, have a look at the 2020 evidence review with consensus-based guideline from the *German-Speaking Society of Neuropediatrics*, as it is the most up-to-date publication on the topic.[24] Here, there is an "open recommendation" about the use of these electrodiagnostic studies (ie, "no proof of, or insufficient evidence for a net benefit; or benefit unclear because of non-viable evidence or a lack of applica-bility"). However, these studies are certainly of value when confirming the diagnosis after initial treatment in order to gain greater diagnostic certainty (ie, open recommen-dation), or to identify the pathophysiologic variants that are of prognostic significance. For example, it is very useful to know that a patient has acute motor axonal neuropa-thy, characterized by pure motor neurologic deficit; or, acute motor sensory axonal neuropathy in which sensory fibers are also involved; or, Miller-Fisher syndrome.[5,23,24,29,30] Miller-Fisher syndrome is the least common type of pediatric GBS, again with a broad differential diagnosis, and is characterized by ophthalmople-gia, ataxia, and areflexia. Facial and lower cranial nerve involvement, limb weakness, respiratory failure, and mild sensory involvement may occur in various combinations.[31]

Neuromuscular Junction Abnormalities

The acquired NMJ disorders resulting in respiratory failure and ICU admission can be categorized as those conditions involving the presynaptic, synaptic, or postsynaptic component of the junction (see **Table 1**). (Whether this categorization will remain useful is debatable. See later section on *neonatal respiratory distress syndrome* and the range in presynaptic, synaptic, or postsynaptic proteins causing the same congenital myasthenia phenotype.) Nevertheless, the discussion points highlighted in later dis-cussion focus on particular examples. Aside from the notes, it is also important to remember that there are many types of toxin exposures affecting the NMJ that have been described around the world. Sadly, the ICU clinician must also be aware of the potential for chemical-biological terrorism and its impact on children.[32] It is beyond the scope of this review to give an update on nerve agents, but it is worth reading about the NMJ effects of the organophosphorus nerve agents that act by inhibiting acetylcholinesterase irreversibly, for example, Sarin (G-series B, O-isopropyl methyl-phosphonofluodidate),[33,34] and Novichok.[35,36]

Botulism

Botulism is a rare, neurotoxin-mediated, life-threatening disease characterized by *flaccid descending* paralysis. It starts with the cranial nerves and progresses to extremity weakness and respiratory failure.[37] The anaerobic, gram-positive bacterium *Clostridium botulinum* (occasionally *Clostridium baratii and Clostridium butyricum*) produces a neurotoxin that prevents acetylcholine release at the NMJ. Irrespective of route of exposure (eg, infant intestinal botulism, food-borne botulism, wound botulism, and adult intestinal toxemia), the clinical neurologic picture is stereotypical. There are, however, 2 challenges to the diagnosis of botulism. First, timeliness of diagnosis in infants in whom the first symptom is constipation, rapidly followed by paralysis, which starts cranially and then descends. Early diagnosis is required for effective timing of human-derived botulism immune globulin intravenous (BIG-IV) treatment. Second, in pediatric patients up to the adolescent age group, there is the problem that the condition may be confused with other diagnoses, such as myasthenia gravis (MG), poisonings and intoxications, GBS, and poliomyelitis.[38] Therefore, think of this diagnosis when considering the diagnosis of MG or GBS.

Early supportive ICU management with mechanical ventilation is a main component of the treatment of botulism, particularly in the infantile form. Historically, potential or theoretic medical treatments have included use of equine serum trivalent botulism antitoxin, BIG-IV, plasma exchange, 3,4-diaminopyridine, and guanidine. However, a 2019 Cochrane review found only "low- and moderate-certainty evidence supporting the use of BIG-IV in infant intestinal bolulism."[39] There is a single randomized controlled trial of infants receiving early treatment (ie, within 72 hours of hospital admission with acute paralysis consistent with infant botulism) with BIG-IV.[40] It shows reduced mean length of hospital stay (the primary efficacy outcome measure) from 5.7 to 2.6 weeks (*P*<.001), and reduced mean duration of mechanical ventilation by 2.6 weeks (*P*=.01). The time course of intervention is now extended beyond 72 hours because of information from subsequent observational studies.

Tick paralysis

Ticks are obligate hematophagous ectoparasites of various animals, including humans, and are abundant in temperate and tropical zones around the world. In the United States, during April to June, tick paralysis is most common in the Pacific Northwest, Rocky Mountain states, and the southeast part of the country. At least 40 kinds of ticks can cause tick paralysis, and the symptoms depend on the species. After the female tick attaches to the host, it secretes a salivary neurotoxin into the bloodstream that spreads and is able to impair acetylcholine release at the motor endplate. Symptoms start with tingling and sometimes muscle pain, and there may be paralysis that starts in the lower limbs and ascends, potentially causing diaphragmatic respiratory failure. Therefore, a sound rule is that GBS should not be diagnosed in a child without first looking very carefully for a tick. In fact, in a comparative analysis of US and Australia public health reporting data (1946–2014 and 1904–2009, respectively), more recent reporting periods in the United States show early misdiagnosis of tick paralysis as GBS.[41] Of note, removal of the tick should restore the child to normal strength.

Transplacental autoimmune myasthenia gravis

For the purpose of this narrative review, consider autoimmune MG (AIMG) as an acquired disease. AIMG may present in the congenital form when a mother with MG gives birth to a floppy baby who has been paralyzed by the transplacental diffusion of antibodies against the adult form of the NMJ. After birth, this antibody transfer ceases, and the neonate will recover over a period of weeks. It is rare for the mother not to have been known to have MG, and therefore, the condition should present no diagnostic difficulty.

A more confusing diagnostic situation occurs when a child is born with arthrogryposis and the Pena-Shokeir phenotype,[42] with transplacental transfer of antibodies against various antigens in the NMJ, including the nicotinic acetylcholine receptor[43,44] or muscle-specific kinase or lipoprotein receptor-related protein 4.[45]

Muscle Disease

It is very rare for an acute muscle disease (eg, myositis and/or rhabdomyolysis) in a pediatric patient to be sufficiently severe to result in thoracic pump-related respiratory failure. It is more likely that acquired muscle disease has developed during a critical illness, and results in weakness and prolonged "weaning" from mechanical ventilation.

In the early days of research into acquired neuromuscular disease in adults with critical illness, muscle biopsy in patients with ICU admission longer than 7 to 10 days demonstrated high yield of acquired tissue abnormalities.[46] There were many possible causes of such findings, but subsequent research has shown that having excluded the prolonged NMJ effects of neuromuscular blocking agents (NMBA) in hepatic or renal failure, drug toxicities, and nutritional deficiencies, we are left with the possibility of so-called intensive care unit–acquired weakness (ICUAW) owing to critical illness myopathy (CIM) and/or polyneuropathy (CIP).[47]

Critical illness myopathy, critical illness polyneuropathy, and intensive care unit–acquired weakness

The prevalence of ICUAW resulting from CIM, CIP, or a combination of the 2 may be 45% or higher in critically ill adults.[47] The condition is well characterized, and the modifiable risk factors include hyperglycemia and the severe endocrinological stress response of critical illness; use of medications such as beta-agonists, aminoglycosides, corticosteroids, and steroid-based NMBA like vecuronium; and illness such as sepsis complicated by acute respiratory distress syndrome, or multiple organ dysfunction syndrome (MODS).[48]

The evidence for ICUAW in pediatric patients with critical illness is not as robust as the evidence in adults with critical illness, and it appears to be an unusual occurrence. The authors of 3 single-center, population-based, pediatric ICU studies have examined the epidemiology of ICUAW, and it is important to consider the data. One study, based in a major referral center in Canada, used the UK Medical Research Council (MRC) muscle strength scale to screen and grade, over a 12-month period, 830 pediatric cases who had been on the ICU for more than 24 hours.[49] Patients underwent NCS and EMG if the MRC scale grade was less than or equal to 4 (ie, at best, muscle contraction with some resistance) in any 1 muscle group. Fourteen of 830 patients (1.7%, 95% CI, 1.0%–2.8%) were considered weak by this criterion and, in these cases, MODS occurred in 11, and sepsis occurred in 9. Most of these pediatric patients had received NMBA, corticosteroids, and aminoglycosides (see earlier discussion). The EMG/NCS was myopathic in 4 children, normal in 2 children, showed a compressive neuropathy in 1 child, and showed a mild demyelinating polyneuropathy in 1 child. A second study, from Egypt, also used the MRC scale to screen for weakness in a pediatric ICU population, but in this instance, the focus was on 105 children who had been admitted for longer than 7 days.[50] Thirty-four of 105 (32%, 95% CI, 24%–42%) of these longer-stay pediatric patients had significant weakness on MRC sum score (ie, <48 when assessing muscle power from 3 movements in each limb, scored 0–5, giving a potential maximum score of 60). Of these 34 children, 29 had electrophysiology features suggestive of axonal polyneuropathy. Similar to the Canadian study,[49] sepsis was the most common underlying condition in those with weakness and CIM/CIP; it occurred in 23 of 34 cases (68%, 95% CI, 51%–81%). A third study from an ICU in India selected 97 children over a period of 12 months, who met certain age (2–12 years) and severity-of-illness (ie, high pediatric risk of mortality score >20 for >24 hours) criteria.[51] These patients underwent daily electrophysiology studies (median of 3 days), and out of 380 observations, there was not a single case that met CIM/CIP criteria (0%, 95% CI, 0%–0.8%). What is worth noting about these studies is the difference in patient selection, or pretest probability, and the relationship to prevalence of abnormal clinical and electrophysiology findings. The study from Egypt[50] was the only study that used a similar selection process to historical adult studies.[47,48] Perhaps the unusual occurrence of ICUAW and CIM/CIP in pediatric ICU patients is simply explained by the fact that prolonged ventilation, 7 to 10 days, is an unusual occurrence.[52]

In contrast to the pediatric ICU population-based studies,[49–51] when the focus is on pediatric cases of sepsis, a single-center cohort of 32 pediatric patients mechanically ventilated for longer than 7 days found evidence of polyneuropathy (most commonly axonal neuropathy) in 29 (91%, 95% CI, 76%–97%), and there was also evidence of weakness with MRC sum scores in the range of 36 to 41.[53] Most of these patients also had been treated with steroids and NMBA.

Taking together all these pediatric studies, there is certainly some likelihood of weakness and CIM/CIP in those patients requiring mechanical ventilation for at least 7 days after ICU admission, particularly in those with sepsis. However, there is a discrepancy between the prevalence of ICUAW in the pediatric versus adult ICU, and there still is not an explanation. Of note, close inspection of the studies also raises the question of whether CIM, CIP, and ICUAW, other than in severe sepsis, are really postpubertal phenomena. Last, in the pediatric population, weakness is not always equivalent to the presence of CIP/CIM, so it is best not to label patients as having such an abnormality without having performed the appropriate electrophysiological investigations.

RECOGNIZING THE ATYPICAL OR OUTLIER PATTERN OF GENETIC RESPIRATORY NEUROMUSCULAR DISEASE IN THE INTENSIVE CARE UNIT PATIENT

There is sufficient epidemiologic evidence to support the notion that time course of acute respiratory failure necessitating invasive respiratory support is predicable. That is, in general, depending on which part of the respiratory tract is primarily involved in an illness (upper airway to lower-respiratory tract, or global), there is an expected time limit to the need for invasive support and ICU admission.[52] The outliers are those patients with unexplained prolonged ICU admission. There is a discussion about prolonged ICU admission in the above section on ICUAW, but this metric is also an important measure for recognizing the patient with possible previously unappreciated or undiagnosed genetic disease causing respiratory failure. Therefore, in every patient with a prolonged course of mechanical ventilation, it is important to ask, "why is this patient still needing this support?" Then, to think about the follow-up questions, such as:

- *Is there a problem with weaning mechanical ventilation?* If so, what is the cause? Is there isolated weakness in the diaphragm or is there general weakness of the thoracic pump?
- *Is there a problem that became evident at the time of attempting to remove the endotracheal tube?* If so, what was the time course, and is there a problem with bulbar control and/or airway protection reflexes?

Table 3
Genetic neuromuscular disorders disclosed by an acute respiratory phenotype

Respiratory Phenotypes	Examples in the Differential Diagnosis
Neonatal respiratory distress	• Congenital muscular dystrophy: Walker-Warburg syndrome • Congenital myopathy: Myotubular or nemaline myopathy • Congenital myasthenic syndromes (see text)
Later onset of respiratory failure with diaphragm involvement	• Spinal muscular atrophy type 1: Werdnig-Hoffman disease • Charcot-Marie-Tooth: Early myopathy, areflexia, respiratory distress, and dysphagia (EMARDD an autosomal recessive disorder; pathogenic variants in multiple epidermal growth factor-like domains 10 [*MEGF10*] gene) • SMARD (spinal muscular atrophy with respiratory distress; see text)
Bulbar motor dysfunction	• Brown-Vialetto-Van Laere syndrome: Pathogenic variant in the riboflavin solute carrier 52 (*SLC52A2*, *SLC52A3*) and ubiquitin 1 (*UBQLN1*) genes • Fazio-Londe syndrome: Also due to pathogenic variant in *SLC52A3* gene • Worster Drought: X-linked or autosomal dominant • Spinal and bulbar muscular atrophy: Kennedy disease (X-linked recessive with ↑trinucleotide [cytosine-adenine-guanine] repeats in the androgen receptor)

Based on the answers to these questions, it follows that there are 3 *respiratory* phenotypes in the ICU that should alert the clinician to possible unappreciated neuromuscular disease. These clinical presentations are neonatal onset respiratory distress out of proportion to any lung pathologic condition; or a later onset with respiratory insufficiency and failure with predominantly diaphragmatic weakness; or bulbar motor dysfunction (**Table 3**). These phenotypes are discussed later and illustrate contemporary understanding and diagnostic strategy. Like the acquired patterns of neuromuscular disease with respiratory failure, the approach is multidisciplinary with the addition of genetic expertise and genomic testing. However, in contrast here, there is a strong argument that after a thorough history and detailed clinical examination that the diagnostic strategy is different. We are now at the point in which "given the option of genetic testing, traditional testing such as EMG, NCS and muscle/nerve biopsy are not the first-line diagnostic tests."[54]

Neonatal (First Month) Respiratory Distress

The working definition of the *neonatal respiratory distress syndrome* phenotype used in several studies is the *presence of peripheral hypotonia and/or arthrogryposis and the absence of neurologic central signs in children who experience respiratory distress during the first month of life*.[55] When this pattern is present without sufficient pulmonary pathologic condition to explain why such an infant is on a mechanical ventilator, the differential diagnosis is wide (see **Table 3**) and, as of 2021, it is known that many genes may be involved.

As an example of the complexity and range in diagnoses, consider the neonatal respiratory distress phenotype with early-onset NMJ and congenital myasthenic syndromes (CMS).[56] In 2019, understanding of the various types of CMS was that the syndrome involved defects in genes encoding for 8 presynaptic proteins, 4 synaptic proteins, 15 postsynaptic proteins, and 5 proteins that undergo glycosylation. In regard to the reported cases with respiratory insufficiency, pathogenic variants were evident in genes encoding components of the following sites:

1. Presynaptic: The acetylcholine and vesicle formation machinery, such as the solute carrier family 18, member A3 (*SLC18A3*), and synaptobrevin homolog 1 (*SYB1*)
2. Synaptic proteins: The collagen-like tail subunit of asymmetric acetylcholinesterase (*COLQ*) and laminin subunit beta 2 (*LAMB2*)
3. Postsynaptic: Acetylcholine receptor subunits, such as the cholinergic receptor nicotinic beta 1 subunit (*CHRNB1*), the cholinergic receptor nicotinic epsilon subunit (*CHRNE*); or components of the acetylcholine receptor-clustering pathway (ie, muscle specific kinase, *MUSK*; unconventional myosin IXA, *MYO9A*; low density lipoprotein receptor-related protein 4, *LRP4*; receptor associated protein of the synapse, *RAPSN*); and, a postsynaptic sodium channel (ie, sodium voltage-gated channel alpha subunit A, *SCN4A*).

The diversity in these findings is interesting and may change how we think about NMJ disorders as new genetic treatments become available. The findings also have significant impact on the optimal approach to molecular genetic testing,[54–56] hence the need for a multidisciplinary expertise, including geneticists, and the availability of approved diagnostic gene panels, exome sequencing with copy number variant analysis, or genome sequencing.[54]

Later-Onset Diaphragmatic Presentation of Respiratory Insufficiency

In adults and the older child, there is literature on previously unsuspected hereditary or genetic conditions that result in phrenic nerve-related diaphragmatic dysfunction with respiratory insufficiency, for example, hereditary neuralgic amyotrophy.[6,57] There is also a "diaphragmatic" presentation in the much younger infant. For example, an entity to be aware of is *Spinal Muscular Atrophy with Respiratory Distress* (SMARD), in which the patient typically first presents for ICU management at aged 6 weeks to 6 months.[58]

SMARD is a rare autosomal recessive motor neuron disorder. In its most common form, there may have been intrauterine growth restriction, with a birth weight less than the third percentile, and subsequent discharging home from the newborn nursery without event.[59] Then, at around 3 months of age the infant presents because of breathing difficulty. Investigation may reveal an abnormality of the diaphragm, which may be unilateral and suggestive of a diaphragmatic eventration. A common scenario is for the baby to then have a surgical repair, during which it is found that the muscle is very thin. When the infant returns to the ICU for postoperative mechanical ventilation, weaning from the mechanical ventilator proves to be impossible, and the infant becomes ventilator-dependent. SMARD1 is caused by homozygous or compound heterozygous pathogenic variants in the gene encoding immunoglobulin μ-binding protein 2 (*IGHMBP2*). SMARD2 has been described in a single case with a similar phenotype to SMARD1 and is caused by an X-linked recessive pathogenic variant in the gene encoding the LAS1-like ribosomal biogenesis protein (*LAS1L*).[60]

Bulbar Motor Dysfunction

Bulbar motor dysfunction syndromes can present with respiratory disturbance at any age, but typically from 6 months onwards. These are rare conditions. However, such patients will be seen in the ICU, and it is always worth thinking about bulbar causes at the time of "failed endotracheal tube extubation." There is a broad differential diagnosis (see **Table 3)** and, in general, there is a history of dysphagia or noisy breathing, and some neurologic deficits (may be underappreciated). One condition is worth mentioning here because it provides a good illustration of gene discovery leading to new treatments. The Brown-Vialetto-Van Laere syndrome is an autosomal recessive disorder involving pontobulbar motor neurons (ie, cranial nerves VII, IX, X, XI, and XII). In some cases, it is caused by pathogenic variants in the solute carrier 52-A2 and 52-A3 (*SLC52A2*, *SLC52A3*) genes, which encode for the riboflavin (vitamin B_2) transmembrane transporters RFVT2 and RFVT3, respectively.[58] Gene discovery has resulted in a therapeutic strategy with, in this instance, supplementation with high-dose riboflavin.

CLINICS CARE POINTS

- Have a structured approach to the care and assessment of the infant or child with rapid onset of neuromuscular paralysis or weakness.
- Carry out a thorough history and examination.
- Ask yourself whether there is a recognizable pattern of acquired neuromuscular disease.
- In the absence of a readily recognizable pattern, consider the atypical or outlier pattern of genetic respiratory neuromuscular disease.

DISCLOSURE

The author has nothing to disclose.

REFERENCES

1. Bolton CF, Chen RC, Wijdicks EFM, et al. Neurology of breathing. Philadelphia: Butterworth-Heinemann; 2004.
2. Wijdicks EFM. The neurology of acutely failing respiratory mechanics. Ann Neurol 2017;81:485–94.
3. Darras BT, Jones HR. Neuromuscular problems of the critically ill neonate and child. Semin Pediatr Neurol 2004;11:147–68.
4. Yates K, Festa M, Gillis J, et al. Outcome of children with neuromuscular disease admitted to paediatric intensive care. Arch Dis Child 2004;89:170–5.
5. Harrar DB, Darras BT, Ghosh PS. Acute neuromuscular disorders in the pediatric intensive care unit. J Child Neurol 2020;35:17–24.
6. Serrano MC, Rabinstein AA. Causes and outcomes of acute neuromuscular respiratory failure. Ann Neurol 2010;67:1089–94.
7. Pitt MC. Nerve conduction studies and needle EMG in very small children. Eur J Paediatr Neurol 2012;16:285–91.
8. Kang PB, McMillan HJ, Kuntz NL, et al. Utility and practice of electrodiagnostic testing in the pediatric population: an AANEM consensus statement. Muscle & Nerve 2020;61:143–55.

9. DeBolt C, Vogt M, for Council of State and Territorial Epidemiologists. Revision to the standard case definition, case classification, and public health reporting of acute flaccid myelitis. Interim-20-ID. Available at: https://cdn.ymaws.com/www.cste.org/resource/resmgr/ps/positionstatement2020/Interim-20-ID-04_AFM_Final.pdf.

10. World Health Organization WHO/V&B/03.01. WHO-recommended standards for surveillance of selected vaccine-preventable diseases. Poliomyelitis 2003; 2008:31–4.

11. Bao J, Thorley B, Isaacs D, et al. Polio—the old foe and new challenges: an update for clinicians. J Paediatr Child Health 2020;56:1527–32.

12. Marx A, Glass JD, Sutter RW. Differential diagnosis of acute flaccid paralysis and its role in poliomyelitis surveillance. Epidemiol Rev 2000;22:298–316.

13. Sabin AB, Ward R. The natural history of human poliomyelitis: I. Distribution of virus in nervous and non-nervous tissues. J Exp Med 1941;73:771–93.

14. Sabin AB, Ward R. The natural history of human poliomyelitis: II. Elimination of the virus. J Exp Med 1941;74:519–29.

15. Ford DJ, Ropka SL, Collins GH, et al. The neuropathology in wild-type mice inoculated with human poliovirus mirrors human paralytic poliomyelitis. Microb Pathog 2002;33:97–107.

16. Teoh H-L, Mohammad SS, Britton PN, et al. Clinical characteristics and functional motor outcomes of enterovirus 71 neurological disease in children. JAMA Neurol 2016;73:300–7.

17. Parrotta E, Kister I. The expanding clinical spectrum of myelin oligodendrocyte glycoprotein (MOG) antibody associated disease in children and adults. Front Neurol 2020;11:960.

18. Beh SC, Greenberg BM, Frohman T, et al. Transverse myelitis. Neurol Clin 2013; 31:79–138.

19. Greenberg B, Plumb P, Cutter G, et al. Acute flaccid myelitis: long-term outcomes recorded in the CAPTURE study compared with paediatric transverse myelitis. BMJ Neurol Open 2021;3:e000127.

20. Centers for Disease Control and Prevention. Case definitions for AFM. CDC. https://www.cdc.gov/acute-flaccid-myelitis/hcp/case-definitions.html. Assessed 1st August, 2021.

21. Murphy OC, Messacar K, Benson L, et al. Acute flaccid myelitis: cause, diagnosis, and management. Lancet 2021;397:334–46.

22. Ide W, Melicosta M, Trovato MK. Acute flaccid myelitis. Phys Med Rehab Clin N Am 2021;32:477–91.

23. Levison LS, Thomsen RW, Markvardsen LK, et al. Pediatric Guillain-Barre syndrome in a 30-year nationwide cohort. Pediatr Neurol 2020;107:57–63.

24. Korinthenberg R, Trollmann R, Felderhoff-Muser U, et al. Diagnosis and treatment of Guillain-Barre syndrome in childhood and adolescence: an evidence- and consensus-based guideline. Eur J Paediatr Neurol 2020;25:5–16.

25. Martins MM, Medronho RA, Cunha AJLAD. Zika virus in Brazil and worldwide: a narrative review. Paediatr Int Child Health 2021;41:28–35.

26. Schober ME, Pavia AT, Bohnsack JF. Neurologic manifestations of COVID-19 in children: emerging pathophysiologic insights. Pediatr Crit Care Med 2021;22: 655–61.

27. Siracusa I, Cascio A, Giordano S, et al. Neurological complications in pediatric patients with SARS-CoV-2 infection: a systematic review of the literature. Ital J Pediatr 2021;47:123.

28. Akcay N, Menentoglu ME, Bektas G, et al. Axonal Guillain-Barre syndrome associated with SARS-CoV-2 infection in a child. J Med Virol 2021;93(9):5599–602.

29. Kalita J, Kumar M, Misra U. Prospective comparison of motor axonal neuropathy and acute inflammatory demyelinating polyradiculopathy in 140 children with Guillain-Barre syndrome in India. Muscle & Nerve 2018;57:751–65.
30. Agarwal E, Bhagat A, Srivastava K, et al. Clinical and electrodiagnostic factors predicting prolonged recovery in children with Guillain-Barre syndrome. Indian J Pediatr 2021. https://doi.org/10.1007/s12098-021-03804-7 (Online ahead of Print).
31. Zuccoli G, Panigrahy A, Bailey A, et al. Redefining the Guillain-Barre spectrum in children: neuroimaging findings of cranial nerve involvement. AJNR Am J Neuroradiol 2011;32:639–42.
32. Chung S, Baum CR, Nyquist A-C, et al. Chemical-biological terrorism and its impact on children. Pediatrics 2020;145:e20193750.
33. Rotenberg JS, Newmark J. Nerve agent attacks on children: diagnosis and management. Pediatrics 2003;112:648–58.
34. Abou-Donia MB, Siracuse B, Gupta N, et al. Sarin (GB, O-isopropyl methylphosphonofluoridate) neurotoxicity: critical review. Crit Rev Toxicol 2016;46:845–75.
35. Hulse EJ, Haslam JD, Emmett SR, et al. Organophosphorus nerve agent poisoning: managing the poisoned patient. Br J Anaesth 2019;123:457–63.
36. Steindl D, Boehmerle W, Korner R, et al. Novichok nerve agent poisoning. Lancet 2021;397:16–22.
37. Rao AK, Sobel J, Chatham-Stephens K, et al. Clinical guidelines for diagnosis and treatment of botulism, 2021. MMWR Recomm Rep 2021;70:1–30.
38. Griese SE, Kisselburgh HM, Bartenfeld MT, et al. Pediatric botulism and use of equine botulinum antitoxin in children: a systematic review. Clin Infect Dis 2017;66(suppl 1):S17–29.
39. Chalk CH, Benstead TJ, Pound JD, et al. Medical treatment for botulism. Cochrane Database Syst Rev 2019;4:CD008123.
40. Arnon SS, Schechter R, Maslanka SE, et al. Human botulism immune globulin for the treatment of infant botulism. N Engl J Med 2006;354:462–71.
41. Diaz JH. A comparative meta-analysis of tick paralysis in the United States and Australia. Clin Toxicol (Phila) 2015;53:874–83.
42. Adam S, Coetzee M, Honey EM. Pena-Shokeir syndrome: current management strategies and palliative care. Appl Clin Genet 2018;11:111–20.
43. Brueton LA, Huson SM, Cox PM, et al. Asymptomatic maternal myasthenia as a cause of the Pena-Shokeir phenotype. Am J Med Genet 2000;92:1–6.
44. Vincent A, Newland C, Brueton L, et al. Arthrogryposis multiplex congenita with maternal autoantibodies specific for a fetal antigen. Lancet 1995;346:24–5.
45. Gilhus NE, Hong Y. Maternal myasthenia gravis represents a risk for the child through autoantibody transfer, immunosuppressive therapy and genetic influence. Eur J Neurol 2018;25:1402–9.
46. Coakley JH, Nagendran K, Honavar M, et al. Preliminary observations on the neuromuscular abnormalities in patients with organ failure and sepsis. Intensive Care Med 1993;19:323–8.
47. Vanhorebeek I, Latronico N, Van den Berghe G. ICU-acquired weakness. Intensive Care Med 2020;46:637–53.
48. Yan T, Li Z, Jiang L, et al. Risk factors for intensive care unit-acquired weakness: a systematic review and meta-analysis. Acta Neurol Scand 2018;138:104–14.
49. Banwell BL, Mildner RJ, Hassall AC, et al. Muscle weakness in critically ill children. Neurology 2003;61:1779–82.
50. Mahmoud AT, Tawfik MAM, El Naby SAA, et al. Neurophysiological study of critical illness polyneuropathy and myopathy in mechanically ventilated children;

additional aspects in paediatric critical illness comorbidities. Eur J Neurol 2018; 25:991-e76.

51. Kasinathan A, Sankhyan N, Muralidharan J, et al. Evaluation of pediatric critical illness neuropathy/myopathy in pediatric intensive care unit. Pediatr Neurol 2017;21(S1):E207.

52. Tasker RC. Gender differences and critical medical illness. Acta Paediatr 2000; 89:621–3.

53. Shubham S, Dhochak N, Singh A, et al. Polyneuropathy in critically ill mechanically ventilated children: experience from a tertiary care hospital in north India. Pediatr Crit Care Med 2019;20:826–31.

54. Chikkannaiah M, Reyes I. New diagnostic and therapeutic modalities in neuromuscular disorders in children. Curr Probl Pediatr Adolesc Health Care 2021; 51(7):101033.

55. Francois-Heude M-C, Walter-Louvier U, Espil-Taris C, et al. Evaluating next-generation sequencing in neuromuscular diseases with neonatal respiratory distress. Eur J Neurol 2021;31:78–87.

56. Finsterer J. Congenital myasthenic syndromes. Orphanet J Rare Dis 2019;14:57.

57. Turk M, Weber I, Vogt-Ladner G, et al. Diaphragmatic dysfunction as the presenting symptom in neuromuscular disorders: a retrospective longitudinal study of etiology and outcome in 30 German patients. Neuromuscul Disord 2018;28:484–90.

58. Teoh HL, Carey K, Sampaio H, et al. Inherited paediatric motor neuron disorders: beyond spinal muscular atrophy. Neural Plast 2017;2017:6509493.

59. Pitt M, Houlden H, Jacobs J, et al. Severe infantile neuropathy with diaphragmatic weakness and its relationship to SMARD1. Brain 2003;126:2682–92.

60. Butterfield RJ, Stevenson TJ, Xing I, et al. Congenital lethal motor neuron disease with a novel defect in ribosome biogenesis. Neurology 2014;82:1322–30.

Uncommon Etiologies of Shock

Shilpa Narayan, MD, Tara L. Petersen, MD, MSEd*

KEYWORDS

- Cardiogenic shock • Distributive shock • Hypovolemic shock • Obstructive shock
- Dissociative shock

KEY POINTS

- Broad classifications of shock are defined based on physiologic response to a variety of insults. There is significant overlap across these classifications. All etiologies share the common failure to provide sufficient energy to meet metabolic demands.
- Rare causes of distributive shock include adrenal crisis and calcium channel blocker toxicity. Both may result in a shock state that is refractory to conventional resuscitative therapies and thus requires a high index of suspicion to promote early and directed resuscitative management.
- Systemic capillary leak syndrome (SCLS) is a rare etiology of hypovolemic shock. It is characterized by episodes of severe hypotension, hemoconcentration, and hypoalbuminemia.
- Acute myocardial infarction (AMI) is the most common cause of cardiogenic shock (CS); however, non–AMI-related CS is becoming more common, and thus recognition of CS in other disease states is vital.
- Dyshemoglobinemias may result in dissociative shock because of the inability of the hemoglobin molecule to release oxygen at the tissue level. In these circumstances, tissue perfusion is adequate, but oxygen delivery is impaired.

INTRODUCTION

Shock is a state in which the cardiovascular system fails to adequately deliver the required substrates to maintain tissue homeostasis and cellular metabolism.[1,2] Without correction, reversible cellular damage rapidly progresses to irreversible injury and may lead to multiorgan failure and/or death. It is imperative to recognize and intervene on a patient in undifferentiated shock, while efficiently working on identifying the etiology to reverse the shock state. In some cases, rare causes of shock occur, and the purpose of this review is to provide a resource for consideration in patients with unclear etiology of shock physiology. For the purposes of this article, we have

The Medical College of Wisconsin, 9000 W. Wisconsin Avenue, MS B550B, Milwaukee, WI 53226, USA
* Corresponding author.
E-mail address: tpetersen@mcw.edu

Crit Care Clin 38 (2022) 429–441
https://doi.org/10.1016/j.ccc.2021.11.009
0749-0704/22/© 2021 Elsevier Inc. All rights reserved.

differentiated shock into 4 broad categories, including distributive, cardiogenic, hypo-volemic, and dissociative (**Table 1**). Presentations of shock often manifest with char-acteristics of one or many of the aforementioned categories.

Distributive Shock

Distributive shock, also known as vasodilatory shock, occurs when there is severe pe-ripheral vasodilatation leading to redistribution of blood flow away from vital organs, such as the brain, heart, and kidneys, leading to poor delivery of required substrates to these systems. The most common causes of distributive shock include septic shock and anaphylaxis. Spinal cord injury leading to neurogenic shock is another form that should be rapidly recognized in trauma patients. Vasodilatory shock is also seen in the systemic inflammatory response syndrome (SIRS), which is most commonly associated with sepsis; however, noninfectious etiologies of SIRS must be considered as listed in **Box 1**.[3] We will focus the rest of this section on rarer causes of distributive shock, which include adrenal failure or exposure to vasodilatory drugs. Systemic capillary leak syndrome (SCLS) is an entity with features of distributive shock that will be further detailed in the hypovolemic shock section.

Table 1
Etiologies of shock

Category of Shock	Common Etiologies Examples	Rare Etiologies
Distributive	Sepsis Toxic shock syndrome Anaphylaxis SIRS Neurogenic shock	Adrenal insufficiency MIS-C Drug exposures • Barbiturates • Phenothiazines • Antihypertensives
Hypovolemic	Dehydration • Inadequate intake • Gastrointestinal losses • Renal losses • Integumentary losses (such as burns, Stevens Johnson Syndrome, insensible losses) Hemorrhage	SCLS
Cardiogenic	Myocardial infarction Congestive heart failure Cardiomyopathy Myocarditis Dysrhythmias	Valvular disease MIS-C Postcardiac surgery Postcardiac arrest Dynamic outflow tract obstruction Thyrotoxicosis • Pericardial tamponade • Critical aortic stenosis • Tension pneumothorax • Pulmonary embolism
Dissociative	Carbon monoxide poisoning	Methemoglobinemia Sulfhemoglobinemia Cyanide toxicity

Abbreviation: MIS-C, multisystem inflammatory syndrome in children associated with COVID-19 infection; SCLS, systemic capillary leak syndrome; SIRS, systemic inflammatory response syndrome.

Box 1
Noninfectious causes of systemic inflammatory response syndrome (SIRS)
Postoperative
Cardiovascular disease
Trauma
Postcardiac arrest
Autoimmune disorders
Vasculitis
Pancreatitis
Burns

Adrenal crisis

Epidemiology and pathophysiology. Adrenal crisis is characterized by an acute, rapid deterioration leading to hypotension and distributive shock in those with adrenal insufficiency (AI). Owing to the nonspecific symptoms of AI, diagnosis of AI is often delayed, and adrenal crisis may be the first presentation of undiagnosed AI. In a cross-sectional study utilizing a patient questionnaire and medical records, less than 30% of women and 50% of men with AI were diagnosed within 6 months of the onset of symptoms. Up to two-thirds of patients in this study experienced prior misdiagnosis. The incidence of adrenal crisis in undiagnosed AI is not known; however, in those with known primary or secondary AI, there is an incidence of 6.3 crises per 100 patient-years.[4–6] Adrenal crisis is a life-threatening emergency. Clinicians should consider AI at the etiology of distributive shock in fluid-refractory and vasopressor-refractory shock. In a chronic cortisol deficient state, alpha-1 receptor expression in arterioles is downregulated, leading to vasoplegia and distributive shock.[7] See **Table 2** for a list of common etiologies of AI and precipitating factors of adrenal crisis.[8]

Assessment and management. In addition to a distributive shock state, other common signs and symptoms include weakness, fever, anorexia, nausea, vomiting, abdominal pain, fever, hypoglycemia, electrolyte derangements, confusion, and coma. These signs and symptoms are vague and overlap with some of the findings typical of septic shock. A task force from the Endocrine Society Clinical Guidelines Subcommittee recommends the immediate administration of parenteral hydrocortisone 100 mg or 50 mg/m^2 for children in suspected or confirmed cases of AI presenting in crisis or distributive shock.[9] Treatment should not be delayed to obtain diagnostic testing, which is adrenocorticotropic hormone (ACTH) stimulation testing. Random serum cortisol, ACTH, aldosterone, dehydroepiandrosterone-sulfate, and renin can be obtained before administration of hydrocortisone and may aid if the diagnosis of AI in a patient is unknown.[8] Continuous or scheduled intermittent dosing of hydrocortisone is often needed after an initial bolus dose and may be tapered to maintenance dosing over 24 to 72 hours once patient stabilizes.[10]

Calcium channel blocker toxicity

Pathophysiology. Vasodilatory shock secondary to overdose of calcium channel blocker (CCB) agents is a result of decreased peripheral vascular resistance and direct peripheral arterial vasodilatation. CCBs also inhibit the influx of calcium in myocardial cells, thus also having negative inotropic and chronotropic effects. Owing to this mechanism of action, management is often refractory to typical management

Table 2
Causes and risk factors for AI

Causes of AI	Risk Factors for Adrenal Crisis
Primary AI:	Gastrointestinal illness
• Autoimmune diseases and syndromes (eg, autoimmune polyglandular syndrome types 1 and 2)	Infection
	Perisurgical
	Physical stress
• Infections (tuberculosis, AIDS, fungal)	Psychological stress
• Metastasis	Pregnancy
• Congenital adrenal hyperplasia	Thyrotoxicosis
• Adrenomyeloneuropathy/leukodystrophy	
• Adrenal hemorrhage or removal	
Secondary AI:	Diabetes mellitus (types I and II)
• Pituitary tumor	Premature ovarian failure
• Other tumors (craniopharyngioma, meningioma)	Hypogonadism
• Pituitary surgery, radiation, infiltration	
• Head trauma	
• Long-term exogenous glucocorticoid use	

strategies of distributive shock. Sustained-release formulations are more commonly associated with severe CCB toxicity because of the delay of onset of symptoms and duration of effect.

Assessment and management. The mainstay of treatment begins with supportive care and gastrointestinal (GI) decontamination. However, if the patient progresses toward distributive shock, limited fluid resuscitation followed by the use of vasopressor support that provides inotropic, chronotropic, and vasoconstrictor properties is indicated. High-dose insulin infusions as a positive inotrope with a glucose infusion to maintain normoglycemia are also recommended. Intravenous calcium infusions have also shown some benefits. Extracorporeal support may have to be considered.[11] In severe cases, there is evolving literature to support the use of methylene blue (nitric oxide inhibitor) in CCB poisoning.[11,12]

Hypovolemic Shock

Hypovolemic shock, the most common type of shock in infants and children,[13] ensues when intravascular volume loss reaches a critical level. This results in diminished cardiac preload and reduced macrocirculation and microcirculation leading to inadequate organ perfusion. The most common causes of hypovolemic shock include dehydration and hemorrhage, both of which have numerous common and unique inciting mechanisms reported in the literature. There are a few rare causes of hypovolemic shock outside of decreased fluid intake, increased GI losses, skin/insensible losses, renal losses, and hemorrhage. Here we highlight a rare syndrome with a hallmark of dramatic intravascular fluid depletion with resultant development of hypoperfusion/shock.

Systemic capillary leak syndrome
First described by Clarkson and colleagues,[14] SCLS is a rare condition characterized by a dysfunctional inflammatory response and endothelial disruption leading to transient episodes of severe hypovolemia due to increased capillary permeability. This results in plasma extravasation and vascular collapse accompanied by hemoconcentration and hypoalbuminemia.[15] Notably, SCLS can be found in the literature under the categorization of both hypovolemic and distributive shock as the extravasation of fluid and

proteins from the intracellular space into the interstitial space results in profound intra-vascular volume depletion (hypovolemic shock) while the inflammatory response can mimic the clinical presentation of sepsis (distributive shock). The exact cause of vascular hyperpermeability is unclear, though it is postulated to be the result of a cytokine-mediated response leading to apoptosis of the endothelium.[14,15]

Epidemiology and pathophysiology. In the most recent epidemiologic review of SCLS, Druey and colleagues reported fewer than 500 cases of idiopathic SCLS since its original description in 1960. Notably, given the rarity of this condition, its mimicry of more common illnesses such as severe sepsis, and its high mortality without treat-ment, SCLS is likely underdiagnosed and thus underreported.[16] Most cases have been reported in middle-aged adults, although cases in children as young as 5 months old have been published.[17,18] Among patients who survive an initial attack, at least 70% are alive 5 years after diagnosis.[19]

Both primary (idiopathic) and secondary causes of SCLS have been described. Although the mechanistic understanding of idiopathic SCLS is still nascent, the work-ing hypothesis invokes an exaggerated microvascular endothelial response to surges of otherwise routinely encountered inflammatory mediators.[16]

Attacks of idiopathic SCLS usually demonstrate 3 phases. A prodromal phase, which is often reported as "flu-like" symptoms, including fatigue, nausea, and myalgia. The acute, or extravasation phase, develops over 1 to 4 days and is characterized by the presence of hypoalbuminemia, hypotension due to intravascular fluid losses, and resultant hemoconcentration.[19] This hemoconcentration may assist in differentiating SCLS from other causes of shock.[20] A recovery phase (also referred to as the fluid recruitment phase) ensues after several days and is characterized by the return of fluid into the intravascular space and subsequent diuresis.[19] Frequency of attacks ranges from a single episode in a lifetime to several attacks per year. In one series of 25 pa-tients, the median number of attacks per year was 3.[20]

The spectrum of diseases associated with secondary SCLS includes viral infections such as influenza and COVID-19,[21–25] hematologic malignancies, and medical treat-ments such as chemotherapy or therapeutic growth factors.[20]

Assessment and management. SCLS is a diagnosis of exclusion and is made when a patient presents with intravascular hypovolemia, generalized edema, and the triad of hypoalbuminemia, hypotension, and hemoconcentration without an otherwise identifi-able alternative cause.

Initial management of shock secondary to SCLS is aimed at resuscitative efforts, including securing the airway, correcting hypoxemia, and restoring perfusion using a strategy of conservative fluid administration and intravenous vasoactive agents as indicated. Upon stabilization, treatment is then directed toward the prevention of com-plications from fluid overload, including pulmonary edema and compartment syn-drome. Nearly all patients will require diuretic therapy during this phase, and some may require renal replacement therapy.[15,16]

Cardiogenic Shock

Cardiogenic shock (CS) is a clinical syndrome of decreased end-organ perfusion and hypoxia due to diminished cardiac output. It is seen in pathology causing a primary car-diac insult, and unfortunately continues to carry a high mortality rate in the range of 30% to 50% despite advances in cardiac interventions.[26,27] Presenting signs and symptoms of CS include hypotension, tachycardia, altered mental status, diminished peripheral perfusion, peripheral and pulmonary edema, jugular venous distention, lactic acidosis, and oliguria. Arrhythmias are also common. Although many trials have provided parameters to define CS, it is important to remember CS is a clinical diagnosis and thus specific hemodynamic parameters are not required to diagnose and treat CS.[28] For the purposes of this review, obstructive etiologies of poor cardiac output are included as a subcategory of CS and will be discussed in this section.

Epidemiology and pathophysiology

In CS, a primary insult causes decreased cardiac output because of ineffective stroke volume, leading to hypotension and poor end-organ perfusion. Initially, there is compensatory peripheral vasoconstriction causing a normal-high systemic vascular resistance (SVR) state with persistent hypotension. Without intervention, there will be a progressive shift into a vasodilatory state and low SVR state that subsequently leads to end-organ injury and/or failure, worsening acidosis, and severe dysfunction of cellular respiration.[28] Previously, up to 80% of CS cases were attributed to acute myocardial infarction (AMI). Although AMI remains the leading etiology of CS, a multicenter study published by the Critical Care Cardiology Trials Network in 2019 reviewing medical admissions to the CICU found that only 30% of CS patients were due to AMI. Other leading etiologies included ischemic cardiomyopathy in 18% of patients and nonischemic cardiomyopathy in 28%. Less commonly, cardiac causes of CS not related to myocardial dysfunction were seen in 17% of the patients, and there were unidentified causes in 7% of patients. The reduction in the incidence of AMI and increased prevalence of advanced heart failure are some of the contributing factors of this shift in epidemiology. It is important to note that up to two-thirds of the patients with CS unrelated to AMI in this study had underlying heart failure.[29]

Assessment and management

The diversity of pathophysiology of the rare non-AMI causes of CS is presented in **Table 3**.[28,30]

Obstructive shock

Another subtype of CS is poor cardiac output due to dynamic outflow tract obstruction, also referred to as obstructive shock. In obstructive shock, there is interference with left ventricular (LV) cardiac output even though the intrinsic myocardial function and intravascular volume status are within normal range. Obstructive shock can be due to intracardiac or extracardiac obstruction, on either the pulmonary or systemic side. We will discuss, in detail, some of the entities leading to this form of shock.

Epidemiology and pathophysiology. The incidence of obstructive shock is unknown; however, it is considered to be a rare form of shock. Disease states causing both decreased diastolic filling and decreased ventricular preload include vena cava compression syndrome, tension pneumothorax, pericardial tamponade, and high PEEP (increased mean airway pressure) in ventilated patients. Increased right ventricular afterload causing decreased preload can be caused by pulmonary arterial embolus, severe pulmonary hypertension, or space-occupying mediastinal masses. Obstruction to LV outflow is caused by high systemic afterload, such as in aortic dissections, critical aortic stenosis, or extracardiac masses. All of these entities share the common feature of a rapid and critical drop in both cardiac output and perfusion to all organ systems.[31,32]

Diagnosis and treatment. Presenting symptoms are similar to those mentioned earlier in this section on CS and include tachycardia, hypotension, altered mental status, oliguria, tachypnea, and other signs of end-organ failure. Owing to compensatory mechanisms, hypotension may not be as prominent initially; however, given the rapid

Table 3
Causes and management of nonmyocardial infarction cardiogenic shock

Etiology	Clinical Causes, Features, and Pathophysiology	Management
Valvular Disease	• Decompensation of known valvular heart disease • Ischemic injury leading to valvular rupture • Infective endocarditis • Critical aortic stenosis	• Consider surgical intervention • Identify precipitating factors • Mechanical cardiac support may be needed
Postcardiac Surgery	• Due to cytokine release after CPB • Associated with longer CPB and pre-existing comorbidities • Often presents as vasodilatory cardiogenic shock due to inflammatory state • Consider dynamic LV obstruction vs RV dysfunction	• Early identification crucial • Correction of reversible parameters (electrolytes, tamponade, others) • Minimize excess catecholamine administration • Medically optimize myocardial contractility and output while minimizing increasing SVR • Consider mechanical cardiac support early
Postcardiac arrest	• Global myocardial stunning causing pump failure • Myocardial ischemia-reperfusion injury exacerbates oxidative stress, cytokine release, and microthrombi formation • Worse in delayed initiation of CPR, longer duration of CPR, nonshockable rhythms, older age, and pre-existing comorbidities	• Medically optimize myocardial contractility and output while minimizing increasing SVR • Consider mechanical cardiac support early
• Thyrotoxicosis or "thyroid storm"	• Causes severe LV dysfunction through direct effect on the myocardium • High clinical suspicion needed in patients with a history of endocrinologic symptoms or disorders and/or exposure to medications associated with thyroid disease	• Limited data available • Beta-blockade may exacerbate cardiogenic shock • Therapeutic plasma exchange to reduce thyroid hormone levels may be effective • Mechanical cardiac support to allow for LV recovery

Abbreviations: CPB, cardiopulmonary bypass; CPR, cardiopulmonary resuscitation; LV, left ventricle; RV, right ventricle; SVR, systemic vascular resistance.

progression of obstructive shock, a high index of suspicion and movement toward intervention is critically important. Treatment should target the underlying etiology and is specific to each entity.[31,32]

Dissociative Shock

Dissociative shock is a rare category of shock and results from the inability of the hemoglobin molecule to release oxygen at the tissue level. In these circumstances, tissue perfusion is adequate, but cellular oxygen delivery is impaired. This shift of the oxyhemoglobin dissociation curve results in failure to deliver enough oxygen to meet tissue metabolic demands. Some may note the following disease entities do not classically fit into the classification of "shock," given the presence of preserved circulation/perfusion. Although perfusion is not always compromised in these cases, the resultant acute cellular oxygen deficiency caused by the acquired dyshemoglobinemias warrants mention within the discussion of shock, given the associated unique diagnostic and treatment considerations.

Carboxyhemoglobinemia (carbon monoxide poisoning)

Carbon monoxide (CO) poisoning is the most frequently encountered acquired dyshemoglobinemia. Smoke inhalation is responsible for most unintentional cases. Other potential sources of exposure include poorly ventilated combustion engines, including motor vehicles, water pipe smoking, and poorly functioning heating systems.[33–36] The clinical findings of CO poisoning are both nonspecific and highly variable. Symptoms range from headache (most common), malaise, nausea, and dizziness to arrhythmias, confusion, and eventually coma. Notably, although a "cherry red" appearance of the skin and lips is classically described as an indicator of CO poisoning, this is not seen in all cases of acute poisoning and thus is considered an insensitive sign.[37]

Treatment of carbon monoxide poisoning is directed at removal from the source, cardiorespiratory support/resuscitation and 100% supplemental oxygen via a non-breather mask or endotracheal tube. There is controversy surrounding the utilization of hyperbaric oxygen (HBO) therapy to decrease the incidence and severity of delayed neurocognitive deficits. Expert guidelines surrounding the use of HBO have been published and consultation with a medical toxicologist or regional poison control center is encouraged whenever HBO therapy is being considered.[33–35]

Acquired methemoglobinemia

Epidemiology and pathophysiology. Methemoglobin (MetHb) is a form of hemoglobin that has been oxidized, changing the heme configuration from the ferrous (Fe2+) state to the ferric (Fe3+) state. MetHb has an impaired ability to bind oxygen and thus results in diminished tissue oxygen delivery. The consequences of MetHb depend on whether it is chronically or acutely increased. Individuals with acute toxic methemoglobinemia can suffer severe hypoxia with resultant end-organ dysfunction leading to death.[38]

Most cases of methemoglobinemia are acquired and result from exposure to medications or environmental toxins (**Table 4**).[38] Although acquired methemoglobinemia is uncommon, it is important to note that infants are thought to be at the highest risk as they have lower baseline MetHb-reductase levels and altered oxygen-hemoglobin dissociation properties.[39]

Assessment and management. Methemoglobinemia should be suspected in patients with unexplained cyanosis or hypoxia that does not resolve with supplemental oxygen. Symptoms may range from mild cyanosis, dyspnea, headache, fatigue, and irritability to lethargy, shock, severe respiratory depression, coma, seizures, and death.[40] Classically, MetHb will cause chocolate-brown discoloration of blood that does not resolve upon oxygenation, which can be a key-diagnostic feature. Typically, the severity of symptoms correlates with the MetHb level. MetHb levels above 30% to 40% can be life-threatening. In some cases, toxicity may be exacerbated by pre-existing conditions such as cardiac disease or coexistent glucose-6-phosphate dehydrogenase (G6PD) deficiency.

Identification of an exposure history along with observation of blood color via phlebotomy sample should result in a high index of suspicion and prompt further diagnostic testing, including co-oximetry and arterial blood gas sampling (normal Pao_2) with methemoglobin level testing.

Management includes discontinuation of exposure, supplemental oxygen, and supportive/resuscitative care. Those with severe symptoms and/or MetHb levels above

Table 4
Examples of chemicals and medications that may cause acquired methemoglobinemia

Chemicals/Substances	Medications
Acetanilide *In varnishes, dyes, rubber*	Aminosalicylic acid
Anilines *In dyes, red wax crayons*	Bismuth subnitrates
Antifreeze	Clofazimine
Benzene derivatives *Solvents*	Chloroquine
Chlorates and chromates *Used in industrial, chemical synthesis*	Dapsone
Hydrogen peroxide	Local anesthetics: sprays/creams such as benzocaine (found in teething ointments), lidocaine, and prilocaine
Naphthalene *Used in mothballs*	Menadione
Naphthoquinone *Used in chemical synthesis*	Metoclopramide
Nitrates and nitrites *Can be found in foods, well water* *Foods include almonds,* *sorghum, cassava (tapioca),* *beans, bamboo shoots*	Methylene blue [a]
Nitrobenzene *Solvent*	Nitric oxide
Paraquat *Used in herbicides*	Nitroglycerin
Resorcinol *Used in wood extraction and resin*	Phenacetin
	Phenazopyridine HCl Phenytoin Primaquine Rasburicase Rifampin Quinones Silver nitrate Sulfonamides

[a] Although methylene blue is a treatment for methemoglobinemia, it is an oxidant and may worsen the clinical status of individuals with G6PD deficiency. Notably, in high doses, methylene blue can paradoxically increase methemoglobinemia.

30% are treated with methylene blue or ascorbic acid. It is important to note that methylene blue is an oxidant and thus should not be used in patients with G6PD because of the risk of hemolytic anemia. For such individuals, ascorbic acid is the preferred treatment modality. Exchange transfusion and HBO should be considered for patients who are unresponsive to initial treatment.[38]

Sulfhemoglobinemia
Epidemiology and pathophysiology. Sulfhemoglobinemia is a very rare condition that can result from exposure to any substance containing a sulfur atom with the ability to bind hemoglobin. The resultant sulfhemoglobin (SulfHb) is a stable, green-pigmented

molecule, which constitutes less than 1% of normal hemoglobin in vivo. SulfHb is made by the oxidation of the iron in hemoglobin to a ferric state which cannot bind oxygen. Notably, the formation of the sulfhemoglobin moiety is irreversible, lasting the lifetime of the erythrocyte. Environmental chemicals and medications that have been linked to producing sulfhemoglobinemia include acetanilide, phenacetin, nitrates, nitroglycerine, trinitrotoluene, metoclopramide, methylene blue, and sulfur compounds.[39]

Assessment and management. Patients present in a similar fashion to those with methemoglobinemia (cyanosis, normal Pao_2). Notably, multiwavelength co-oximetry does not accurately distinguish SulfHb from MetHb. Specialized biochemical testing is available in only a few centers across the world, thus the ability to obtain results quickly is limited. Unlike methemoglobin formation, which is reversible with the antidote methylene blue, sulfhemoglobin formation has no known antidote. Thus, the lack of response to methylene blue can provide a diagnostic clue while awaiting biochemical testing results and should, in severe cases, prompt consideration of alternative therapies such as exchange transfusion.[41,42]

Cyanohemoglobinemia (cyanide toxicity)
Epidemiology and pathophysiology. Cyanide toxicity is rare. According to the Toxic Exposure Surveillance System of the American Association of Poison Control Centers, there were 283 single-substance human exposures to nonrodenticide cyanide in 2019, inclusive of 2 fatalities.[43] Cyanide toxicity may result from a broad range of exposures, including combustion of products containing carbon and nitrogen during domestic fires (most common), industrial (mining, plastic manufacturing), medical (prolonged infusions of nitroprusside), diet (cyanogenic glycosides found in fruit pits/seeds) and acts of bioterrorism. Cyanide toxicity results in cellular hypoxia via poisoning of the electron transport chain. The resultant anaerobic metabolism leads to the formation of lactic acid and the development of an anion gap metabolic acidosis. In addition, cyanohemoglobin is unable to transport oxygen and thus exacerbates tissue hypoxia.[44]

Assessment and management. Clinical findings depend on the amount, duration, and route of exposure. Cardiovascular and central nervous system dysfunction are most prominent and include initial tachycardia and hypertension followed by bradycardia, hypotension, and dysrhythmias as well as headache, confusion, vertigo, loss of consciousness, and seizures. Other hallmark clinical features include flushing ("cherry-red" appearance) of the skin caused by a high venous oxyhemoglobin concentration because of the impairment of oxygen utilization by tissues. Although classically described, it is important to note that this sign is present in the minority of patients with cyanide toxicity.[45]

As with all uncommon entities, diagnosis requires clinicians to maintain a high index of suspicion based on history and presentation. Diagnostic testing should include routine laboratory evaluation including general chemistries and arterial blood gas sampling to assess for anion gap acidosis as well as a serum lactate and, if possible, a central venous blood gas (to assess for diminished venous-arterial Po_2 gradient). Blood cyanide concentrations may not correlate with toxicity and results are often not available in time to guide acute management. Evaluation for concurrent toxicities, such as carbon monoxide and methemoglobinemia, is also an important consideration. Treatment includes resuscitation, decontamination, and antidote administration directed at the binding of cyanide, induction of methemoglobinemia, and use of sulfur donors. It is recommended that clinicians should seek consultation from a medical toxicologist or regional poison center in these cases.[44–46]

SUMMARY

Disease classification within discrete shock categories is often difficult because of variation in clinical presentation and physiologic response to therapy over time. Patients often present with mixed shock pictures and thus close monitoring and re-evaluation are paramount to both the resuscitation and postresuscitation phases of management. Likewise, although most patients will ultimately be diagnosed with common etiologies of shock, clinicians must continue to rely on a thorough history and focused physical examination as key features can promote higher indices of suspicion for uncommon diseases where timely recognition can significantly alter management and clinical outcomes.

CLINICS CARE POINTS

- Distributive shock is the leading cause of shock in adult patients. Adrenal crisis and calcium channel blocker toxicity are rare causes of distributive shock that require rapid identification and medical intervention to reverse the process.

- Systemic capillary leak syndrome (SCLS) is a rare etiology of hypovolemic shock. It is characterized by episodes of severe hypotension, hemoconcentration, and hypoalbuminemia.

- Acute myocardial infarction (AMI) is the most common cause of cardiogenic shock (CS); however, non–AMI-related CS is becoming more common, and thus recognition of CS in other disease states is vital.

- Dyshemoglobinemias may result in dissociative shock because of the inability of the hemoglobin molecule to release oxygen at the tissue level. In these circumstances, tissue perfusion is adequate, but oxygen delivery is impaired.

DISCLOSURE

The authors have nothing to disclose.

REFERENCES

1. Vincent J-L, De Backer D. Circulatory shock. N Engl J Med 2013;369(18): 1726–34.
2. Nadel S, Kissoon NT, Ranjit S. Recognition and initial management of shock. In: Nichols DG, editor. Rogers' textbook of pediatric intensive care. 4th edition. Philadelphia: Lippincott Williams & Wilkins; 2008. p. 372–5, chap 26.
3. Dulhunty JM, Lipman J, Finfer S. Does severe non-infectious SIRS differ from severe sepsis? Intensive Care Med 2008;34(9):1654–61.
4. Tompkins MG, Bissell BD, Sowders V, et al. Inclusion of adrenal crisis in the differential diagnosis of distributive shock. Am J Health Syst Pharm 2020;77(6):415–7.
5. Bleicken B, Hahner S, Ventz M, et al. Delayed diagnosis of adrenal insufficiency is common: a cross-sectional study in 216 patients. Am J Med Sci 2010;339(6):525–31.
6. Hahner S, Loeffler M, Bleicken B, et al. Epidemiology of adrenal crisis in chronic adrenal insufficiency: the need for new prevention strategies. Eur J Endocrinol 2010;162(3):597–602.
7. Smith N, Lopez RA, Silberman M. Distributive shock. StatPearls publishing. Available at: https://pubmed.ncbi.nlm.nih.gov/29261964/.
8. Puar THK, Stikkelbroeck NMML, Smans LCCJ, et al. Adrenal crisis: still a deadly event in the 21st century. Am J Med 2016;129(3):339.e1-9.

9. Bornstein SR, Allolio B, Arlt W, et al. Diagnosis and treatment of primary adrenal insufficiency: an endocrine society clinical practice guideline. J Clin Endocrinol Metab 2016;101(2):364–89.

10. Bancos I, Hahner S, Tomlinson J, et al. Diagnosis and management of adrenal insufficiency. Lancet Diabetes Endocrinol 2015;3(3):216–26.

11. Graudins A, Lee HM, Druda D. Calcium channel antagonist and beta-blocker overdose: antidotes and adjunct therapies. Br J Clin Pharmacol 2016;81(3): 453–61.

12. Warrick BJ, Tataru AP, Smolinske S. A systematic analysis of methylene blue for drug-induced shock. Clin Toxicol 2016;54(7):547–55.

13. Smith L, Alcamo A, Carcillo J, et al. Shock states. In: Fuhrman B, Zimmerman J, editors. Pediatric critical care. 6th edition. Philadelphia: Elsevier Saunders; 2021. p. 352–62, chap 34.

14. Clarkson B, Thompson D, Horwith M, et al. Cyclical edema and shock due to increased capillary permeability. Am J Med 1960;29:193–216.

15. Druey KM, Greipp PR. Narrative review: the systemic capillary leak syndrome. Ann Intern Med 2010;153(2):90–8.

16. Druey KM, Parikh SM. Idiopathic systemic capillary leak syndrome (Clarkson disease). J Allergy Clin Immunol 2017;140(3):663–70.

17. Karatzios C, Gauvin F, Egerszegi EP, et al. Systemic capillary leak syndrome presenting as recurrent shock. Pediatr Crit Care Med 2006;7(4):377–9.

18. Bozzini MA, Milani GP, Bianchetti MG, et al. Idiopathic systemic capillary leak syndrome (Clarkson syndrome) in childhood: systematic literature review. Eur J Pediatr 2018;177(8):1149–54.

19. Dhir V, Arya V, Malav IC, et al. Idiopathic systemic capillary leak syndrome (SCLS): case report and systematic review of cases reported in the last 16 years. Intern Med 2007;46(12):899–904.

20. Kapoor P, Greipp PT, Schaefer EW, et al. Idiopathic systemic capillary leak syndrome (Clarkson's disease): the Mayo clinic experience. Mayo Clin Proc 2010; 85(10):905–12.

21. Case R, Ramaniuk A, Martin P, et al. Systemic capillary leak syndrome secondary to coronavirus disease 2019. Chest 2020;158(6):e267–8.

22. Beber A, Dellai F, Abdel Jaber M, et al. Systemic capillary leak syndrome triggered by SARS-CoV2 infection: case report and systematic review. Scand J Rheumatol 2021;1–3. https://doi.org/10.1080/03009742.2021.1917145.

23. Ebdrup L, Druey KM, Druey K, et al. Severe capillary leak syndrome with cardiac arrest triggered by influenza virus infection. BMJ Case Rep 2018;08:2018doi.

24. Lawrence JL, Hindi H. Capillary leak syndrome aggravated by influenza type A infection. Cureus 2018;10(4):e2554.

25. Sousa A, Len O, Escolà-Vergé L, et al. Influenza A virus infection is associated with systemic capillary leak syndrome: case report and systematic review of the literature. Antivir Ther 2016;21(2):181–3.

26. Vahdatpour C, Collins D, Goldberg S. Cardiogenic shock. J Am Heart Assoc 2019;8(8):e011991.

27. Berg DD, Bohula EA, Morrow DA. Epidemiology and causes of cardiogenic shock. Curr Opin Crit Care 2021;27(4):401–8.

28. Chioncel O, Parissis J, Mebazaa A, et al. Epidemiology, pathophysiology and contemporary management of cardiogenic shock – a position statement from the Heart Failure Association of the European Society of Cardiology. Eur J Heart Fail 2020;22(8):1315–41.

29. Berg DD, Bohula EA, Van Diepen S, et al. Epidemiology of shock in contemporary cardiac intensive care units. Circ Cardiovasc Qual Outcomes 2019;12(3). https://doi.org/10.1161/circoutcomes.119.005618.
30. Modarresi M, Amro A, Amro M, et al. Management of cardiogenic shock due to thyrotoxicosis: a systematic literature review. Curr Cardiol Rev 2020;16(4): 326–32.
31. Standl T, Annecke T, Cascorbi I, et al. The nomenclature, definition and distinction of types of shock. Deutsches Aerzteblatt Online 2018. https://doi.org/10.3238/arztebl.2018.0757.
32. Kumar A, Parrillo JE. Shock: classification, pathophysiology, and approach to management. In: Parrillo J, Dellinger RP, editors. Critical care medicine: principles of diagnosis and management in the adult. Philadelphia: Elsevier Inc; 2008. p. 379–422, chap 22.
33. Ernst A, Zibrak JD. Carbon monoxide poisoning. N Engl J Med 1998;339(22): 1603–8.
34. Weaver LK. Carbon monoxide poisoning. Crit Care Clin 1999;15(2):297–317, viii.
35. Rose JJ, Wang L, Xu Q, et al. Carbon monoxide poisoning: pathogenesis, management, and future directions of therapy. Am J Respir Crit Care Med 2017; 195(5):596–606.
36. Nguyen V, Salama M, Fernandez D, et al. Comparison between carbon monoxide poisoning from hookah smoking versus other sources. Clin Toxicol (Phila) 2020; 58(12):1320–5.
37. Harper A, Croft-Baker J. Carbon monoxide poisoning: undetected by both patients and their doctors. Age Ageing 2004;33(2):105–9.
38. Kaminecki I, Huang D. Methemoglobinemia. Pediatr Rev 2021;42(3):164–6.
39. Easley R, Brady K, Tobias J. Hematologic emergencies. In: Nichols D, editor. Rogers' textbook of pediatric intensive care. 4th edition. Philadelphia: Lippincott Williams & Wilkins; 2008. p. 1730–3, chap 101.
40. Cortazzo JA, Lichtman AD. Methemoglobinemia: a review and recommendations for management. J Cardiothorac Vasc Anesth 2014;28(4):1043–7.
41. Lu HC, Shih RD, Marcus S, et al. Pseudomethemoglobinemia: a case report and review of sulfhemoglobinemia. Arch Pediatr Adolesc Med 1998;152(8):803–5.
42. Aravindhan N, Chisholm DG. Sulfhemoglobinemia presenting as pulse oximetry desaturation. Anesthesiology 2000;93(3):883–4.
43. Gummin DD, Mowry JB, Beuhler MC, et al. 2019 annual report of the American association of poison control centers' national poison data system (NPDS): 37th annual report. Clin Toxicol (Phila) 2020;58(12):1360–541.
44. Vogel SN, Sultan TR, Ten Eyck RP. Cyanide poisoning. Clin Toxicol 1981;18(3): 367–83.
45. Parker-Cote JL, Rizer J, Vakkalanka JP, et al. Challenges in the diagnosis of acute cyanide poisoning. Clin Toxicol (Phila) 2018;56(7):609–17.
46. Huzar TF, George T, Cross JM. Carbon monoxide and cyanide toxicity: etiology, pathophysiology and treatment in inhalation injury. Expert Rev Respir Med 2013; 7(2):159–70.

Genetic Defects that Predispose to Serious Viral Infections

James Verbsky, MD, PhD

KEYWORDS

- Primary immune deficiency • Viral infections • Toll-like receptors
- RIG-like receptors • Combined immune deficiency • Innate immunity
- Adaptive immunity

KEY POINTS

- Primary immune deficiencies can present with only viral infections, or with viral infections in the setting of other infectious disease.
- There are over 400 genetic defects causing immune deficiencies, and sequencing panels are a rapid way to screen for these defects.
- Early detection of primary immune deficiencies can lead to interventions to prevent further infectious pathology.

Abbreviations	
PIDD	primary immune deficiency disorder
RIPK1	receptor interacting serine/threonine kinase 1
TRIF	TIR domain-containing adaptor inducing interferon-beta

INTRODUCTION

A protective immune response to viruses involves both the innate and adaptive immune systems. Viruses are first detected when cells recognize evolutionarily conserved viral molecular patterns, such as viral DNA or RNA, via cell surface and intracellular receptors. This recognition initiates an inflammatory response as well as other mechanisms that attempt to limit the early spread of the virus until a specific adaptive immune response against the virus is generated.[1] This response is complex, involving a variety of receptors and inflammatory proteins, with 2 of the more essential steps being the production of interferon proteins and subsequent interferon stimulation that limit the replication of viruses, particularly in nonhematopoietic cells.[2] Innate

Medical College of Wisconsin, 8701 Watertown Plank Road, Milwaukee, WI 53226, USA
E-mail address: jverbsky@mcw.edu

Crit Care Clin 38 (2022) 443–453
https://doi.org/10.1016/j.ccc.2021.11.012
0749-0704/22/© 2021 Elsevier Inc. All rights reserved.

immune antigen presentation cells, such as dendritic cells, then present the viral antigens to T and B lymphocytes in secondary lymphoid organs such as lymph nodes and mucosal-associated lymphoid tissue. The adaptive immune response then generates virus-specific T cells (ie, cytotoxic CD8 T cells), which are essential to clearing infected cells, and virus-specific CD4 helper T cells and B cells, which produce antibody that can neutralize free viral particles.

Defects in innate viral sensors lead to very specific viral susceptibility with an otherwise normal immune response to other pathogens, whereas adaptive immune defects generally vary in the spectrum and severity of infections. For example, defects in the Toll-like receptor 3 (TLR3) pathway have a limited viral susceptibility pattern consisting primarily of recurrent herpes simplex virus (HSV) infections affecting only the brain; these disorders are discussed further in this article. Cell-mediated or combined immune defects that involve the development and/or function of T cells can result in a wide susceptibility to viruses with significant severity and furthermore typically result in additional susceptibility to bacterial, fungal, and opportunistic pathogens (eg, *Cryptosporidium*, *Pneumocystis*). Humoral immune defects, which affect B-lymphocyte development and/or antibody production, result in significant susceptibility to encapsulated bacteria, as well as a somewhat isolated susceptibility to enteroviral infections.[3]

CLINICAL AND LABORATORY EVALUATION OF A PATIENT WITH SEVERE, UNUSUAL, OR RECALCITRANT VIRAL INFECTIONS

When confronted with a patient with severe or recurrent viral infections, a careful history and examination should establish the types of viruses, extent of organ involvement, and history of infections with other pathogens. Combined immune deficiencies affecting T and B cells often result in susceptibility to a variety of pathogens, including opportunistic pathogens. Suggestive findings on examination such as microcephaly, ataxia, telangiectasias, or pigmentary defects in the setting of viral infections can direct one to specific diagnoses (eg, ataxia-telangiectasia, Nijmegen breakage syndrome, Chediak-Higashi syndrome).

A family history of infections or malignancy, or the death of family members in childhood, can be informative. The onset and types of other infections is useful because each PIDD can have a specific set of infectious susceptibilities. Physical examination findings can also help point to a specific diagnosis. With respect to inheritance patterns, PIDDs with viral susceptibility can be autosomal recessive, X-linked recessive, or autosomal dominant and can vary from neonatal to adult onset. The most severe defects tend to present in the first year of life and are usually autosomal recessive or X-linked recessive disorders. Inquiring about malignancy is essential, as T- and B-cell receptor generation requires DNA repair enzymes, and DNA repair defects can result in combined immune deficiency and increased predisposition of malignancies such as lymphoma.

The initial diagnostic laboratory evaluation should include a broad immune deficiency workup consisting of the following:

- Immunoglobulin G, A, M, and E quantification
- Specific vaccine titers (eg, tetanus and pneumococcus) in individuals previously vaccinated against these pathogens to assess whether a response was generated
- Lymphocyte subset enumeration, including T-, B-, and natural killer (NK) cell counts as well as memory and naïve T-cell percentages
- T-cell mitogen assay

- In some cases, NK cytotoxicity studies can be helpful to evaluate cytotoxic T-cell function

The results of this screen can help narrow the differential diagnosis. For example, lack of B lymphocytes and immunoglobulins in a male patient with disseminated enteroviral infection would highly suggest X-linked agammaglobulinemia. *Pneumocystis* infection in a patient with an elevated immunoglobulin M (IgM) and low IgG is a classic presentation of X-linked hyper-IgM syndrome. However, often there are no laboratory findings specific for each immune deficiency.

ADVANCED TESTING FOR PRIMARY IMMUNE DEFICIENCY DISORDERS WITH VIRAL SUSCEPTIBILITY

Next-generation sequencing has allowed for a dramatic increase in identification of distinct, genetically mediated PIDDs with viral susceptibility, with more than 400 genetic defects identified that are associated with immune deficiency.[4] Challenges in optimizing testing strategies remain. Different PIDDs can have overlapping features or variable penetrance, making prediction of a likely diagnosis—and therefore ordering of a specific single-gene test or limited gene panel test—difficult. Furthermore, such specific molecular testing for these disorders is often not commercially available or is only performed in specialized or research laboratories. In addition, many factors can affect functional immune testing, and few functional tests are diagnostic for specific PIDDs. Next-generation sequencing panels and exome sequencing are able to evaluate hundreds of PIDD genes rapidly and are more cost-effective than serial immune testing. Given the ability to evaluate more genes simultaneously in a more cost-effective manner, genetic testing should be sent earlier during the evaluation of a patient with unusual, severe, or opportunistic infections. However, finding a damaging genetic defect may not be sufficient for diagnosis, requiring correlation of clinical findings as well as functional testing before making a definitive diagnosis. In a way, the evolving role of a clinical immunologist is to determine if the clinical features of a patient fit the genetic defect detected by next-generation sequencing panels.[5]

PRIMARY IMMUNE DEFICIENCY DISORDERS WITH VIRAL SUSCEPTIBILITY DUE TO INNATE IMMUNE DEFECTS

Innate viral sensors are essential for the initial detection of a viral pathogen and include Toll-like receptors, the retinoic acid–inducible gene I-like receptors, the nucleotide oligomerization domain (NOD)-like receptors (also called NACHT, LRR, and PYD

Table 1
Innate immune sensors to viruses

Receptor	Viral Ligand	Signaling Molecules	Transcription Factor
TLR3	dsRNA	TRIF>RIP1>TRAF6>TAK1>IKKA/B	NF-κB family
		TRIF>TRAF3>TBK1	IRF3/IRF7
TLR7, TLR8	ssRNA	MYD88>IKKA/B	NF-κB family
TLR9	CpG DNA	MYD88>IKKA/B	NF-κB family
RIG-I/MDA5	dsRNA	MAVS>TBK1	IRF3/IRF7
STING	DNA	IKKA/B>NF-κB	NF-κB family
		TBK1>IRF3/7	IRF3/IRF7

Abbreviations: CpG, 5'-phosphate-G-3'; ssRNA, single-stranded RNA; dsRNA, double-stranded RNA.

domain proteins), and cytosolic DNA sensors.[1] Activation of these receptors by specific viral molecules leads to inflammatory cytokine and interferon production, although the mechanisms and pathways used by each differ. Defects in specific receptors, their signal transducing proteins, or the downstream transcriptional responses can lead to viral susceptibility (**Table 1**).

Recurrent Herpes Encephalitis, Human Papilloma Viruses, and Other Innate Immune Defects

Herpes encephalitis is classically a disease of newborns. If the disease becomes recurrent or presents at a later age, a PIDD should be considered. Over the past decade the use of next-generation sequencing has led to the discovery of pathogenic variants in several genes involved in the TLR3 pathway that result in recurrent herpes encephalitis. Approximately 5% of patients with herpes encephalitis have defects in TLR3 signaling.[1]

All TLRs use the MYD88 and IRAK4 proteins to ultimately activate NF-κB, except for TLR3, which is unable to recruit MYD88. TLR3 can use an alternative pathway that includes TRIF, TRAF6, and RIP1 to activate NF-κB. TLR3 can also use TRAF3, TBK1, and IRF3 and IRF7 to activate transcription of interferons. Type 1 interferons bind interferon receptors that signal through the JAK/STAT signaling pathway, and STAT proteins bind to IRF9, subsequently activating interferon-responsive genes.[6]

Genetic defects in this pathway result in recurrent herpes encephalitis (**Table 2**).[7–11] The fact that they do not suffer systemic HSV infections is thought to be related to the importance of the TLR3 pathway in limiting viral spread in neurons, whereas immune cells use redundant sensing pathways to respond to the virus. Functional testing of the TLR3 pathway is limited to research laboratories, namely because TLR3 defects can be missed when peripheral blood is tested; patient fibroblasts are necessary.[7] Genetic testing is the mainstay of diagnosis of these disorders. Recurrence is common and potentially neurologically devastating, highlighting the importance of establishing the diagnosis.

Other viral susceptibility is seen with TLR and JAK/STAT pathway defects (see **Table 2**). In addition, defects in this pathway can lead to susceptibility to other infections. For example, IRF7 defects were reported in a case of severe influenza infection.[12] IRF9 deficiency was associated with a variety of viral susceptibilities including influenza, symptomatic infection after MMR vaccination, VZV, RSV, and enterovirus.[13] IKBKG (ie, NF-κB essential modifier or NEMO) is required for NF-κB activation and genetic males with hypomorphic IKBKG variants can have a variety of viral infections such as HSV encephalitis, influenza, cytomegalovirus (CMV) and

Table 2
Genetic defects associated with specific viral susceptibility

HSV Encephalitis	HHV8	HPV	Influenza
TLR3	STIM1	CXCR4	IRF7
UNC93 B		EVER1/EVER2	IRF9
TRIF		DOCK8	
TRAF3		IKBKG	
TBK1			
IKBKG			

Abbreviations: HHV, human herpes virus; HPV, human papilloma virus; HSV, herpes simplex virus.

Epstein-Barr virus (EBV).[14,15] These patients also have susceptibility to a variety of mycobacterial and opportunistic pathogens and exhibit ectodermal dysplasia, with failure to sweat, abnormal skin, and conical teeth. STAT1 defects can also lead to fungal and mycobacterial susceptibility, because STAT1 is involved in interferon gamma (IFN-γ) signaling as well.[16]

ADAPTIVE (T- OR B-CELL) DEFECTS THAT RESULT IN SUSCEPTIBILITY TO VIRAL INFECTIONS

Although the innate immune system is critical to sensing viruses, clearance of virus requires the adaptive immune system. Virus-specific CD4 T cells are necessary to activate B lymphocytes to produce effective antiviral immunoglobulins and to support cytotoxic CD8 T-cell activation and differentiation. CD8 T cells express cytotoxic granules that can kill virally infected cells and malignant cells and are essential for the clearance of a viral infection as well as the maintenance of immunologic memory to prevent further infections. Virus-specific antibodies can neutralize extracellular virus and are elaborated by plasma cells. Disorders of adaptive immunity typically exhibit a broad range of infectious susceptibilities in addition to viruses. Humoral or antibody disorders classically involve bacterial sinopulmonary infections with encapsulated organisms. T-cell disorders result in variable susceptibility to other opportunistic infections including fungi, mycobacteria, *Pneumocystis*, and *Cryptosporidium*.

Humoral Immune Defects with Viral Susceptibility

B-lymphocyte, or humoral, immune defects are characterized by defective antibody production with preserved cell-mediated immunity. The classic presentation of humoral PIDDs is recurrent and potentially severe respiratory tract infections with bacterial pathogens, in particular encapsulated bacteria. *Haemophilus* and *Streptococcus* infections are common. These patients are usually not susceptible to most viral infections because T-cell function is preserved. However, these individuals are susceptible to a few types of viruses because antibodies do help neutralize extracellular viruses. For example, disseminated enteroviral infections can occur and can be severe and chronic. Chronic meningoencephalitis has been reported.[17] Polio virus or live vaccine–associated polio infections can also occur[18]; this is less of a concern with the inactivated poliovirus vaccine. Rhinovirus infections have also been reported. Most of these viral infections improve with the institution of immunoglobulin replacement.

Humoral PIDDs typical exhibit very low IgG, IgA, and IgM levels as well as poor vaccine responses. Several PIDDs with predominant humoral defects have been described and include the following:

- X-linked agammaglobulinemia is the prototypic humoral PIDD due to a defect of the Bruton tyrosine kinase (BTK) gene.[19] In addition to low antibody levels, flow cytometry classically shows a lack of B lymphocytes because BTK is required for B-cell development. Staining for the BTK protein can be done on monocytes or platelets, as these cell types also express BTK. Staining for BTK protein in maternal carriers can be informative; all B cells will express BTK, whereas only half of monocytes will express the protein.
- Other defects in B-cell development can occur and result in autosomal recessive agammaglobulinemia (IGLL1, IGHM). These are typically detected by sequencing.
- Activation-induced cytidine deaminase and uracil N-glycosylase deficiency are 2 humoral immune defects with a hyper-IgM phenotype (ie, low IgA and IgG,

elevated IgM). These genes are expressed in B cells and are involved in B-cell class switching.

- CD40 and CD40L defects also exhibit a hyper-IgM phenotype with low IgG and IgA. These patients are also susceptible to opportunistic infections including *Pneumocystis* and *Cryptosporidium*.

Common variable immune deficiency (CVID) is a complex PIDD with several monogenic causes as well as polygenic inheritance. CVID is likely the most common humoral immune defect. Diagnosis is based on low antibody levels and poor vaccine responses after a period of normal immune function. Although diagnosis is based on defective antibody responses, sometimes there can be T-cell defects as well. A variety of infections have been demonstrated in CVID.[20] The classic presentation is that of recurrent sinopulmonary bacterial infections, but some viral infections (eg, CMV, norovirus, papilloma virus) can also be problematic. Atypical bacteria such as *Mycoplasma* can also cause disease. Certain autoimmune disorders are more frequently encountered (eg, granulomatous disease, autoimmune cytopenias), and the risk of malignancy is also increased. Single gene defects have been reported in up to 30% of affected patients, with representative genes including *CTLA4* and *LRBA*.[21]

Combined Immune Defects with Prominent Viral Susceptibility

Combined immune defects also occur due to defects in T-cell development or function. Because T cells are necessary for B-cell function, T-cell defects can also result in poor antibody function and thus a combined immune deficiency. Some disorders also affect B-cell development. The hallmark of combined immune defects is susceptibility to many pathogens, including viruses, fungi, mycobacteria, and other opportunistic pathogens.[22]

Severe Combined Immunodeficiency

Severe combined immunodeficiency (SCID) is the most severe PIDD and is characterized by a complete deficiency of T lymphocytes due to genetic defects affecting their development or survival. SCID has the highest susceptibility to viral infections as well as other opportunistic infections.[23,24] Early onset pneumonitis can be seen due to a variety of viruses, including CMV. Varicella, either wild type or vaccine associated, can occur, as can vaccine-associated infections with measles, mumps, and rubella. Rotavirus infections can be prolonged and severe in SCID, and vaccine-associated rotavirus infections have also been reported. SCID also is associated with hypogammaglobulinemia, either due to lack of B cells or due to defective T-cell regulation of B cells, with resultant bacterial infections. A variety of opportunistic infections can also occur; examples include mycobacteria leading to disseminated infections (including following Bacille Calmette-Guérin vaccination), fungal infections, *Pneumocystis*, and *Cryptosporidium*.

Early detection of SCID is critical to survival of affected infants, as chronic infections can lead to worse outcomes during hematopoietic stem cell transplantation (HSCT), the main therapeutic option for SCID.[25] Patients with SCID detected prenatally or by family history have a much better survival advantage after HSCT compared with those who are detected later; this is likely due to the acquisition of infections that are difficult to clear once maternal antibodies wane. Fortunately, newborn screening for SCID is now implemented in all of the United States and many other countries.[26] The newborn screening program for SCID quantifies T-cell receptor excision circles (TRECs) from newborn screening cards. TRECs are generated during T-cell receptor gene rearrangement and do not replicate as cells divide. Thus, the presence of TRECs is reflective of the number of naïve T cells in the circulation; this is important because maternal lymphocytes can engraft and expand in infants, and defective T-cell development can lead to abnormal T cells that are autoreactive and expand *in vivo*. However, in both of these cases the TRECS will be low.

Once an abnormal test is found, infants should be evaluated immediately with appropriate infectious precautions to confirm the diagnosis. Confirmatory testing by enumerating lymphocyte subpopulations is necessary to confirm the diagnosis.

T, B, and NK cell counts are determined as are the percentage of naïve and memory T cells. T-cell counts in SCID are typically less than 200 cells/μL, and mitogenic responses are abnormal. Once detected, preventive measures, including parenteral immunoglobulin administration and anti-infective prophylaxis against *Pneumocystis*, fungi, and herpes viruses, are instituted to keep infants healthy before transplant. Additional infection control measures include testing breastfeeding mothers for CMV, limiting visitors and sick contact, instituting strict handwashing procedures, and using boiled water for formula. Genetic testing, often via rapid sequencing panels that can evaluate nearly all known causes of SCID efficiently, is sent to confirm the diagnosis but in certain cases is not necessary.[27] Genetic testing can also aid in determining the conditioning protocol used during HSCT.

With newborn screening the survival of infants with SCID has improved, as most infants with SCID are detected at birth. A few PIDDs, however, can lead to delayed onset of an SCID phenotype, such as ADA1 deficiency. In addition, certain groups, such as Amish, Mennonite, and native American populations, have a higher rate of SCID; some populations may defer newborn screening. Thus, one of the most important questions to ask when an infant presents with unusual infections is whether they were screened for SCID.

Combined Immune Deficiencies Presenting with Viral Infections

Combined immunodeficiencies (CIDs) share many similarities with SCID but tend to be somewhat less severe and present later in life. CIDs typically have more T cells than SCID and may not be picked up on newborn screening. The pattern of infections is similar to SCID, but is of less severity, and a broad range of viruses has been reported.[22] In addition, autoimmune complications are common in these disorders. These disorders can loosely be grouped into several pathophysiologic mechanisms:

- Hypomorphic defects in genes known to cause SCID can also cause CIDs, such as *RAG1/RAG2*.
- Defects in lymphocyte signaling pathways (eg, *LCK*, *ZAP70*, *PI3KCD*, *BCL10*, *IKBKB*)
- Defects in molecules involved in T- and B-cell interactions (CD40, CD40L, ICOS, IL21R)
- T-cell receptor recombination and DNA repair defects (*RAG1*, *RAG2*, *DCLRE1C*, *NHEJ1*, *LIG4*, *PRKDC*)
- Defects in thymic development (22q11 deletions syndrome, CHARGE)

The diagnosis of these disorders is largely through sequencing panels, as the number of PIDDs with features of combined immunodeficiency is currently greater than 75 and is increasing.[5] DNA sequencing panels allow for the rapid evaluation of dozens of CIDs. However, correlation of clinical and immunologic testing is necessary to confirm that a genetic defect is consistent with the clinical features. There may be clues to the diagnosis based on the pattern of infections, immunologic testing results, and associated physical examination findings (implicated genes are noted in parentheses):

Table 3
Primary immune deficiency disorders with Epstein-Barr virus susceptibility

Disease	Genes	Associated Features
XLP1	SAP	Lymphoma, hypogammaglobulinemia
XLP2	XIAP	Hypogammaglobulinemia, colitis
HLH	PRF	
	UNC13D	
	STX11	
	STXBP3	
	LYST	Chediak-Higashi syndrome, pigment defects
	RAB27	Griscelli syndrome, pigment defects
EBV viremia	ITK	—
	MAGT1	
	CD27	

*Abbreviations:*HLH, hemophagocytic lymphohistiocytosis; XLP, X-linked lymphoproliferative syndrome.

- EBV infection and its associated lymphoproliferative disorder are seen with a variety of genetic defects (eg, *XIAP, SH2D1A, CD27, ITK*) (**Table 3**).
- Antibody testing may reveal high IgM levels with low levels of IgG and IgA, a pattern sometimes referred to as the hyper-IgM phenotype. This phenotype is classically thought to be due to CD40/CD40L defects, but other defects may occur (eg, *PI3KCD, PIK3R1, MSH6, PMS2*).
- Severely elevated IgE levels are seen in several CIDs (*STAT3, IL6R, IL6ST, DOCK8*).
- Ectodermal dysplasia (ie, lack of sweat, conical teeth) is seen in disorders affecting NF-κB activation (*IKBKG, NFKBIA, IKBKB*).
- Microcephaly and abnormal facies can be a sign of DNA repair defects (*NBS1, LIG4, NHEJ1*).
- Ataxia and telangiectasias are seen with ATM defects
- Thrombocytopenia and bleeding disorders are seen in Wiskott-Aldrich syndrome and related disorders (*WASP, WIPF1, ARPC1B*).
- Short stature can be seen in a variety of CIDs (*RMRP, SMARCAL1, STAT5b*).

The evaluation and treatment of patients with suspected CID is similar to that of patients with SCID. Antibody levels, vaccine titers, and lymphocyte subpopulation analysis can provide clues to the diagnosis. Treatment of these disorders varies. If severe enough, HSCT may be warranted. Other treatments include immunoglobulin replacement and antiviral antibiotic prophylaxis.

Hemophagocytic Lymphohistiocytosis

After development and activation of T lymphocytes in the setting of a viral infection, cytotoxic T lymphocytes are required to kill virally infected cells and clear the virus; this must be done without bystander damage to neighboring uninfected cells to prevent widespread immune pathology. This highly specific killing is accomplished by the granule exocytosis pathway. A properly activated CD8 T cell binds to virally infected cells and forms an immune synapse with the target cell. Signaling molecules then activate the CD8 T cells, and granules containing perforin and granzymes are transported along microtubules and released into the immune synapse. Perforin facilitates uptake of the granule components into the target cells, where granzymes activate apoptotic pathways in the target cells. Defects in any step of this pathway can lead to HLH.[28]

Patients with genetic defects causing HLH seem healthy at birth and will pass newborn screening for SCID. Because the generation of cytotoxic granules requires the LYST protein and movement of granules requires proteins such as RAB27a, proteins that are also important in melanosomes, these patients may present with features of albinism. HLH is often triggered in the first several years of life following infection with certain viruses, such as EBV, CMV, HHV6, and parvovirus, and this leads to activation and expansion of CD8 cytotoxic lymphocytes, but these cells are unable to kill the virally infected cells. This leads to persistent activation and expansion of these cells, which also produce several inflammatory cytokines such as IFN-γ. High levels of IFN-γ in particular activate macrophages, which then cause inflammation and tissue destruction. This leads to hepatitis, central nervous system inflammation, pancytopenia with hemophagocytes in the marrow or lymphoid tissue, and disseminated intravascular coagulation due to tissue factor expression by activated macrophages. The diagnosis of HLH is made either by identifying a genetic defect known to cause HLH or by fulfilling 5 of the following 8 diagnostic criteria:

- Fever
- Splenomegaly
- Cytopenia affecting at least 2 cell lines (hemoglobin <9 mg/dL, platelets <100,000/mcL neutrophils <100/mcL)
- Hypofibrinogenemia (<150 mg/dL) OR hypertriglyceridemia (fasting triglyceride >177 mg/dL)
- Low NK activity
- Significantly elevated ferritin levels (>500 ng/mL)
- Elevated (>2400U/mL) soluble CD25 levels (ie, a marker of widespread T-cell activation)
- Hemophagocytosis in the bone marrow, lymph nodes, spleen, or liver

Treatment of HLH occurs in 2 phases. The first consists of treating the immune-mediated pathology, leading to organ dysfunction so that patients can eventually undergo the second phase, HSCT. This first goal is typically achieved via a multipronged approach that includes treatment with the cytotoxic agent, etoposide, to kill lymphocytes and activated macrophages, cyclosporine A or FK506 to inhibit T-cell activation, and dexamethasone to kill T cells and block cytokine transcription. Additional treatment modalities include intrathecal methotrexate to treat and/or prevent central nervous system involvement; newer agents have been proposed, such as IFN-γ neutralizing antibodies or JAK/STAT inhibitors. The ultimate treatment of HLH is the HSCT, as HLH is a fatal disease that may recur even if the initial inflammatory phase is suppressed.

SUMMARY

Severe, recurrent, or unusual infections with viruses can be a sign of a primary immunodeficiency. A careful history and physical examination can reveal clues to the diagnosis. Some immune defects produce susceptibility to very specific viral infections, whereas others show susceptibility to viral infections as well as many other infectious organisms. Newborn screening for SCID should prevent many severe infections with viral pathogens, as patients with this severe immune defect are detected at birth. Genetic testing with sequencing panels has become a key diagnostic tool to diagnose a patient with a primary immunodeficiency. Confirmatory functional testing and correlation with clinical findings is essential when evaluating genetic defects that are found with sequencing. Treatment of these disorders varies greatly but can include immunoglobulin replacement, antiviral prophylaxis, and even hematopoietic stem cell transplantation. An intensivist must consider primary immune deficiencies when confronted with a patient with severe or unusual viral infections.

CLINICS CARE POINTS

- Early detection of immune defects that result in viral infections can improve long term outcomes.
- Genetic sequencing panels are a rapid and efficient way to screen for primary immune deficiencies.
- Some primary immune deficiencies, such as HLH, need to be considered early to prevent significant morbidity or mortality.

REFERENCES

1. Carty M, Guy C, Bowie AG. Detection of viral infections by innate immunity. Biochem Pharmacol 2021;183:114316.
2. Schoggins JW. Interferon-stimulated genes: what do they all do? Annu Rev Virol 2019;6(1):567–84.
3. Ruffner MA, Sullivan KE, Henrickson SE. Recurrent and Sustained viral infections in primary immunodeficiencies. Front Immunol 2017;8:665.
4. Tangye SG, Al-Herz W, Bousfiha A, et al. Human Inborn Errors of immunity: 2019 Update on the Classification from the International union of immunological Societies Expert Committee. J Clin Immunol 2020;40(1):24–64.
5. Bousfiha A, Jeddane L, Picard C, et al. Human Inborn Errors of immunity: 2019 Update of the IUIS Phenotypical Classification. J Clin Immunol 2020; 40(1):66–81.
6. Mogensen TH. IRF and STAT transcription factors - from basic Biology to roles in infection, protective immunity, and primary immunodeficiencies. Front Immunol 2019;9(3047).
7. Zhang SY, Jouanguy E, Ugolini S, et al. TLR3 deficiency in patients with herpes simplex encephalitis. Science (New York, NY) 2007;317(5844):1522–7.
8. Sancho-Shimizu V, Pérez de Diego R, Lorenzo L, et al. Herpes simplex encephalitis in children with autosomal recessive and dominant TRIF deficiency. J Clin Invest 2011;121(12):4889–902.
9. Casrouge A, Zhang SY, Eidenschenk C, et al. Herpes simplex virus encephalitis in human UNC-93B deficiency. Science (New York, NY) 2006;314(5797):308–12.
10. Pérez de Diego R, Sancho-Shimizu V, Lorenzo L, et al. Human TRAF3 adaptor molecule deficiency leads to impaired Toll-like receptor 3 response and susceptibility to herpes simplex encephalitis. Immunity 2010;33(3):400–11.
11. Herman M, Ciancanelli M, Ou YH, et al. Heterozygous TBK1 mutations impair TLR3 immunity and underlie herpes simplex encephalitis of childhood. J Exp Med 2012;209(9):1567–82.
12. Ciancanelli MJ, Huang SX, Luthra P, et al. Infectious disease. Life-threatening influenza and impaired interferon amplification in human IRF7 deficiency. Science (New York, NY) 2015;348(6233):448–53.
13. Hernandez N, Melki I, Jing H, et al. Life-threatening influenza pneumonitis in a child with inherited IRF9 deficiency. The J Exp Med 2018;215(10):2567–85.

14. Zonana J, Elder ME, Schneider LC, et al. A novel X-linked disorder of immune deficiency and hypohidrotic ectodermal dysplasia is allelic to incontinentia pigmenti and due to mutations in IKK-gamma (NEMO). Am J Hum Genet 2000; 67(6):1555–62.
15. Courtois G, Smahi A, Reichenbach J, et al. A hypermorphic IkappaBalpha mutation is associated with autosomal dominant anhidrotic ectodermal dysplasia and T cell immunodeficiency. The J Clin Invest 2003;112(7):1108–15.
16. Dupuis S, Jouanguy E, Al-Hajjar S, et al. Impaired response to interferon-alpha/beta and lethal viral disease in human STAT1 deficiency. Nat Genet 2003;33(3): 388–91.
17. Winkelstein JA, Marino MC, Lederman HM, et al. X-linked agammaglobulinemia: report on a United States registry of 201 patients. Medicine 2006;85(4):193–202.
18. Mamishi S, Shahmahmoudi S, Tabatabaie H, et al. Novel BTK mutation presenting with vaccine-associated paralytic poliomyelitis. Eur J Pediatr 2008;167(11): 1335–8.
19. Bearden D, Collett M, Quan PL, et al. Enteroviruses in X-linked agammaglobulinemia: Update on Epidemiology and Therapy. J Allergy Clin Immunol In Pract 2016;4(6):1059–65.
20. Oksenhendler E, Gérard L, Fieschi C, et al. Infections in 252 patients with common variable immunodeficiency. Clin Infect Dis 2008;46(10):1547–54.
21. de Valles-Ibáñez G, Esteve-Solé A, Piquer M, González-Navarro EA, Hernandez-Rodriguez J, Laayouni H, González-Roca E, Plaza-Martin AM, Deyà-Martínez Á, Martín-Nalda A, et al. Evaluating the genetics of common variable immunodeficiency: Monogenetic Model and beyond. Front Immunol 2018;9:636.
22. Al-Herz W, Essa S. Spectrum of viral infections Among primary immunodeficient children: report from a National registry. Front Immunol 2019;10:1231.
23. Gennery AR, Cant AJ. Diagnosis of severe combined immunodeficiency. J Clin Pathol 2001;54(3):191–5.
24. Crooks BNA, Taylor CE, Turner AJL, et al. Respiratory viral infections in primary immune deficiencies: significance and relevance to clinical outcome in a single BMT unit. Bone Marrow Transplant 2000;26(10):1097–102.
25. Buelow BJ, Routes JM, Verbsky JW. Newborn screening for SCID: where are we now? Expert Rev Clin Immunol 2014;10(12):1649–57.
26. Routes J, Verbsky J. Newborn screening for severe combined immunodeficiency. Curr Allergy Asthma Rep 2018;18(6):34.
27. Dvorak CC, Haddad E, Buckley RH, et al. The genetic landscape of severe combined immunodeficiency in the United States and Canada in the current era (2010-2018). J Allergy Clin Immunol 2019;143(1):405–7.
28. Verbsky JW, Grossman WJ. Hemophagocytic lymphohistiocytosis: diagnosis, pathophysiology, treatment, and future perspectives. Ann Med 2006;38(1):20–31.

Moving?

Make sure your subscription moves with you!

To notify us of your new address, find your **Clinics Account Number** (located on your mailing label above your name), and contact customer service at:

Email: journalscustomerservice-usa@elsevier.com

800-654-2452 (subscribers in the U.S. & Canada)
314-447-8871 (subscribers outside of the U.S. & Canada)

Fax number: 314-447-8029

Elsevier Health Sciences Division
Subscription Customer Service
3251 Riverport Lane
Maryland Heights, MO 63043

*To ensure uninterrupted delivery of your subscription, please notify us at least 4 weeks in advance of move.